ACUPUNCTURE CASE HISTORIES FROM CHINA

ACUPUNCTURE CASE HISTORIES FROM CHINA

EDITED BY

Chen Jirui, M.D. and Nissi Wang, M.Sc.

EASTLAND PRESS   Seattle

© 1988 by Eastland Press, Incorporated,
P.O. Box 12689, Seattle, Washington, 98111.
All rights reserved.

Library of Congress Catalog Card Number: 88-80070
International Standard Book Number: 0-939616-07-6
Printed in the United States of America.

Photolithoprinted by Cushing-Malloy, Incorporated,
Ann Arbor, Michigan, 1988.
Book design by Catherine L. Nelson.
Brush calligraphy by Kou Hoi-Yin.

Table of Contents

CHAPTER ONE: General Internal Medicine (continued)

CHAPTER TWO: Neurological Disorders

CHAPTER THREE: Pain

CHAPTER FOUR: Disorders of the Eyes, Ears, Nose and Throat

CHAPTER FIVE: Disorders of the Skin

CHAPTER SIX: Women's Disorders

CHAPTER SIX: Women's Disorders (continued)

CHAPTER SEVEN: Children's Disorders

INDICES

Foreword

The practice of Chinese medicine in the west has a great potential which only recently has begun to be tapped. Areas in which further progress is needed include the expansion of the scope of acupuncture therapy to include basic physical and emotional disorders (both in out-patient and in-patient settings), incorporation of Chinese diagnostic procedures (including pulse and tongue analysis) into the normal history and physical exam, and the integration of regular preventative Chinese medical treatment into western health-care. Any one of these applications would have a significant impact on the health of people in the west, and the health-care systems that serve us. However, real progress is possible only if practitioners of acupuncture undergo a rigorous education that includes a thorough presentation of traditional Chinese medical theory, as well as an intensive and comprehensive clinical training.

In the past, the level of theoretical understanding of Chinese medicine among western practitioners of acupuncture has been unsatisfactory and incomplete. For a variety of reasons, however, this is beginning to change. Perhaps chief among these is the increasing number of authoritative translations of Chinese medical texts, both ancient and modern, into English. This growth in the accessible literature, and the increasingly cosmopolitan nature of the acupuncture community, has led to a heightened appreciation and acceptance among western acupuncturists of the multiplicity of theories and practices that comprise Chinese medicine. This process involves an awareness that no one theoretical framework is right or wrong to the exclusion of others; rather, each of them must be understood so that they can be utilized in appropriate circumstances. Along with this greater open-mindedness is the beginning of impartial and meticulous investigations into the validity of the various theories and their practical applications. Such research will be an important factor in determining which aspects of a medical system originating in ancient China are applicable to conditions in the modern west.

While there has been progress in understanding the theoretical bases of Chinese medicine, the problem of high quality clinical training remains. There are now only a very limited number of highly experienced clinical instructors in the west. Although it is expected that their numbers will increase, at the present time this situation seriously affects the quality of students graduating from many of the schools.

It is for this reason that *Acupuncture Case Histories from China* is a particularly valuable contribution to the advance of acupuncture in the west. Comprised of analyzed case histories from prominent practitioners in China, it fills a major gap in the literature. This book will therefore be useful both to students during their clinical training, as well as to established practitioners who wish to improve their clinical skills. Because of the wide variety of clinical conditions represented in this volume, it should also help to stimulate further research into the applications of acupuncture. Hopefully, this will lead to the incorporation of acupuncture therapy in the treatment of many more patients, and expand its use in the hospital environment.

There is much that is obscure in the ancient classics of Chinese medicine, just as there is much controversy among modern schools of acupuncture. Only through careful study and analysis of the texts, and the treatment of large numbers of patients in diverse environments, will it become possible to discern those aspects of Chinese medicine which are relevant to contemporary practice. *Acupuncture Case Histories from China* will serve as a stepping-stone to future progress.

JEREMY ROSS
BRISTOL, UNITED KINGDOM
January, 1988

Contributors

Xu Yizhi, M.D. CHONGQING INSTITUTE OF TRADITIONAL CHINESE MEDICINE

Quan Ruxian, M.D. GREATER ENCYCLOPEDIA OF CHINA

Li Rongde, M.D. BEIJING INSTITUTE OF OPHTHALMOLOGY

Sun Shushen, M.D. BEIJING INSTITUTE OF OPTHALMOLOGY

Lu Shoukang, M.M. CHINESE ACADEMY OF TRADITIONAL CHINESE MEDICINE

Zheng Qiwei, M.M. CHINESE ACADEMY OF TRADITIONAL CHINESE MEDICINE

Li Yang, M.M. CHINESE ACADEMY OF TRADITIONAL CHINESE MEDICINE

Ji Xiaoping, M.M. CHINESE ACADEMY OF TRADITIONAL CHINESE MEDICINE

INTRODUCTION

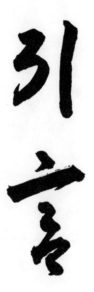

Introduction

One important resource that has been missing from the literature on Chinese medicine in the west is the case history. From their teachers and textbooks, students can learn the general principles of Chinese medicine, how to differentiate one syndrome from another, locate points, insert needles and apply moxibustion. However, because Chinese medicine is a medicine of particulars, only through the medium of the case history can a student learn how the principles of Chinese medicine are actually applied in a particular case. It is therefore an indispensable adjunct to personal study and clinical training.

The case histories in this book were contributed by several prominent acupuncturists in China. Each case reflects the thought processes and methodology of the individual practitioner in treating a particular patient. Because of the flexibility of acupuncture therapy, and the unique style of each practitioner, it should come as no surprise to the reader that some cases with very similar diagnoses are treated differently.

Throughout the text, numerous references are made to special point classifications and specific techniques of needling and moxibustion. To avoid confusion, and to assist the reader in better understanding the cases in this book, we have provided a general discussion of these points and techniques later in the introduction.

FREQUENCY OF TREATMENT

All of the cases in this book were drawn from the records of acupuncture practitioners in the People's Republic of China, where the health care system is socialized. This allows patients to undergo treatment inexpensively, and on a frequent basis. The discussion of the frequency of treatment below should therefore be viewed in this context, and is intended only to provide the reader with very general guidelines.

For acute infectious diseases, acupuncture is usually administered once daily. However, if the disease is severe, treatment may be as often as 2-3 times daily. For those conditions which have a predictably short course (e.g., the common cold), a course of therapy need not be instituted. For conditions with a protracted course (e.g., acute viral hepatitis), a course of therapy consisting of 5-7 days may be instituted, with 1-2 days' rest between courses. The needles are generally retained from 30-60 minutes during each session.

For acute noninfectious disorders (e.g., cholecystitis, sprains, etc.), needling may be administered once daily, or twice daily if particularly severe. The needles are usually retained from 20-40 minutes, and the length of a course of therapy is the same as that for acute infectious diseases.

For chronic conditions, both infectious and noninfectious, the frequency of treatment is determined on the basis of individual circumstances. In general, needling is administered once every other day, and during convalescence, twice a week. The needles are retained from 20-30 minutes. A course of therapy is generally comprised of 10-15 treatments, with 3-5 days' rest between courses.

TREATING THE INDIVIDUAL

As in prescribing herbs and western drugs, the manner and method of acupuncture therapy should be tailored to the individual. The age and physical characteristics of the patient, as well as the nature of the disease itself, must be taken into consideration.

Because the Qi and Blood in children under the age of 10 are not fully developed, needling should be shallow, using #32 or #34 gauge needles, with little if any manipulation. If the child can remain still, the needles may be retained for a short period of 10 minutes or so.

For elderly or very weak patients whose Qi and Blood are diminished, needling should generally be shallow, with little manipulation. The needles may be retained for about 20 minutes

To obtain the needle sensation when treating obese patients, the needles must usually be inserted more deeply than when treating thin patients. For patients who are robust, obese, or whose sensitivity to needling is diminished, the needles should be of larger gauge (#28 or #30), and needle ma-

nipulation should be stronger, with retention from 20-40 minutes.

There are certain special factors to consider when treating women. During pregnancy, those points which facilitate menstrual flow and invigorate the Blood, such as LI-4 *(he gu),* Sp-6 *(san yin jiao),* B-60 *(kun lun)* and B-67 *(zhi yin),* should not be treated in order to prevent miscarriage. In addition, during the first trimester, points on the lower abdomen should not be needled. After the first trimester, points on both the lower abdomen as well as the lower back should be avoided.

There is much controversy among practitioners in China concerning needling during menstruation. This controversy is reflected in a few of the cases reported in chapter 6, inasmuch as the cases were contributed by different practitioners. Some believe that when treating non-gynecological problems, if the points being used influence the Womb or menses, treatment should be discontinued so as not to interfere with the natural physiological process of menstruation. This would be true, for example, of such points as Sp-6 *(san yin jiao)* and LI-4 *(he gu),* and points on the lower abdomen and lower back. If these points are needled during menstruation, it is possible that excessive bleeding will occur. Other practitioners, however, believe that there are no adverse reactions to needling during menstruation because acupuncture is regulatory in effect, and acts to balance the physiologic processes.

THE ACUPUNCTURE PRESCRIPTION

The successful treatment of a disease with acupuncture therapy depends in large measure upon the prescription, i.e., the selection and combination of points. The choice of prescription is based on the differentiation of syndromes in accordance with the principles of Chinese medicine, and on the functions and special characteristics of individual points.

Selecting Points

Point selection is guided primarily by the theory of the channels, in that points are generally chosen from those channels which are affected, directly or indirectly, by a disease. There are three methods of point selection: local, remote, and symptomatic.

Local points: Local refers to the vicinity of the pain or distress. All acupuncture points may be used to treat conditions located in their vicinity. Local points are most often chosen to treat superficial or localized conditions. For example, B-1 *(jing ming)* in the vicinity of the eye may be chosen for eye diseases, and SI-19 *(ting gong)* in the vicinity of the ear for ear diseases.

Remote points: Remote refers to a site which is distant from the location of the disorder, usually below the elbow or knee. Remote points may be selected from a channel corresponding to the affected area or Organ, or from an exterior-interiorly related channel. For example, either S-36 *(zu san li)*, which is a Stomach channel point located on the lower leg, or Sp-4 *(gong sun)*, which is a Spleen channel point located on the foot, may be chosen as remote points in the treatment of stomachache. This is because the Stomach and Spleen channels are exterior-interiorly related.

Symptomatic points: Symptomatic point selection is a method of choosing points for systemic conditions. This method differs from local and remote point selection methods, which are based on the distance of the points from the location of the disease. Instead, symptomatic point selection is based on the functions of individual points. For example, in treating a fever of excess due to an external pathogenic influence,

GV-14 *(da zhui)*, LI-4 *(he gu)* or LI-11 *(qu chi)* may be chosen because of their fever-reducing functions.

Although each of these three methods of point selection may be used individually, more often they are combined to enhance the therapeutic effect.

Combining Points

Among the numerous methods of combining points in a prescription, only those which are commonly used today, and which are mentioned in the cases in this book, will be described here.

Combining Yang channel points with Yin channel points: This method is based on the Yin-Yang, interior-exterior relationships of the Organs and their channels. For a condition affecting a Yang channel, points on its corresponding Yin channel can be chosen, or vice versa. Alternatively, points on both the Yang channel and its paired Yin channel can be combined. For example, to treat coughing, L-9 *(tai yuan)* on the Lung channel (Yin) can be combined with LI-4 *(he gu)* on the Large Intestine channel (Yang). The combination of source and connecting points (see below) on paired channels is another example of this method.

Combining points on the front with points on the back: This method combines points on the chest and abdomen with points on the back, and is used in treating diseases of the Organs. The combination of associated points on the back with alarm points on the chest and abdomen (see below) is representative of this method.

Combining points above with points below: This method combines points on the arms and above the waist with points below the waist. For example, in treating acute pain of the lower back, GV-26 *(ren zhong)* above can be combined with GV-1 *(chang qiang)* below. Another application of this method is the use of points on the lower part of the body for conditions on the upper part of the body, and vice versa. For example, G-41 *(zu lin qi)* and G-37 *(guang ming)* on the lower leg can be used in treating eye disorders. A combination of the upper and lower confluent points of the eight miscellaneous channels (see below) is yet another example of this method.

Combining points on the left with points on the right: This method is based on the bilateral orientation of the channels and points, and may be applied in either of two ways: by needling points on one side of the body for a disorder on the opposite side, or by combining points on the same side with those on the opposite side.

Combining the alarm points with the associated points of the back: The alarm points (also known as the *mu* points) are sites on the chest and abdomen where the Qi of each of the Organs gathers. The associated points (also known as the back-*shu* points) are sites on the back through which the Qi of each of the Organs flows. Each Organ possesses its own alarm and associated points (Tables 1 and 2). Experience has shown that when disease affects an Organ, its alarm or associated point will become sensitive, or will reflect other changes, such as redness. These points thus also have diagnostic value.

The alarm and associated points may be combined to treat disease in their corresponding Organs. For example, if the Gall Bladder is affected, its alarm point, G-24 *(ri yue)*, and its associated point, B-19 *(dan shu)*, can be chosen. The alarm and associated points can also be used individually to treat disease affecting the sensory organs with which each of their corresponding Yin and Yang Organs is associated. For example, the ear is the external 'opening' of the Kidney. For diseases of the ear, the associated point of the Kidney, B-23 *(shen shu)*, may therefore be selected.

TABLE 1.
Associated Points of the Back

ORGAN	ASSOCIATED POINT
Lung	B-13 *(fei shu)*
Pericardium	B-14 *(jue yin shu)*
Heart	B-15 *(xin shu)*
Liver	B-18 *(gan shu)*
Gall Bladder	B-19 *(dan shu)*
Spleen	B-20 *(pi shu)*
Stomach	B-21 *(wei shu)*
Triple Burner	B-22 *(san jiao shu)*
Kidney	B-23 *(shen shu)*
Large Intestine	B-25 *(da chang shu)*
Small Intestine	B-27 *(xiao chang shu)*
Bladder	B-28 *(pang guang shu)*

TABLE 2.
Alarm Points

ORGAN	ALARM POINTS
Lung	L-1 *(zhong fu)*
Pericardium	CV-17 *(tan zhong)*
Liver	Liv-14 *(qi men)*
Heart	CV-14 *(ju que)*
Gall Bladder	G-24 *(ri yue)*
Stomach	CV-12 *(zhong wan)*
Spleen	Liv-13 *(zhang men)*
Triple Burner	CV-5 *(shi men)*
Kidney	G-25 *(jing men)*
Small Intestine	CV-4 *(guan yuan)*
Large Intestine	S-25 *(tian shu)*
Bladder	CV-3 *(zhong ji)*

Combining source and connecting points: Each of the primary channels has a source point which is located on or near the wrist or ankle (Table 3). The source points are those sites to which the source Qi of the channels flows, and is retained. These points are closely associated with the Triple Burner because source Qi resides there and influences the functioning of the Organs. The source points are therefore used to treat diseases of the Organs.

TABLE 3.
The Twelve Source Points

CHANNEL	SOURCE POINT
Lung	L-9 (tai yuan)
Pericardium	P-7 (da ling)
Heart	H-7 (shen men)
Spleen	Sp-3 (tai bai)
Liver	Liv-3 (tai chong)
Kidney	K-3 (tai xi)
Large Intestine	LI-4 (he gu)
Triple Burner	TB-4 (yang chi)
Small Intestine	SI-4 (wan gu)
Stomach	S-42 (chong yang)
Gall Bladder	G-40 (qiu xu)
Bladder	B-64 (jing gu)

TABLE 4.
The Fifteen Connecting Points

CHANNEL	CONNECTING POINT
Lung	L-7 (lie que)
Pericardium	P-6 (nei guan)
Heart	H-5 (tong li)
Spleen	Sp-4 (gong sun)
Liver	Liv-5 (li gou)
Kidney	K-4 (da zhong)
Conception	CV-15 (jiu wei)
Great Connecting Channel of the Spleen	Sp-21 (da bao)
Bladder	B-58 (fei yang)
Large Intestine	LI-6 (pian li)
Triple Burner	TB-5 (wai guan)
Small Intestine	SI-7 (zhi zheng)
Stomach	S-40 (feng long)
Gall Bladder	G-37 (guang ming)
Governing	GV-1 (chang qiang)

The connecting points (also known as the *luo* points) are those sites at which the connecting channels branch off from the primary channels, connecting them with their respective interior-exteriorly related channels. In addition to the twelve connecting points of the primary channels, there are also connecting points for the Conception and Governing vessels, and for the Great Connecting channel of the Spleen (Table 4). The connecting points are used for diseases which affect both of the interior-exteriorly related primary channels.

The source and connecting points may either be used individually, or in combination. When they are used in combination, the source point of the channel which is primarily affected by a disease is combined with the connecting point of its interior-exteriorly related channel. The source point is termed the 'host', and the connecting point is termed the 'guest'. For example, in the treatment of a disease which primarily affects the Heart channel, H-7 *(shen men)*, the source point (or 'host') of the Heart channel, may be combined with SI-7 *(zhi zheng)*, the connecting point (or 'guest') of the interior-exteriorly related Small Intestine channel.

Combining confluent points of the eight miscellaneous channels: Each of the eight miscellaneous channels has a point of confluence with one of the primary channels on the extremities (Table 5). These points may be used individually to treat diseases of the miscellaneous channels. More commonly, they are used in tandem to treat a disorder

TABLE 5. Confluent Points of the Eight Miscellaneous Channels

PRIMARY CHANNEL	CONFLUENT POINT	MISCELLANEOUS CHANNEL
Spleen	Sp-4 (gong sun)	Penetrating
Pericardium	P-6 (nei guan)	Yin Linking
Small Intestine	SI-3 (hou xi)	Governing
Bladder	B-62 (shen mai)	Yang Heel
Gall Bladder	G-41 (zu lin qi)	Girdle
Triple Burner	TB-5 (wai guan)	Yang Linking
Lung	L-7 (lie que)	Conception
Kidney	K-6 (zhao hai)	Yin Heel

in a particular region of the body, by combining a confluent point on a lower extremity with one on an upper extremity. For example, L-7 *(lie que)*, the confluent point of the Conception vessel on the arm, may be combined with K-6 *(zhao hai)*, the confluent point of the Yin Heel channel on the leg, to treat disorders of the throat and chest.

Special Points

In addition to the various point combinations mentioned above, there are other special groups of points with unique functional attributes which are commonly used in the clinic.

Five Transport Points: These points are located below the elbows and knees. Each of the primary channels has five transport points (also known as *shu* points), the well, gushing, transporting, traversing and uniting points (Table 6). Using the imagery of moving water, the five names describe the development of the flow of Qi in the channels. The well point is the source of channel Qi; the gushing point is where the Qi begins to flow; the transporting point is where the flow of Qi deepens; the traversing point finds the Qi flowing vigorously; and the uniting point is where the Qi converges.

The well points are used in treating diseases of the Organs, particularly fullness in the epigastric and hypochondriac regions. The gushing points are used when a disease causes a change in the complexion, or when fever is present. The transporting points are used in treating protracted conditions, heaviness of the body, and joint pain. The traversing points may be needled for conditions which affect the sound of the voice, or for coughing with dyspnea, accompanied by fever and chills. The uniting points may be used for bleeding, for diseases of the Stomach caused by improper diet, or for diarrhea.

The five transport points may also be used in conjunction with the mother-son, tonifying-draining method. In the mutual generation cycle of the five phases, the 'mother' generates the 'son'. In the *Classic of Difficulties* (chapter 69), this concept was correlated with the tonifying-draining method: "For deficiency, tonify the mother; for excess, drain the son." Here, the terms 'mother' and 'son' refer both to the channels, and to the transport points on the channels. Thus, for a condition of deficiency, the 'mother' point of the affected channel, or the 'mother' point of its 'mother' channel, should be tonified. Conversely, for a condition of excess, the 'son' point of the affected

TABLE 6. The Five Transport Points

CHANNEL	WELL	GUSHING	TRANSPORTING	TRAVERSING	UNITING
Lung	L-11 *(shao shang)*	L-10 *(yu ji)*	L-9 *(tai yuan)*	L-8 *(jing qi)*	L-5 *(chi ze)*
Pericardium	P-9 *(zhong chong)*	P-8 *(lao gong)*	P-7 *(da ling)*	P-5 *(jian shi)*	P-3 *(qu ze)*
Heart	H-9 *(shao chong)*	H-8 *(shao fu)*	H-7 *(shen men)*	H-4 *(ling dao)*	H-3 *(shao hai)*
Spleen	Sp-1 *(yin bai)*	Sp-2 *(da du)*	Sp-3 *(tai bai)*	Sp-5 *(shang qiu)*	Sp-9 *(yin ling quan)*
Liver	Liv-1 *(da dun)*	Liv-2 *(xing jian)*	Liv-3 *(tai chong)*	Liv-4 *(zhong feng)*	Liv-8 *(qu quan)*
Kidney	K-1 *(yong quan)*	K-2 *(ran gu)*	K-3 *(tai xi)*	K-7 *(fu liu)*	K-10 *(yin gu)*
Large Intestine	LI-1 *(shang yang)*	LI-2 *(er jian)*	LI-3 *(san jian)*	LI-5 *(yang xi)*	LI-11 *(qu chi)*
Triple Burner	TB-1 *(guan chong)*	TB-2 *(ye men)*	TB-3 *(zhong zhu)*	TB-6 *(zhi gou)*	TB-10 *(tian jing)*
Small Intestine	SI-1 *(shao ze)*	SI-2 *(qian gu)*	SI-3 *(hou xi)*	SI-5 *(yang gu)*	SI-8 *(xiao hai)*
Stomach	S-45 *(li dui)*	S-44 *(nei ting)*	S-43 *(xian gu)*	S-41 *(jie xi)*	S-36 *(zu san li)*
Gall Bladder	G-44 *(qiao yin)*	G-43 *(xia xi)*	G-41 *(zu lin qi)*	G-38 *(yang fu)*	G-34 *(yang ling quan)*
Bladder	B-67 *(zhi yin)*	B-66 *(zu tong gu)*	B-65 *(shu gu)*	B-60 *(kun lun)*	B-40 *(wei zhong)*

channel, or the 'son' point of its 'son' channel, should be drained.

Each of the Organs (and its associated channel) corresponds to one of the five phases: the Liver and Gall Bladder to wood; the Heart and Small Intestine to fire; the Spleen and Stomach to earth; the Lung and Large Intestine to metal; and the Kidney and Bladder to water. Similarly, each of the five transport points on the channels corresponds to one of the five phases. On the Yin channels, the well point corresponds to wood; the gushing point to fire; the transporting point to earth; the traversing point to metal; and the uniting point to water. On the Yang channels, the well point corresponds to metal; the gushing point to water; the transporting point to wood; the traversing point to fire; and the uniting point to earth.

Application of the mother-son, tonifying-draining method in conjunction with the five transport points is illustrated by the following example. The Large Intestine and its channel correspond to metal, and the Bladder and its channel to water. Because water follows metal in the generation cycle of the five phases, the Bladder channel is the 'son' in relation to the Large Intestine channel, which is the 'mother'. On the Large Intestine channel itself, the gushing point, LI-2 *(er jian)*, corresponds to water, and is therefore the 'son' point on the 'mother' channel. On the Bladder channel, the gushing point, B-66 *(zu tong gu)*, also corresponds to water, and is therefore the 'son' point on the 'son' channel. Thus, for a condition of excess affecting the Large Intestine channel, either of these 'son' points could be needled to drain the excess.

Eight Meeting Points: Each of the eight meeting points (also known as the influential points) is especially effective for treating the particular aspect of the body with which it is associated (Table 7). For example, if the sinews are affected, then G-34 *(yang ling*

quan), the meeting point of the sinews, may be needled. Or if a Yang Organ is diseased, then CV-12 *(zhong wan),* the meeting point of the Yang Organs, may be needled.

TABLE 7.
The Eight Meeting Points

ORGAN	MEETING POINT
Yin Organs	Liv-13 *(zhang men)*
Yang Organs	CV-12 *(zhong wan)*
Qi	CV-17 *(tan zhong)*
Blood	B-17 *(ge shu)*
Sinews	G-34 *(yang ling quan)*
Blood vessels	L-9 *(tai yuan)*
Bones	B-11 *(da zhu)*
Marrow	G-39 *(xuan zhong)*

Accumulating Points: These are points where the Qi and the Blood of a channel flow and accumulate. (They are also known as cleft points.) Each of the primary channels, as well as the Yin and Yang Linking channels, and Yin and Yang Heel channels, has an accumulating point (Table 8). There are thus 16 accumulating points in all. The accumulating points are used to treat various acute diseases. For example, for an acute Stomach condition, the accumulating point of the Stomach, S-34 *(liang qiu),* may be needled.

Four Dominant Points: There are four points, S-36 *(zu san li),* B-40 *(wei zhong),* L-7 *(lie que)* and LI-4 *(he gu),* which are commonly used for treating diseases of different regions of the body above the waist. The particular regions of the body for which each point is indicated are summarized in the following rhyme from the Ming dynasty classic, *Gatherings from Outstanding Acupuncturists:* "The Stomach and abdomen belong to *zu san li,* / the back is *wei zhong's* territory. / For the head and neck, *lie que* should be sought after, / and for the face and mouth, to *he gu* refer."

TABLE 8.
The Sixteen Accumulating Points

CHANNEL	ACCUMULATING POINT
Lung	L-6 *(kong zui)*
Pericardium	P-4 *(xi men)*
Heart	H-6 *(yin xi)*
Large Intestine	LI-7 *(wen liu)*
Triple Burner	TB-7 *(hui zong)*
Small Intestine	SI-6 *(yang lao)*
Stomach	S-34 *(liang qiu)*
Gall Bladder	G-36 *(wai qiu)*
Bladder	B-63 *(jin men)*
Spleen	Sp-8 *(di ji)*
Liver	Liv-6 *(zhong du)*
Kidney	K-5 *(shui quan)*
Yin Linking	K-9 *(zhu bin)*
Yang Linking	G-35 *(yang jiao)*
Yin Heel	K-8 *(jiao xin)*
Yang Heel	B-59 *(fu yang)*

Lower Uniting Points: The lower uniting points (also known as the lower sea points) are located on the lower extremities where the channels of the Yang Organs unite with the Yang channels of the leg (Table 9). These points are therefore indicated for diseases of the Yang Organs. For example, to treat diseases of the Gall Bladder, G-34 *(yang ling quan),* the lower uniting point of the Gall Bladder, may be needled.

TABLE 9. Lower Uniting Points of the Six Yang Organs

ORGAN	LOWER UNITING POINT
Stomach	S-36 *(zu san li)*
Large Intestine	S-37 *(shang ju xu)*
Small Intestine	S-39 *(xia ju xu)*
Bladder	B-40 *(wei zhong)*
Triple Burner	B-39 *(wei yang)*
Gall Bladder	G-34 *(yang ling quan)*

S-36 *(zu san li)* is the uniting point of the Stomach channel. Since the lower uniting points are used for treating diseases of the Organs, S-36 *(zu san li)* is thus indicated for all types of Stomach and intestinal conditions. B-40 *(wei zhong)* is the lower uniting point of the Bladder channel. In addition to regulating the Bladder and controlling urination, B-40 *(wei zhong)* is indicated for pain of the back and lower back. L-7 *(lie que)* is the connecting point of the Lung channel, which connects with the Large Intestine channel. L-7 *(lie que)* is also one of the confluent points of the eight miscellaneous channels, joining with the Conception vessel, which traverses the face. L-7 *(lie que)* is thus indicated for diseases of the head, neck and face. LI-4 *(he gu)* is the uniting point of the Large Intestine channel, and is indicated for diseases of the Large Intestine. In addition, because the face is traversed by the Large Intestine channel, LI-4 *(he gu)* is also indicated for disorders of the head, face and sensory organs.

NEEDLING METHODS

Experience has shown that for acupuncture therapy to be effective the patient must feel the needle sensation, often referred to as 'obtaining Qi'. This sensation will differ from individual to individual, and has been variously described as one of numbness, soreness or distention that may spread, or be conducted, in a certain direction. If after needle insertion the sensation arrives quickly, the treatment will generally be effective. If the sensation is retarded, the treatment will be less effective. If there is no sensation at all, the treatment will usually be ineffective. This phenomenon is described in the *Ode of the Golden Needle:* "Rapid Qi, rapid effect; slow Qi, slow effect." Therefore, if the sensation is absent or slow in arriving, the reasons must be analyzed. The practitioner should first reassess the needle location, depth and angle. If these are found to be correct, then the method of needle manipulation should be reevaluated, because it is through manipulation that the needle sensation is obtained and conducted.

In choosing the method of needle manipulation, the practitioner must decide according to his or her own experience. Again, there are few set rules. With many practitioners, when they discover that a particular method is effective for treating a certain condition, they will continue to use that method in ensuing cases, thus making it their specialty.

Following is a discussion of the various needling methods used in the cases in this book to obtain and conduct the needle sensation.

Methods of Stimulation

The methods described in this section are used to obtain Qi after the needle has been inserted. The two basic techniques are raise-thrusting and twirling.

Raise-thrusting: This method involves inserting the needle to the appropriate depth, and then repeatedly raising and thrusting the needle. In general, a strong needle sensation is elicited when the amplitude is large, and the frequency is rapid. Conversely, a small amplitude and reduced frequency elicits a mild needle sensation.

Twirling or rotating: After the needle has been inserted to the appropriate depth, it is twirled back and forth. A strong needle sensation is elicited when the arc is large, and the twirling is rapid. A mild needle sensation results when the arc is small, and the twirling is slow. In twirling the needle, the arc should be between 180-360°. The needle should not be rotated in one direction only, which will cause the fibrous muscle tissue to 'catch' on the needle, producing pain.

Raise-thrust and twirling manipulation are generally used together, and are the most frequently utilized forms of stimulation. In addition, there are a number of supplementary methods which are utilized to hasten the arrival of Qi, and to strengthen the needle sensation.

'Following' is used when Qi is not obtained, but the needle is in the proper location for the point. This method involves lightly pressing the skin along the channel of the point being needled. The aim is to stimulate the flow of Qi in the channel so that Qi will be obtained at the point.

'Flicking' is applied when the needle sensation is weak. With the needle inserted, the handle of the needle is lightly flicked with the fingers. This will cause the needle to vibrate so that the sensation of Qi is strengthened.

'Scraping' is a method of strengthening and spreading the needle sensation. With the needle inserted, the tail of the needle is pressed lightly with the thumb to hold the needle steady. Using the nail of the index or middle finger of the same hand, the needle is then scraped. Alternatively, the index or middle finger may be used to steady the needle, and the scraping is applied with the nail of the thumb. Another variation is to use the nails of the thumb and index finger to scrape the handle from bottom to top, in a spiral manner.

Tonifying and Draining

An important component of needling methodology are the techniques of tonifying (strengthening) and draining (reducing), which are based on ancient medical principles. In the *Miraculous Pivot* (chapter 10) it is written: "Diseases of excess should be drained, and diseases of deficiency should be tonified." And in the *Thousand Ducat Prescriptions* it is written: "When needling is applied, tonifying and draining should be the principal techniques that are used first."

Tonifying means to strengthen the normal Qi so that diminished function is restored. Draining means to promote the expulsion of pathogenic influences or excess, again to restore normal bodily function.

Tonifying and draining are accomplished through different needle manipulation techniques. Through long experience, ancient practitioners developed many such techniques. Today only seven of these are commonly used in the clinic.

Balanced tonifying-draining: Raise-thrust and twirling manipulation are administered evenly. This is the most commonly used technique, by means of which both tonifying and draining are accomplished at the same time. This technique was used in many of the cases reported in this book, regardless of whether the condition was one of deficiency or excess. Many practitioners in China believe that unless the condition is severely deficient or excessive in nature, balanced tonifying-draining manipulation should be adequate to resolve the problem.

Twirling (rotating): For tonifying, the degree of rotation is small, the force used is slight, the twirling is slow, and the duration of manipulation is short. For draining, the degree of rotation is large, the force used is strong, the twirling is rapid, and the duration of manipulation is long. Some practitioners add a directional dimension to the twirling: for tonifying, the needle is rotated with force to the left, and for draining, to the right.

Raise-thrust: For tonifying, the needle is first inserted superficially, and then deeply. The needle is thrust forcefully and raised gently, with small amplitude, slow frequency, and a short duration of manipulation. For draining, the needle is first inserted deeply, and then raised to a superficial level. The needle is thrust gently and raised forcefully, with large amplitude, rapid frequency, and a longer duration of manipulation.

Slow-quick: For tonifying, the needle is inserted slowly, with little twirling, and is then quickly withdrawn. For draining, the needle is inserted quickly, with much twirling, and is then slowly withdrawn.

Directing the needle: For tonifying, the needle is pointed in the direction of channel flow. For draining, the needle is pointed against channel flow.

Respiration: For tonifying, the needle is inserted as the patient exhales, and withdrawn as the patient inhales. For draining, the needle is inserted as the patient inhales, and withdrawn as the patient exhales.

Opening and covering: For tonifying, after the needle is withdrawn, the needle hole is pressed with the finger to retain the Qi. For draining, the needle is agitated while it is withdrawn, and the needle hole is not pressed, which allows the pathogenic influences to escape.

Combined Needling Methods

These are techniques which combine tonifying and draining manipulation with techniques for moving Qi.

'Burning the mountain' and 'cooling the sky' are tonifying and draining techniques in which the insertion and withdrawal of the needle is accomplished in stages. Because three different depths are required, these techniques are appropriate only for points located in fleshy areas of the body.

'Burning the mountain' is a tonifying technique. The needle is first inserted to a superficial level, and is then advanced to a middle, and finally to a deep level. At each level, the needle is forcefully thrust, and gently raised, nine times. When these manipulations are completed, the needle is raised again to the superficial level. The procedure may be repeated until the patient experiences a warm or burning sensation, either locally or spreading along the channel. This technique is used for treating syndromes of Cold or deficiency.

'Cooling the sky' is a draining technique. As in the previous technique, the insertion and withdrawal of the needle is accomplished in three stages, and at three levels. The needle is first inserted to a deep level, and is then raised to a middle, and finally to a superficial level. At each level, the needle is gently thrust, and forcefully raised, six times. The procedure is repeated until a sensation of coolness is experienced. This technique is used for treating syndromes of intense Heat.

Because the sensation produced by these techniques is strong, they should be used with discretion. If the appropriate sensation is not elicited after a few repetitions, the technique should be discontinued until the next session. Both of these methods can be combined with other tonifying or draining techniques (respiration, opening and covering, etc.) in order to strengthen the therapeutic effect.

'Yin hidden in Yang' and 'Yang hidden in Yin' are combined methods of tonifying and draining. They are used for treating syndromes of both deficiency and excess. The needles are manipulated at two levels, superficial and deep.

For 'Yin hidden in Yang', the emphasis is on tonification: tonifying manipulation is followed by draining manipulation. The needle is first inserted to a superficial level, and is then forcefully thrust, and gently raised, nine times. The needle is then advanced to the deep level where draining is performed by gently thrusting, and forcefully raising the needle six times.

For 'Yang hidden in Yin', the emphasis is on draining: draining manipulation is followed by tonifying manipulation. The needle is first inserted to a deep level where it is gently thrust, and forcefully raised, six times. The needle is then withdrawn to a superficial level where it is forcefully thrust, and gently raised, nine times.

Retaining the Needles

After a needle has been inserted and manipulated, it may either be removed or retained in place. The purpose of retaining a needle is to strengthen the needling effect, as well as to allow further manipulation. There are no fixed rules concerning the duration of needle retainment, although some general guidelines were provided earlier in this introduction. Practitioners should use their judgment and experience in this respect.

SPECIAL NEEDLING METHODS

Joining Points

This is a method whereby the needle penetrates under the skin from one point to another. In effect, the points are 'joined' with the needle.

When needling in superficial tissue such as the face, transverse insertion is used. For other areas, slanted insertion is utilized. On the extremities, a point on one aspect may be joined with a point on the other aspect, e.g., P-6 *(nei guan)* with TB-5 *(wai guan)*. In some cases, more than two points may be joined during the same treatment: a point is joined first in one direction with another point; the needle is then partially withdrawn, and redirected to join with a third point.

This method is useful for treating patients who are apprehensive about the use of many needles. It strengthens the stimulation, and permits treatment of a large area with a single needle.

Cutaneous Needling

The cutaneous needle is also known as the 'plum blossom' or 'seven star' needle, as five to seven short needles are embedded in the head of the instrument. By tapping the skin along the channels, over points or other areas, the flow of Qi and Blood is stimulated.

For patients of robust constitution, or who are suffering from diseases of excess, strong stimulation may be used until very slight bleeding appears. Suitable areas for treatment include the back, buttocks and other, more muscular regions of the body.

Mild stimulation is used for children, persons of weak constitution, and for those suffering from diseases of deficiency. The needle is tapped until the skin becomes red and moist. Mild stimulation is suitable for areas such as the face, where the muscle tissue is thin.

Many types of disease may be treated with cutaneous needling. It is particularly effective for various skin disorders, including numbness of the skin. High blood pressure, insomnia and headache may also be treated with this method.

Pyramid Needling (Bloodletting)

In a number of cases reported in this book, the pyramid (tri-ensiform) needle was used for bloodletting. This method may be performed at acupuncture points or superficial veins, or at the sites of sprains, contusions and boils (early stages only). When utilizing this method, the skin is first cleaned thoroughly with alcohol. The skin is then pricked with the pyramid needle, and a few drops of blood are squeezed out. The skin is then swabbed again with alcohol.

The functions of bloodletting are to open the orifices and expel Heat, invigorate the flow of Blood to remove stasis, and to clear the channels. It is particularly useful for diseases of excess and of Heat, or for diseases of Cold excess. Conditions such as loss of consciousness, high fever, Wind-stroke, sore throat, redness and swelling of the eye, protracted painful obstruction, erysipelas, and numbness of the toes and fingers may all be treated with bloodletting.

The following items should be noted when using bloodletting:

• Because this type of therapy causes considerable pain, the patient must be positioned securely, and encouraged to cooperate with the practitioner. Precau-

tions against fainting should be taken.

• When pricking, the motion must be swift, accurate and shallow. Arteries must be avoided, and only a few drops of blood should be let during one treatment.

• Patients of weak constitution or with deficiency of Blood and Qi, as well as individuals with bleeding disorders, should not undergo this method of treatment.

• The frequency of bloodletting is largely a matter of discretion. In general, bloodletting may be administered once daily, with 3-5 treatments comprising one course of therapy. For acute conditions, however, treatment may be administered twice daily.

Piercing Therapy

Piercing therapy is a technique whereby the skin is pierced open and flaxen-like tissue fibers underneath are severed. The instrument used may be a large-gauge needle, pyramid needle, surgical scalpel, dental probe or hypodermic needle.

In general, this method is performed on eruptions of the skin that are associated with certain diseases. Such eruptions are often found on the back, particularly in the vicinity of the associated points of the back along the Bladder channel, since these are the locations to which the Qi of the Organs flows. However, eruptions may occur in other areas as well.

The eruptions usually appear as pinhead-sized papules, and may be red, pink, brown or grayish white. These eruptions must be distinguished from moles, angiomas, folliculitis and other skin pigmentations.

The procedure is performed in the following manner. The area to be treated is first disinfected with alcohol or iodine. A small, superficial incision is made, approximately 2-3mm in length. About 2-3 fibers of the underlying fibrous tissue are picked up and severed with the instrument. The wound is then dressed and covered with a bandage.

A surgical scalpel may be used to make the incision after local anesthetization. A needle is then inserted into the wound to sever the fibers.

The following precautions should be observed:

- Sterile technique must be strictly followed. To prevent infection, the patient should be advised to keep the wound dry.

- The patient should lie down during the procedure in order to avoid fainting, and should rest afterward.

- Pregnant women and individuals with heart conditions or bleeding disorders should not undergo this procedure.

- Piercing therapy is performed only once at a site, and should not be repeated.

MOXIBUSTION

Moxibustion is a method by which moxa *(Artemisia vulgaris)* with or without other herbs are burned on or above the skin, usually over acupuncture points. The heat that is produced is conducted through the channels so that the flow of Qi and Blood is stimulated, the normal Qi is strengthened, and pathogenic influences are eliminated. Moxibustion may be used alone for conditions that cannot be effectively treated by acupuncture, or it may be used in conjunction with needling in order to enhance the therapeutic effect.

Only the most commonly used forms of moxibustion will be discussed here. The two general methods are moxa cone and moxa stick moxibustion.

Moxa Cone Moxibustion

In this type of moxibustion, the moxa wool is shaped tightly into cones of various sizes. Depending on the strength of the patient's constitution and the nature of the disease, the size and number of cones used will differ. In general, for robust individuals and in the early stages of disease, more and larger cones should be used than for very young, weak or elderly patients, or for protracted conditions. When applying moxibustion to the head, face and chest, the cones should be fewer in number and smaller in size than for areas of deeper tissue, such as the back and abdomen.

There are two types of moxa cone moxibustion, direct and indirect.

Direct moxibustion: With this method, the cone is placed directly over the acupuncture point and burned. The scarring or pustulating variety of direct moxibustion is performed by allowing the cone to be completely consumed, so that the skin is cauterized and a blister is raised. About one week following the treatment, a pustule will develop, after which a scar will form. Because of the intense pain produced by this method, it is only used on patients who are of strong constitution. Scarring moxibustion is generally used for chronic disorders such as asthma, consumptive conditions and scrofula.

The non-scarring method of direct moxibustion produces intense heat in the skin, but without causing a blister. When the burning cone begins to cause pain, it is quickly removed with forceps or tweezers, and a new cone is burned in its place. This method is used for treating syndromes of Cold or deficiency.

Indirect moxibustion: With this method, a medium is placed between the burning cone and the skin. Depending on the condition to be treated, different mediums may be selected, the most common being ginger and garlic.

Ginger. A slice of fresh ginger 2-3cm in diameter and 2-3mm thick is used. Several tiny holes are first punctured into the slice, which is then placed over the point. A moxa cone is burned on top of the slice until the patient feels pain from the heat. The cone—or the entire ginger slice—is removed momentarily, and is then replaced. Additional cones may be burned on the ginger until the underlying skin has become red and moist. Ginger has a warm nature and is capable of dispelling Cold. This medium is therefore used for vomiting, abdominal pain, diarrhea, or joint pain due to Cold.

Garlic. A slice of fresh garlic is prepared in the same manner as described above for ginger, or the garlic may be crushed into a paste and spread on the skin over the point. A moxa cone is then placed on the garlic medium and burned, just as above. Garlic is warm and pungent in nature, and reduces swelling. It is therefore used for scrofula, abdominal masses and non-ulcerated carbuncles.

Salt. The umbilicus is filled with table salt, and a slice of ginger is placed on the salt. A large moxa cone is then placed on the ginger and burned. (If the moxa cone is placed directly on the salt, the salt may ignite and burn the skin.) This method is used for acute abdominal pain accompanied by diarrhea and vomiting, and for Wind-stroke.

Moxa Stick Moxibustion

This type of moxibustion is widely used today because of its convenience. There are two methods, warming and sparrow-pecking.

In warming moxibustion, the burning end of the moxa stick is held about 1-2cm above the selected point for approximately 3-5 minutes, until the skin has become moist and flushed. To ascertain the intensity of the heat at the point, the index and middle fingers of the practitioner's free hand can be placed on either side of the point. The distance of the moxa stick from the skin may then be adjusted accordingly. If the area to be treated is large, a variation of warming

moxibustion called circular moxibustion may be used, whereby the moxa stick is circled around and above the area until the skin becomes flushed.

In sparrow-pecking moxibustion, the burning end of the moxa stick is rapidly moved up and down in a 'pecking' motion above the acupuncture point, without touching the skin. The heat from this method is more direct and intense than that from warming moxibustion, and is therefore suitable for chronic disorders due to Cold.

Warm Needle Moxibustion

This is a technique that combines needling with moxibustion, and is used for conditions that require both forms of therapy. After the needle has been inserted and manipulated, moxa wool is attached to the handle of the needle and burned. Alternatively, a small piece or stub may be cut from a moxa stick and secured to the handle. Aluminum foil may be placed around the needle at the skin in order to catch the ashes.

Moxibustion Cylinder or Box

A moxibustion (or warming) cylinder is a metal container with a handle used to hold burning moxa. The container has several openings at one end to permit the emission of heat. For treating large, flat areas, a flat-bottomed container may be used, and for smaller areas or individual points, a pointed container. During treatment, the container is moved back and forth on the skin with an ironing motion until the area becomes red. This method of moxibustion is suitable for children and the elderly.

Wooden moxibustion boxes are approximately 16cm long, 10cm wide, and 10cm high. A metal screen mesh is fitted into the box, recessed about 6cm from the bottom. One or two slices of a moxa stick, each measuring 3-5cm in length, are ignited at one end and set on the screen. The box is then placed over the area to be treated, where it is left for 10-15 minutes. Because the screen is recessed, the moxibustion box can be placed over an area with or without needles. Suitable areas for this form of moxibustion are the chest, abdomen and back. It is used for such conditions as stomachache, menstrual cramps and back pain.

CONCLUSION

This introduction is intended to help the reader better understand the cases presented in this book. A basic knowledge of the principles of acupuncture and traditional Chinese medicine is assumed. In acupuncture, many diseases can be treated successfully using a variety of methods and point combinations. It should therefore be emphasized that the cases in this book represent only the experiences of a few prominent practitioners, and are not intended to serve as inflexible models for others to follow. Rather, it is hoped that these cases will shed some light on the actual manner and method of acupuncture practice in the People's Republic of China.

Note: *Point Nomenclature*
In this book, the following abbreviations are used for points on the channels, which are based upon the nomenclature adopted by the World Health Organization:

ABBREVIATION	CHANNEL
L-	Lung
LI-	Large Intestine
S-	Stomach
Sp-	Spleen
H-	Heart
SI-	Small Intestine
B-	Bladder
K-	Kidney
P-	Pericardium
TB-	Triple Burner
G-	Gall Bladder
L-	Liver
GV-	Governing
CV-	Conception

The point numbering system is the same as that used in *Acupuncture: A Comprehensive Text,* with the following exceptions on the Bladder channel:

COMPREHENSIVE TEXT	CASE HISTORIES
B-36 *(fu fen)*	B-41 *(fu fen)*
B-37 *(po hu)*	B-42 *(po hu)*
B-38 *(gao huang shu)*	B-43 *(gao huang shu)*
B-39 *(shen tang)*	B-44 *(shen tang)*
B-40 *(yi xi)*	B-45 *(yi xi)*
B-41 *(ge guan)*	B-46 *(ge guan)*
B-42 *(hun men)*	B-47 *(hun men)*
B-43 *(yang gang)*	B-48 *(yang gang)*
B-44 *(yi she)*	B-49 *(yi she)*
B-45 *(wei cang)*	B-50 *(wei cang)*
B-46 *(huang men)*	B-51 *(huang men)*
B-47 *(zhi shi)*	B-52 *(zhi shi)*
B-48 *(bao huang)*	B-53 *(bao huang)*
B-49 *(zhi bian)*	B-54 *(zhi bian)*
B-50 *(cheng fu)*	B-36 *(cheng fu)*
B-51 *(yin men)*	B-37 *(yin men)*
B-52 *(fu xi)*	B-38 *(fu xi)*
B-53 *(wei yang)*	B-39 *(wei yang)*
B-54 *(wei zhong)*	B-40 *(wei zhong)*

The *pin yin* used for CV-17 in this book is *tan zhong,* rather than *shan zhong.* □

CHAPTER ONE
General Internal Medicine

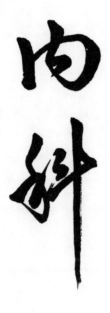

Abdominal Distention from Stagnant Liver Qi

Gǔ Zhàng 鼓胀

Dai, female, 45 years old. The patient's chief complaint was abdominal distention of 2 years'
duration. The condition appeared after a time of extreme emotional stress that resulted in pain
and fullness in the subcostal regions. Ultrasonography, barium meal examination and a liver
function test revealed nothing remarkable. The use of modern and traditional Chinese medi-
cines for 18 months was ineffective. Because the symptoms became more severe, she sought
acupuncture treatment.

The four examinations of traditional Chinese medicine found a markedly distended abdomen which resembled a pregnancy of six to seven months, with a circumference of 100cm. The abdomen was soft and tympanitic, and no mass was palpable. The patient appeared tired and had a sallow complexion. She complained of depression, and stated that she sighed frequently, was irritable and had a poor temper. She had a poor appetite and experienced frequent belching. The abdominal distention was aggravated by anger and intake of food, but was relieved with upward or downward elimination of gas.

Her menstrual periods were irregular and quite painful, with a dark red flow of moderate amount, and her breasts became distended during menstruation. The tongue was pale with a white coating, and the pulse was thin and wiry.

SYNDROME DIFFERENTIATION

In Chinese medicine, abdominal distention is known as 'drum distention' because of the protuberant shape of the abdomen. There are three clinical types of abdominal distention, due to accumulation of Qi, Blood and water respectively. Qi distention is a result of emotional depression and stagnant Liver Qi. Blood distention is usually a complication of Qi distention. Water distention may be caused by damage to the Spleen, such that its function of transporting and distributing nutrients and water is disrupted.

The clinical manifestations of each type of distention are also different. In Qi distention, the skin is elastic upon palpation and is of normal color. The signs and symptoms, which are aggravated by anger, are relieved upon elimination of gas. In Blood distention, the abdomen is hard upon palpation and is more distended, with blue veins standing out over the surface. Masses may be felt under the costal margins, and prickling pain is experienced over those regions. The skin is usually scaly and dry, and the patient has a dark complexion. The tongue is purple, and may sometimes present with red spots. Of all of the abdominal distention syndromes, the abdomen is most distended in the case of water distention. The skin of the abdomen appears smooth and shiny, and is easily pitted with the finger. (It takes some time for the pit to disappear.) There is urinary dysfunction, and there may be edema of the lower limbs. The tongue is often covered with a white, greasy coating.

Based upon the clinical presentation of this patient, the condition was diagnosed as Qi distention due to stagnant Liver Qi. The Liver has the function of smoothing and regulating the flow of Qi and Blood, and exerts a great influence on the function of Qi in the Organs, especially the Spleen. In this case, the Liver failed to function properly, and the Spleen was therefore unable to transport and distribute nutrients and water effectively, resulting in a poor appetite and a bloated feeling after meals. Because of the dysfunction of the Spleen in promoting growth and development, the body became deficient in Qi and Blood, giving rise to symptoms such as fatigue, lassitude and a sallow complexion. And because of the dysfunction of the Stomach in facilitating the downward movement of food, frequent belching resulted. The pale tongue and thin pulse both reflected dysfunction of the Spleen, while the wiry pulse was a sign of Liver involvement. Finally, as a result of dysfunction of the Liver in storing Blood, menstrual disorders and dysmenorrhea occurred.

In summary, this was a case of Qi distention resulting from stagnant Liver Qi, which led to diminished function of the Spleen. Symptoms of both excess due to stagnant Liver Qi, and deficiency due to diminished function of the Spleen in metabolizing nutrients, were present.

TREATMENT

The principles of treatment consisted of soothing the Liver and promoting the functions of the Spleen and Stomach in order to remove the stagnation and resolve the distention. Points on the Liver and Spleen channels were the principal points in the prescription, and both tonifying and draining manipulation were utilized.

Points selected:

CV-17 *(tan zhong)*, CV-12 *(zhong wan)*, Liv-13 *(zhang men)*, P-6 *(nei guan)*, S-36 *(zu san li)*, Sp-6 *(san yin jiao)*, Liv-3 *(tai chong)*, Sp-4 *(gong sun)*

All points were needled once daily, and the needles retained for 20 minutes during each session. One course of treatment consisted of 10 sessions, followed by 2-3 days' rest.

Discussion of points:

Draining manipulation was used at CV-17 *(tan zhong)*, CV-12 *(zhong wan)*, P-6 *(nei guan)* and Liv-3 *(tai chong)*, and tonifying manipulation at the other points. CV-17 *(tan zhong)* was chosen to normalize the flow of Qi, as it is the point associated with Qi among the eight meeting points. CV-12 *(zhong wan)* was selected as a local point. Liv-13 *(zhang men)*, the alarm point of the Spleen, combined with S-36 *(zu san li)* and Sp-6 *(san yin jiao)*, serve to tonify the Spleen and Qi.

P-6 *(nei guan)* and Sp-4 *(gong sun)*, two of the points of confluence of the eight miscellaneous channels, were used to relax the mind, and to remove stagnation. P-6 *(nei guan)* was chosen to regulate the upper Burner, and Sp-4 *(gong sun)* to regulate the lower Burner. When used together, they clear the Triple Burner. Liv-3 *(tai chong)*, the source point of the Liver channel, was combined with Liv-13 *(zhang men)* to soothe the Liver.

RESULTS

No improvement was noted after three courses of treatment. CV-6 *(qi hai)* was then added, and deep insertion (1.5-2.0 units) with longer needles was applied at CV-12 *(zhong wan)* and CV-6 *(qi hai)*. This was in accord with chapter 57 of *Miraculous Pivot,* which teaches that abdominal distention syndromes should be treated promptly, using draining manipulation, and that deep needle insertion should be applied if no effect is noted. This is because Qi is deeply entrenched in the interior, and shallow needle insertion cannot reach the affected area; the stagnation will therefore not be eliminated, nor will the normal flow of Qi be restored.

After one course of treatment with this modified point prescription, the abdominal distention began to improve, as did the other symptoms. After another four courses, the circumference of the abdomen decreased from 100cm to 83cm, the patient's appetite improved, and menstruation returned to normal without any dysmenorrhea. Three more courses with the same set of points were administered to consolidate the effect. Follow-up for one year showed no relapse.

Note: With regard to deep needle insertion, a word of caution may be in order. At CV-12 *(zhong wan)* and CV-6 *(qi hai)*, needle insertion is perpendicular to a depth just *above* the inner lining of the abdominal wall. Penetration of the abdominal cavity must be avoided. Needle manipulation should be limited to twirling, without raising or thrusting. □

Abdominal Distention from Stagnant Liver Qi

Gǔ Zhàng 鼓胀

Song, female, 49 years old. For 5 years the patient often felt tired and weak, and suffered from slight abdominal distention and dryness in the eyes, all of which she paid little attention to. One year ago, the abdominal distention became severe, and she felt general malaise. Her vision became blurred and her appetite was poor. She had slight, generalized edema, scanty urine and a severe headache. Her illness was diagnosed as cirrhosis of the liver. She was treated with traditional Chinese and western medicines, which alleviated the symptoms. Four months ago, however, her condition became aggravated. Her abdomen ballooned with distention to the point that she was unable to lie on her back. She experienced generalized edema, scanty urine, thirst and dizziness. She returned to the hospital. Liver function studies were normal, but an ultrasound scan suggested swelling on the left lobe of the liver with parenchymal damage.

Examination of the patient found her face to be pale. She was listless and spoke in a very low voice. The heart and lungs were normal to auscultation and percussion. Her abdomen was severely distended, measuring 130cm in circumference, and the skin over it shined with tension. Shifting dullness was heard on percussion. The lower border of the liver reached the navel. The liver itself was firm upon palpation, with marked tenderness.

The extremities were cold to the touch and both legs were markedly edematous. The tongue was very swollen and toothmarked, and the coating was slippery in appearance. The pulse was submerged and slippery.

SYNDROME DIFFERENTIATION

The Liver is situated below the costal region and its channel is distributed bilaterally. This Organ 'opens' through the eyes. The patient's condition was due to stagnant Liver Qi, hence the symptoms of pain in the sides, poor appetite, abdominal distention, general malaise and listlessness. Prolonged stagnation of Liver Qi led to stasis of Blood, manifested by pain and hard swelling below the costal regions.

Because the Spleen was 'conquered' by the Liver, Spleen Qi became deficient, which caused insufficiency of nutrients for the production and development of Qi and

Blood. This accounted for the pale complexion and weak voice. The weakening of the Spleen in turn caused insufficiency of Blood in the Liver, depriving the eyes of nourishment, and thus leading to their dryness and to the blurring of vision. The deficiency of Spleen Qi and the weakening of the Spleen's function also resulted in coldness of the extremities, and in the stagnation of Dampness and the failure of water circulation; hence the swollen legs and abdominal distention. The protracted deficiency of Spleen Qi induced deficiency of Kidney Yang, which aggravated all of the above symptoms. The swollen, tooth-marked tongue with a slippery coating, and the submerged, slippery pulse indicated the presence of excess Fluids.

In summary, this was a case of Blood stasis in the Liver due to stagnant Liver Qi, which caused deficiency of Liver Qi and Blood, and in turn led to deficiency of Spleen Qi and Kidney Yang.

TREATMENT

Points on the Liver channel and Conception vessel, as well as the associated points of the back, formed the basis of the prescription. Balanced tonifying-draining manipulation was used, and the needles were retained for 30 minutes during each session. Points on one side of the body (either front or back) were treated first; the needles were then removed, and points on the other side of the body were treated. Acupuncture was administered once daily. Fifteen treatments comprised one course of therapy, with 2-3 days' rest between courses.

Points selected:

S-36 *(zu san li)*, Sp-6 *(san yin jiao)*, Liv-4 *(zhong feng)*, CV-9 *(shui fen)*, CV-6 *(qi hai)*, CV-3 *(zhong ji)*, B-18 *(gan shu)*, B-20 *(pi shu)*, B-23 *(shen shu)*, B-28 *(pang guang shu)*

Discussion of points:

S-36 *(zu san li)*, Sp-6 *(san yin jiao)* and CV-6 *(qi hai)* help replenish Qi and Blood; Sp-6 *(san yin jiao)* also invigorates the Spleen, thus helping to eliminate the Dampness and edema. CV-3 *(zhong ji)*, the alarm point of the Bladder, was chosen to promote diuresis. CV-9 *(shui fen)* is an empirical point used for removing water. Liv-4 *(zhong feng)* was used to treat the stagnant Liver Qi and Blood stasis, and to resolve the edema. B-18 *(gan shu)* and B-20 *(pi shu)* were needled to treat the stagnant Liver Qi, and to invigorate the Spleen. B-23 *(shen shu)* and B-28 *(pang guang shu)* were used to replenish Kidney Yang, and to remove the Dampness and edema.

RESULTS

After two treatments, the volume of urine increased, and the abdominal distention was somewhat mitigated. After fifteen treatments, the volume of urine was further increased. The edema gradually subsided, the patient's appetite improved, and she became more spirited. After thirty treatments, her abdomen measured 91cm in circumference. Her face turned ruddy and the edema in her legs further diminished. After sixty treatments, the ascites disappeared altogether, and the abdomen measured 84cm. The liver was palpable 4cm below the xiphoid process, and 1.5cm below the costal margin; its consistency was soft.

Treatment was continued with the same set of points for another four months to consolidate the therapeutic effect. By that time, the patient's vigor was fully restored. She spoke in a loud, clear voice, moved about freely, and was able to do household chores. Her clinical symptoms had basically disappeared. Altogether, she had been treated for more than five months, and had received a total of one hundred fifty-five treatments. □

Abdominal Distention from Damp-Heat
(Paralytic Ileus)

Gǔ Zhàng 鼓脹

Zhou, male, 36 years old. The patient suffered from a perforated appendix complicated by general peritonitis. He had undergone an appendectomy and peritoneal drainage. Sixteen hours after the operation, abdominal distention was experienced, although flatus was expelled. Two days after the operation, however, no additional gas was passed, and the distention increased. Auscultation found an absence of peristaltic sounds, and X-ray revealed gaseous distention of the intestinal tract. Gastrointestinal decompression by Wangensteen suction and rectal tube was instituted, supplemented with neostigmine. The distention was somewhat diminished, but then increased on the following day, and was complicated by nausea and vomiting. The patient was thereupon referred for acupuncture therapy.

Examination of the patient found that his body temperature was 36.8⁰C. The abdomen was quite distended, but without tenderness or rebound tenderness, and percussion was resonant. Peristaltic sounds could not be heard. The abdominal wound was healed, and the sutures and drainage tubes had been removed. White blood cell count was 8,000/cu mm.

The four examinations of Chinese medicine found a dark, lackluster complexion. The patient was very restless and complained of a bitter taste in the mouth. His mouth was also dry, but he had no desire to drink. His urine output was decreased, and its color was yellow. The tongue was dark red with a greasy, yellow coating. The pulse was submerged and forceful.

SYNDROME DIFFERENTIATION

In Chinese medicine, acute appendicitis is known as Intestinal Abscess, and is ascribed to Damp-Heat which interferes with the flow of Qi and Blood in the Intestines. In severe cases, the Heat may cause putrefaction of Blood and tissue, resulting in total obstruction of the intestinal tract, and severe disruption of Qi dynamics. Surgical intervention may resolve the Damp-Heat; however, the disruption of Qi dynamics may be aggravated by the mechanical disturbances of surgery; hence the abdominal distention.

The functions of the Stomach and Intestines are the digestion of food and the transport of indigestible residue downward.

When the Large Intestine is obstructed, Stomach Qi cannot descend; it therefore flows in the reverse direction, and gives rise to nausea and vomiting.

The patient's symptoms of restlessness, bitter taste in the mouth, scanty, yellow urine, dryness in the mouth without desire to drink, and a yellow, greasy tongue coating were manifestations of the remnants of Damp-Heat in the digestive tract. When Qi is stagnant, the flow of Blood will be inadequate. That is why the face was lackluster and the tongue was dark red in color. The submerged pulse denoted an interior disease, and forcefulness signified excess.

The syndrome was therefore one of disruption of the Qi dynamics of the intestinal tract by Damp-Heat, which resulted in stagnation.

TREATMENT

The principles of treatment were to stimulate the movement of Qi, disperse the stagnation, resolve the Dampness and clear the Heat.

Points selected:

S-25 *(tian shu)*, S-37 *(shang ju xu)*, P-6 *(nei guan)*, S-36 *(zu san li)*

Discussion of points:

S-25 *(tian shu)* and S-37 *(shang ju xu)*, the alarm and lower uniting points respectively of the Large Intestine, were the principal points in the prescription. They were chosen to directly regulate the Qi dynamics of the intestinal tract, and to resolve the remnants of Damp-Heat. P-6 *(nei guan)*, one of the points of confluence of the eight miscellaneous channels, calms the Heart and Spirit, and regulates Qi; in this case, it was used to pacify the Stomach and arrest the vomiting. S-36 *(zu san li)*, the lower uniting point of the Stomach, is traditionally used for distention of the lower abdomen and for

other digestive disorders. Here, it was combined with P-6 *(nei guan)* to pacify the Stomach and arrest the vomiting, and with S-25 *(tian shu)* and S-37 *(shang ju xu)* to relieve abdominal distention.

Draining manipulation was applied at all four points through raise-thrust and twirling techniques. At P-6 *(nei guan)* and S-36 *(zu san li)* the needles were retained for 30 minutes, and at S-25 *(tian shu)* and S-37 *(shang ju xu)* for 2 hours. The needles were retained for this length of time to prolong and strengthen the needle sensation. Once every 15 minutes the needles were manipulated for 5 minutes.

RESULTS

Following the first treatment, the patient was placed under observation. After six hours, the therapeutic effect was not very satisfactory. Although the nausea and vomiting were relieved, the other symptoms were still present. The peristaltic sounds were weak and only occasionally heard.

The point selection was then reassessed. It was determined that S-25 *(tian shu)* and S-37 *(shang ju xu)* should be replaced because both are Stomach channel points, and it was thought that the trauma of surgery had disrupted the flow of Qi in the Stomach channel and rendered these points ineffective. B-25 *(da chang shu)* and B-32 *(ci liao)* were therefore substituted.

B-25 *(da chang shu)* is the associated point on the back for the Large Intestine. It is particularly effective in treating diseases of that Organ. B-32 *(ci liao)* has the effect of regulating Qi and invigorating Blood. Combined with S-36 *(zu san li)*, it is used empirically to treat intestinal distention and acute intestinal obstruction. Furthermore, because B-32 *(ci liao)* is almost at the same level as the large intestine, it may be regarded as a local point. Draining manipulation was used at these two points, and the needles were retained for two hours, with five minutes of manipulation once every fifteen minutes. When B-32 *(ci liao)* was needled, the sensation was felt in the lower abdomen.

Immediately after completion of the second treatment, gas was expelled and sounds of peristalsis were heard. The distention was markedly alleviated. The same points were needled on the following day, and the needles were retained for 30 minutes. Marked diminution in distention associated with peristaltic sounds was noted, and 500ml of liquid diet was given. Eight hours later, the patient had his first bowel movement since the surgery. After a total of only 3 treatments, bowel movement of gas and stool was normal, and food could be taken. Treatment was then discontinued, and the patient was discharged after just 5 days in the hospital. □

Asthmatic Condition
(Bronchial Asthma)

Xiāo Zhèng 哮症

Ji, male, 46 years old. The patient complained of recurrent asthmatic attacks and coughing of 10 years' duration, often precipitated by changes in the weather. He recently suffered a relapse for 2 weeks after a cold. He was short of breath, and was unable to breathe while lying down. There was slight sweating, chills, and white, foamy and watery sputum. His appetite was poor, and his stools were unformed. The tongue was light red with a white, greasy coating. The pulse was submerged, slippery and frail. Auscultation revealed severe rhonchi and wheezing. Chest X-ray was normal. Chinese and western medicines were tried, but were ineffective. The patient thereupon came to the acupuncturist.

SYNDROME DIFFERENTIATION

Bronchial asthma is a paroxysmal allergic disease of the lungs characterized by repeated attacks of wheezing and dyspnea. In traditional Chinese medicine, bronchial asthma falls under the broad category of asthmatic condition, and its etiology is attributed to obstruction by Phlegm.

There are three clinical types of Phlegm obstruction. Cold-Phlegm obstruction of the Lung is caused by invasion of external Cold which draws forth hidden Phlegm *(fú tán)*. Manifestations include frequent attacks after colds, wheezing, foamy, white sputum, a slippery, white tongue coating, and a floating, tight pulse. Heat-Phlegm obstruction of the Lung is induced by Heat and is character-ized by loud and rough wheezing, yellow, sticky and thick sputum, and a red tongue with a yellow, greasy coating. The pulse is slippery and rapid, and the patient feels restless. The third type of Phlegm obstruction is caused by deficiency of Spleen and Kidney Yang, in which Qi fails to transform the Fluids, which then accumulate as Phlegm in the interior. The clinical manifestations include wheezing and shallow, labored breathing, particularly after physical exertion. The tongue is pale and tender in appearance. The pulse is frail, and the patient feels chilly.

In the present case, the patient had suffered from paroxysmal asthmatic attacks for ten years, which caused accumulation of Phlegm in the interior. Upon invasion by external Cold, its combination with the old Phlegm resulted in a sign of Cold-Phlegm obstruction: thin, white and foamy sputum. This condition caused shortness of breath, which prevented the patient from lying down. Aversion to cold was a sign of Yang deficiency. The poor appetite and unformed stools indicated that Cold was not only in the Lung, but had also damaged Spleen Yang. The submerged, slippery and frail pulse also pointed to the presence of Phlegm, and to deficiency of Yang. The diagnosis was accordingly Cold-Phlegm obstruction of the Lung, and deficiency of Spleen Yang.

TREATMENT

The principles of treatment were to warm the Lung and reduce Phlegm, and to strengthen the Spleen and invigorate Spleen Yang.

Points selected:
Moxibustion was administered at B-13 *(fei shu)*, B-43 *(gao huang shu)*, CV-12 *(zhong wan)* and S-36 *(zu san li)*; acupuncture at CV-22 *(tian tu)*, CV-17 *(tan zhong)*, L-7 *(lie que)* and S-40 *(feng long)*

Discussion of points:
B-13 *(fei shu)* is the associated point of the Lung on the back. Treating this point has the effect of ventilating the Lung and relieving asthma. The use of moxibustion strengthens the effect of warming Cold and reducing Phlegm in the Lung. Moxibustion at B-43 *(gao huang shu)* regulates and warms Lung Qi. CV-12 *(zhong wan)* is the alarm point of the Stomach, and S-36 *(zu san li)* is the lower uniting point of the Stomach channel. The Spleen and the Stomach are interior-exteriorly related; hence administering moxibustion at these two points strengthens the Spleen and warms Spleen Yang.
CV-22 *(tian tu)* is an important point for treating asthma. CV-17 *(tan zhong)* is the center of respiration, and is thus effective in treating respiratory diseases. L-7 *(lie que)* is the point of confluence of the Lung channel and Conception vessel, and is effective in clearing the Lung. When these three points are stimulated, asthma and coughing are relieved. S-40 *(feng long)* is an important point for reducing Phlegm, and is used specifically for diseases associated with Phlegm.

B-13 *(fei shu)* and B-43 *(gao huang shu)* were treated bilaterally with indirect moxibustion, using a ginger medium. Ginger is warm in nature and is capable of dispelling Cold. With the patient in a prone position, a slice of ginger was placed over each of the four points, and a small moxa cone was burned on each of the slices. Heat was transmitted through the ginger. When the heat became excessive, the ginger slice was gently removed. Ten moxa cones were used during each session at each of the points. After a cone was consumed, its ashes were removed and another cone was burned on the ginger.

CV-12 *(zhong wan)* and S-36 *(zu san li)* were first needled, and then heated with warm needle moxibustion. CV-22 *(tian tu)* was needled to a depth of 1.5 units along the back of the sternum. As soon as the needle sensation was obtained, the needle was withdrawn. All other points were needled with balanced tonifying-draining manipulation using raise-thrust technique.

RESULTS

The asthma and coughing were improved after daily treatments for ten days, and the patient was able to lie down without difficulty in breathing. However, since the Kidney is the foundation of the innate constitution and controls inspiration, it is difficult to restore the functions of the Lung and Spleen when the Kidney Essence is insufficient. Moxibustion was therefore administered at CV-4 *(guan yuan)* to tonify Kidney Qi.

After another two weeks of daily treatments, all symptoms were markedly improved, and the asthma was basically resolved. The patient no longer felt chilly, his appetite was improved, and his stools were normal. Treatment continued for another week at CV-22 *(tian tu)*, S-40 *(feng long)* and CV-4 *(guan yuan)*, after which the condition was considered to be under control. During a two-year follow-up, there was no recurrence of symptoms. □

Collapse from Roundworms
(Biliary Ascariasis)

Hui Jué 蚘厥

Song, male, 27 years old. The patient, a farmer, suffered paroxysms of upper abdominal colic for 3 days. About 1 week before, the patient had noticed dull pain around the umbilicus, which was partially relieved by pressure. He often regurgitated sour fluids. Four days ago he was given syrup of piperazine to expel worms because ascaris (roundworm) eggs were found in the stools. After expulsion of about 10 adult worms, severe pain was felt to the right of the xiphoid process, which lasted half an hour. Since then, 3-4 paroxysms occurred daily. The pain was described as piercing, from front to back; it was excruciating, and did not respond to analgesics.

Examination found that the patient was pale, and was obviously suffering from severe pain. His abdomen showed no signs of rigidity, but was exquisitely tender in the area to the right of the xiphoid process. The extremities were cold to the touch. The tongue body was pale and the tongue coating was thick, greasy and white. The pulse was thin and wiry.

Laboratory examination showed a white blood cell count of 21,000/cu mm. Differential count of the white blood cells was 23% neutrophils, 70% lymphocytes, 3% eosinophils, 1% basophils and 3% monocytes. The hemoglobin was 12g.

The stools contained many ascaris eggs. The western medical diagnosis was biliary ascariasis, and the traditional Chinese medical diagnosis was collapse *(jué)* from roundworms.

SYNDROME DIFFERENTIATION

The patient had long been infested with worms. Administration of an anthelminthic resulted in partial elimination; however, this disturbed the remaining worms, some of which wandered into the biliary tract, which interfered with the Qi dynamics of the Liver-Gall Bladder system. Obstruction to the flow of Qi gave rise to pain, hence the right hypochondric colic. Disturbance of Liver-Gall Bladder Qi caused adverse flow of Stomach Qi, thus the acid regurgitation. When the pain became extremely intense, symptoms of collapse syndrome were evident: facial pallor, cold extremities and wiry pulse. The thick, greasy, white tongue coating denoted the presence of Dampness in the digestive tract, and the wiry pulse indicated pain.

The syndrome was therefore one of obstruction of Qi in the Liver-Gall Bladder due to roundworms which interfered with the ascending and descending of Qi. Dampness was also present in the digestive tract.

TREATMENT

Points selected:

G-34 *(yang ling quan)*, CV-12 *(zhong wan)*, B-19 *(dan shu)*, G-24 *(ri yue)*, S-36 *(zu san li)*

Treatment was administered once daily, and the needles were retained for 30 minutes during each session.

Discussion of points:

G-34 *(yang ling quan)* is the lower uniting point of the Gall Bladder, and is used in treating diseases of that Organ. It has been found that needling G-34 *(yang ling quan)* relaxes Oddi's sphincter,[1] and enhances the contraction of the gall bladder. It is therefore a commonly-used point for dislodging parasites and suppressing biliary pain. CV-12 *(zhong wan)* is the meeting point of the Yang Organs. Needling this point promotes the ascending and descending of Qi, and regulates the Triple Burner and the six Yang Organs. B-19 *(dan shu)* is the associated point on the back for the Gall Bladder. G-24 *(ri yue)* is the alarm point of the Gall Bladder. Needling these two points facilitates the flow of Gall Bladder Qi, which helps suppress the pain. S-36 *(zu san li)* strengthens the Stomach and Spleen, resolves Dampness and regulates Qi. As a general tonifying point, it is capable of strengthening the normal Qi in order to expel pathogenic influences.

Each of the points was first tonified and then drained, because this condition was one in which signs of both deficiency and excess were present. Deficiency was manifested during the attacks of pain by the facial pallor and cold in the extremities, while excess was manifested by the presence of Dampness and worms.

The sequence of treatment was first to tonify normal Qi, and then to drain the pathogenic influences. Accordingly, at G-34 *(yang ling quan)* the needle was first inserted to a depth of about 0.3 unit, and then manipulated with a tonifying method of raise-thrust and twirling. After the arrival of Qi, the needle was inserted deeper to about 1 unit, and this time draining manipulation was applied through raise-thrust and twirling. The needle sensation was strongly felt as a sense of cold and numbness shooting along the Gall Bladder channel in the direction of the gall bladder. At CV-12 *(zhong wan)* the same method of tonifying followed by draining manipulation was applied; the final needle depth was 1.3 units. Reaction to the needle was one of local distention. B-19 *(dan shu)* was needled with the same method to a final depth of 1 unit. G-24 *(ri yue)* was needled obliquely to a depth of 0.3 unit, and then to 0.5 unit. At S-36 *(zu san li)* the same method was utilized. A strong sensation of cold, distention and soreness moving toward the upper abdomen was obtained.

RESULTS

While the needles were retained during the first treatment session, the pain immediately diminished. Before withdrawing the needles, they were manipulated once again (tonifying followed by draining), and the pain

---

[1] Yun Min, et al. "X-ray observations of biliary tract function following acupuncture." In: "Shanghai Yangpu District Central Hospital, Department of Radiology. Coordination of acupuncture during X-ray in diagnosing gastrointestinal diseases: abstracts from papers delivered at the National Conference on Acupuncture and Moxibustion and Acupuncture Anesthesia." 1979; 42.

almost disappeared. The following day, the patient reported only slight discomfort in the upper right quadrant. He was treated again in the same manner, and the discomfort disappeared upon withdrawal of the needles. Two more treatments were administered to consolidate the effect. Examination of peripheral blood then showed total white blood cell count of 8000/cu mm, and differential count of 65% neutrophils, 26% lymphocytes, 3% eosinophils, 1% basophils and 5% monocytes.

The patient was discharged with complete relief of symptoms. He was advised to take further anthelminthic therapy to expel any remaining worms. □

Constipation

Biàn Bì 便秘

Lin, male, 65 years old. The patient had been bedridden for quite some time, and suffered from chronic constipation, with bowel movements only once every 3-5 days. Even when he had an urgent need to defecate, it required great exertion to do so. He was listless, short of breath on exertion, had weakness of the limbs, and sweated spontaneously. His face, lips and fingernails were pale. The tongue was tender and pale, with a thin coating. The pulse was submerged, thin and without strength.

SYNDROME DIFFERENTIATION

Constipation can refer to hardness of the stools, or to difficult or infrequent defecation. This patient had bowel movements at 3-5 day intervals, which required considerable exertion.

Depending on the signs and symptoms, constipation is of two general types, excess and deficiency. Excess-type constipation can be subdivided into two patterns: congealed Heat in the digestive tract, and stagnant Liver Qi. In addition to constipation, the former pattern may include such symptoms as a sensation of fullness in the stomach, bad breath, thirst and restlessness. The stools are dry and hard and may contain blood. Other symptoms include yellow urine, a yellow and dry tongue coating, and a slippery, forceful pulse. Stagnant Liver Qi, on the other hand, presents with such symptoms as belching, distention in the hypochondriac region, poor appetite, a wiry pulse, and a thin, greasy tongue coating.

Deficiency-type constipation can also be subdivided into two patterns: deficient Qi and Blood, and deficient Yang with replete Yin. The former pattern is primarily encountered in patients after an illness, in women after childbirth, and in the aged. Symptoms include paleness of the face, lips and fingernails, listlessness, weakness of the limbs, shortness of breath on exertion, and spontaneous sweating. Often, much effort is needed to empty the bowels. The tongue is pale with a thin coating, and the pulse is submerged, thin and without force. With deficient Yang and replete Yin, in addition to constipation, other symptoms include coldness of the limbs, a preference for warmth and an aversion to cold, coldness and pain in the abdomen, a white tongue with a moist coating, and a submerged, slow pulse. This pattern is also found primarily in the aged and debilitated.

In this particular patient, the constipation was due to deficient Qi and Blood after a protracted illness in old age. When Qi is deficient, the Large Intestine becomes weak in conveying its contents, and when Blood is deficient, the body Fluids become insufficient to moisten the Large Intestine; constipation results. The listlessness, weakness of the limbs, shortness of breath on exertion, and spontaneous sweating indicated deficiency of Qi, while the pale face, lips and fingernails reflected deficiency of Blood. The paleness of the tongue, and the submerged pulse which was without strength, were also manifestations of Qi and Blood deficiency.

TREATMENT

Since this patient suffered from deficient Qi and Blood, treatment was directed at tonifying the Qi, nourishing the Blood, moistening the Intestines, and releasing the obstruction from the bowels. In Chinese medicine, the Spleen and Stomach are the source for the genesis and transformation of Qi and Blood. Tonifying the Spleen and Stomach therefore replenishes Qi and Blood.

Points selected:
B-20 *(pi shu)*, B-21 *(wei shu)*, S-36 *(zu san li)*, TB-6 *(zhi gou)*, S-37 *(shang ju xu)*

All points were needled bilaterally with tonifying manipulation. Treatment was administered once daily.

Discussion of points:
Because the root problem was deficiency of Qi and Blood, S-36 *(zu san li)*, B-20 *(pi shu)* and B-21 *(wei shu)* were selected. S-36 *(zu san li)* is a general tonification point for the Spleen and Stomach. B-20 *(pi shu)* and B-21 *(wei shu)* are the associated points on the back for the Spleen and Stomach respectively. Tonifying these points therefore strengthens the source of Qi and Blood. TB-6 *(zhi gou)* is an effective point in treating constipation, and can be used for all forms of this disorder.

The lower uniting point of the Large Intestine, S-37 *(shang ju xu)*, is an important point in treating diseases of that Organ. The effectiveness of the lower uniting points in treating diseases of the Yang Organs was first noted in chapter 4 of the *Miraculous Pivot*. In chapter 2, it was also observed that both the Large and Small Intestines pertain to the Stomach. Thus, although both the Large Intestine's lower uniting point, S-37 *(shang ju xu)*, and the Small Intestine's lower uniting point, S-39 *(xia ju shu)*, belong to the Stomach channel, they can be effectively used in treating diseases of the Intestines. Since constipation is a disorder of the Large Intestine, S-37 *(shang ju xu)* was chosen here.

RESULTS

After two treatments, the patient was able to empty his bowels once a day. Although he still experienced some difficulty in passing stools, less exertion was needed than before. After five more treatments, his bowel movements were quite smooth and required little effort. The stools were soft in consistency. Therapy was suspended for five days, after which a second course of seven treatments was administered to consolidate the therapeutic effect. Acupuncture was then discontinued.

On follow-up two months later, the patient's condition had stabilized. He continued to have effortless bowel movements once a day. However, the systemic symptoms persisted because acupuncture had not been administered for a long enough period of time to resolve the root problem of Qi and Blood deficiency. □

Coughing of Blood
(Pulmonary Tuberculosis)

Kǎ Xuè 咯血

Chen, male, 27 years old. The patient was hospitalized about 6 months ago because of massive pulmonary hemorrhage. The diagnosis was pulmonary tuberculosis. After collapse therapy by pneumothorax, the bleeding was arrested, and the patient was discharged after showing some improvement. However, he recently experienced coughing of blood, presumably after undue fatigue. On 2 occasions, blood loss was estimated to be approximately 400ml and 100ml respectively. X-ray showed bilateral infiltrations. Sputum culture was negative. Upon readmission to the hospital, attempts were made to stop the hemorrhage with modern drugs, but to no avail. Because the lesions were bilateral, and pneumothorax was no longer feasible, the patient was referred for acupuncture therapy.

The four examinations of Chinese medicine revealed coughing with expectoration of frothy sputum mixed with much blood, which was bright red in color. There was chest and hypochondriac pain, spontaneous sweating, low-grade afternoon fever and flushed cheeks. The tongue was red and without coating, and the pulse was thin and rapid.

SYNDROME DIFFERENTIATION

Pulmonary tuberculosis is regarded in Chinese medicine as a type of deficiency consumption *(xū láo)*. It is a contagious disease, with a focus of disharmony primarily in the Lung. It is characterized by symptoms of coughing, coughing of blood, flushed cheeks, afternoon fever and night sweats. Clinically, most cases are ascribed to deficient Yin. It is deficient Lung Yin that gives rise to the coughing, coughing of blood, and the pain in the chest and hypochondria. Prolonged deficiency of Lung Yin affects the Kidney, resulting in deficiency of Kidney Yin, which is manifested in night sweats and flushed cheeks. Deficient Yin generates internal Heat, expressed as a low grade fever. A red tongue without coating, and a thin, rapid pulse are further evidence of Fire from deficient Yin.

The diagnosis in this case was accordingly deficient Lung Yin combined with Fire.

TREATMENT

The goal of treatment was to nourish the Lung Yin in order to clear the Lung, suppress the Fire and arrest the bleeding.

Points selected:

L-5 *(chi ze)*, L-10 *(yu ji)*, L-6 *(kong zui)*, LI-11 *(qu chi)*, Sp-6 *(san yin jiao)*, B-17 *(ge shu)*

Sp-6 *(san yin jiao)* was tonified. All other points were drained. Needle manipulation was moderate. After arrival of the needle sensation, the needles were retained for 30 minutes, and manipulated once every 10 minutes.

Discussion of points:

L-5 *(chi ze)* is the uniting point of the Lung channel. This point pertains to water and is thus the 'son' point. Draining this point, according to the rules of 'mother-son', drains Heat from the Lung. It is indicated for coughing of blood and chest pain. L-10 *(yu ji)* is the gushing point of the Lung channel and is used for cooling the Lung. L-6 *(kong zui)* is the accumulating point of the Lung channel. Accumulating points are those at which the Blood and Qi of a channel collect. They are particularly effective in the treatment of acute conditions. In this case, the point was used to treat coughing of blood. The aforementioned three points are traditionally used to cool Heat and arrest bleeding. The combined use of these points has a synergistic effect of cooling the Heat, clearing the Lung, suppressing the Fire and arresting the bleeding.

LI-11 *(qu chi)* is a point on the Large Intestine channel, which is exterior-interiorly related to the Lung channel. LI-11 *(qu chi)* is particularly effective in clearing Heat, specifically Heat in the Lung. Stimulating Sp-6 *(san yin jiao)* strengthens the Spleen and the Kidney. Because the Spleen is the 'mother' Organ of the Lung, stimulating this point nourishes the Yin and clears the Lung. B-17 *(ge shu)* is the meeting point of Blood and is therefore traditionally used in treating both hemorrhagic disorders and stasis of Blood.

RESULTS

After one treatment, the coughing of blood stopped immediately. That night the patient slept soundly. He was observed for ten days, and the coughing of blood did not recur. He was then discharged and advised to recuperate at home. □

Dizziness from Ascendant Liver Yang (Hypertension)

Xuàn Yùn 眩暈

Kong, male, 69 years old. The patient complained of headache, lightheadedness and blurred vision, tinnitus and diminished hearing, fullness in the chest, restlessness, palpitations, insomnia, and weakness in the knees of more than 10 years' duration. The symptoms were aggravated by physical or mental fatigue, and by emotional trauma. His blood pressure was consistently elevated at approximately 200/110mm Hg.

Physical examination revealed an obese patient with a flushed face. His pulse was wiry and rapid, and his tongue was red. Blood pressure was 210/110mm Hg. Ophthalmoscopic exam revealed sclerosis and constriction of the retinal arteries. Rheoencephalography indicated increased tension and decreased elasticity in the vertebral and basilar arteries. The diagnosis was group II hypertension.

SYNDROME DIFFERENTIATION

Dizziness can be caused by ascendant Liver Yang, Phlegm-Dampness or deficiency of Qi and Blood. In this case, the patient's symptoms indicated ascendant Liver Yang as the underlying cause.

The patient had suffered from this condition for over ten years. The condition was aggravated by emotional trauma or mental fatigue. According to Chinese medicine, emotional disturbance and mental exertion depletes Liver Yin and incites Liver Yang, resulting in Yin deficiency and ascendance of Yang. The Liver 'opens' to the outside through the eyes. With deficiency of Liver Yin, the eyes are not properly nourished, and vision may become blurred. Liver Yang flares upward to affect the head and face; hence the flushed face, dizziness and headache. Ascendant Liver Yang also stirs up Heart Fire which affects the upper part of the body, leading to restlessness, fullness in the chest, palpitations and insomnia. A red tongue and a rapid, wiry pulse are signs of Yin deficiency and ascendant Yang. Deficiency of Liver Yin also affects Kidney Yin, leading to symptoms of Kidney Yin deficiency such as tinnitus, diminished hearing, and weakness and soreness in the lower back and knees.

TREATMENT

Since the patient suffered from Liver Yin deficiency with ascendant Liver Yang, treatment was directed at subduing Liver Yang and nourishing Liver Yin, as well as reducing Heart Fire and replenishing Kidney Yin. Supplemental points were chosen according to symptoms.

Selection of points:

Liv-3 *(tai chong)*, K-3 *(tai xi)*, P-7 *(da ling)* and Liv-8 *(qu quan)* were the principal points. LI-11 *(qu chi)* and S-40 *(feng long)* were the supplemental points.

Needling was administered once daily, with ten sessions comprising one course of treatment.

Discussion of points:

Liv-3 *(tai chong)* is the source point of the Liver channel. Draining this point subdues ascendant Liver Yang. Liv-8 *(qu quan)* is the uniting point of the Liver channel. Because it is the water point, and water precedes wood in the generation cycle of the five phases, tonifying this point replenishes Liver Yin. Liv-3 *(tai xi)* is the source point of the Kidney channel. Tonifying this point nourishes Kidney Yin. P-7 *(da ling)* is the source point of the Pericardium channel. Draining this point clears Heart fire. LI-11 *(qu chi)* clears Heat and regulates Qi and Blood.

Even though this patient did not have any obvious manifestations of Phlegm, S-40 *(feng long)* was selected because Phlegm is often present to some extent in cases of ascendant Liver Yang since the Spleen's transporting function is affected. S-40 *(feng long)* is the connecting point of the Stomach channel, joining this channel with the Spleen channel. Because the Spleen is regarded as the source of Phlegm, S-40 *(feng long)* is an effective point in treating this problem.

In this particular case, a tonifying-draining method of manipulation known as 'against-with' *(yìng suí)* was utilized. Needling *against* the channel means that the direction of needle insertion is against the flow of the channel. It is a method of draining. Liv-3 *(tai chong)* on the Liver channel (which flows upward from the foot to the abdomen) was needled in a downward direction through to Liv-2 *(xing jian)*. P-7 *(da ling)* on the Pericardium channel (which flows downward from the chest to the hand) was needled in an upward direction through to P-6 *(nei guan)*. Needling *with* the channel means that the direction of needle insertion is with the flow of the channel. It is a method of tonification. Thus, K-3 *(tai xi)* on the Kidney channel (which flows upward from the foot to the abdomen) was needled in an upward direction through to K-7 *(fu liu)*.

The 'against-with' technique was used at these points because their anatomical locations in superficial tissue precluded the effective use of raise-thrust manipulation. The other points in the prescription, which are located in areas of greater tissue mass, were needled with raise-thrust technique. Liv-8 *(qu quan)* was tonified, while S-40 *(feng long)* and LI-11 *(qu chi)* were drained.

RESULTS

After five sessions, the patient's headache disappeared, and the dizziness, tinnitus and palpitations were ameliorated. His blood pressure, however, was still 200/110mm Hg. After one course of treatment, blood pressure was controlled in the vicinity of 180/110mm Hg, with remission of all symptoms. An ophthalmoscopic exam revealed that the retina remained the same as before treatment. Nevertheless, because the patient was satisfied with the results, treatment was terminated. On follow-up six months later, his blood pressure was stable. □

Dysentery-Like Disorder
(Bacillary Dysentery)

Lì Jí 痢疾

Zhang, male, 25 years old. Four days prior to his visit to the clinic, the patient suffered abdominal pain and diarrhea after eating some food which was probably contaminated. The following morning, blood and pus were noticed in the stool. Various antibiotics and atropine were self-administered, but were ineffective. The patient had over 30 bowel movements daily, mixed with blood and pus. The stools had a fishy odor, and a sticky consistency. The patient also experienced tenesmus, a burning sensation inside the anus, thirst, restlessness and fever. The tongue was deep red with a yellow, greasy coating, and the pulse was soggy and rapid.

Examination found the patient to have an oral temperature of 38.5°C, a pulse rate of 100/minute, and a white blood cell count of 12,000/cu mm. Stool smear showed large amounts of polymorphonuclear lymphocytes, and culture found *Shigella dysenteriae.*

SYNDROME DIFFERENTIATION

Dysentery-like disorders have been described in ancient Chinese medical literature as far back as the 3rd century B.C. *(Simple Questions*, chapter 29). Generally speaking, the acute form of the disease is usually attributed to Damp-Heat resulting from contaminated food. Stagnation of Damp-Heat in the Intestines interferes with the movement of stool, and gives rise to abdominal pain and tenesmus. Fever, thirst, restlessness and a burning sensation in the anus are manifestations of Heat, while the sticky quality and fishy odor of the stools are signs of Dampness. The red tongue and rapid pulse are evidence of Heat, while the yellow, greasy tongue coating and the soggy pulse reflect Dampness.

TREATMENT

The principle of treatment was to remove the Damp-Heat.

Points selected:
LI-11 *(qu chi)*, S-25 *(tian shu)*, S-37 *(shang ju xu)*, LI-4 *(he gu)*
Draining manipulation through raise-thrust and twirling techniques was utilized.

41

After arrival of the needle sensation, the needles were retained for 30 minutes, and manipulated once. Treatment was administered daily.

Discussion of points:

LI-11 *(qu chi)* is the uniting point of the Large Intestine channel and is an important Heat-removing point. LI-4 *(he gu)* is the source point of the Large Intestine channel. The combined use of these two points removes Damp-Heat from the Large Intestine. S-25 *(tian shu)* is the alarm point of the Large Intestine, and S-37 *(shang ju xu)* is the lower uniting point of the same Organ. The combined use of these two points regulates Qi and Blood in the Large Intestine channel. Traditional Chinese medicine holds that in treating bloody, purulent, dysentery-like stools, the removal of Damp-Heat should always be supplemented by the regulation of Qi and Blood. This is because regulating Qi relieves tenesmus, and regulating Blood arrests bleeding, and thus bloody stool.

RESULTS

After the first treatment, the number of bowel movements was reduced by one-half, and after the second treatment, the fever subsided, with remission of other symptoms. After three treatments, bowel function returned to normal and the stools were free of blood and pus. Examination found an oral temperature of 36.7°C, white blood cell count of 8,000/cu mm, and a negative fecal smear. A stool culture taken after the fifth treatment showed no growth of pathogenic organisms. The patient was therefore discharged after seven treatments. He returned two weeks later for a follow-up, and reported no further episodes of diarrhea.

Note: In treating dysentery-like diarrhea, it is important to discern which of the two pathogenic factors, Dampness or Heat, is predominant. If Heat (characterized by blood in the stool) predominates, GV-14 *(da zhui)* and S-44 *(nei ting)* are added to the prescription to enhance removal of the Heat. If Dampness (characterized by pus in the stool) predominates, Sp-6 *(san yin jiao)* and Sp-9 *(yin ling quan)* are added instead. This case, with both blood and pus in the stool, illustrates a pattern in which Dampness and Heat were present in equal measure. Therefore, none of the supplemental points were utilized. ☐

Epigastric Pain and Distention
(Gastroptosis)

Wèi Zhàng Tòng 胃脹痛

Zhang, female, 31 years old. About 6 months ago, the patient, a manual laborer, began suffering from epigastric pain, accompanied by a sensation of distention and sinking of the stomach. Prior to the onset of symptoms, her workload had become very heavy, and she was often fatigued. Her busy schedule caused her to eat irregularly. The symptoms gradually became worse. Her appetite slowly diminished, and she lost weight. Two months ago, the patient underwent a barium meal X-ray which revealed that the lower pole of her stomach was 9cm below the line connecting her anterior superior iliac spines. The tentative diagnosis was gastroptosis. Various treatments with both Chinese and western medicines were attempted, but the results were unremarkable.

Examination found the patient to be pale and emaciated. When lying flat, her abdomen appeared scaphoid in shape. It was soft, felt better when warm, and did not resist pressure. Her tongue was pale and tooth-marked, with a thin, white coating. The pulse was submerged, moderate in rate, and lacked force.

SYNDROME DIFFERENTIATION

Overwork consumes Qi and Blood, while irregular eating hurts the Stomach and Spleen. From the history of this patient it can be surmised that there was deficiency of both the Stomach and Spleen, as well as of Qi and Blood. Because weakness of the Stomach and Spleen disturbs their transporting and transforming functions, there was loss of appetite, and abdominal distention after meals.

A deficiency of the Spleen causes the middle Qi to sink, which in this case affected the Stomach; thus the gastroptosis. Stagnancy in the flow of Qi, from whatever reason, causes pain. In this case, the stagnancy resulted from deficiency, and was therefore relieved by warmth and pressure. The pallor, emaciation, pale and tooth-marked tongue, and the submerged and forceless pulse, were all signs of deficiency of Qi and Blood. The syndrome was therefore one of deficiency of the Spleen and Stomach, associated with deficiency of Qi and Blood.

TREATMENT

Points selected:

CV-12 *(zhong wan)* joined to CV-10 *(xia wan)*; S-21 *(liang men)* joined to S-23 *(tai yi)*; CV-6 *(qi hai)* joined to CV-4 *(guan yuan)*; S-36 *(zu san li)*

Treatment was administered once daily. Ten treatments comprised one course of therapy, with three days' rest between courses. The needles were retained for thirty minutes during each session.

Discussion of points:

CV-12 *(zhong wan)* is the alarm point of the Stomach. When joined to CV-10 *(xia wan)*, the Stomach is strengthened and its Qi is moved so that the distention and pain are resolved. When S-21 *(liang men)* and S-23 *(tai yi)* are joined, the middle Burner is tonified and its Qi is replenished. CV-6 *(qi hai)* tonifies the middle Burner, which is the source of postnatal Qi, while CV-4 *(guan yuan)* tonifies Kidney Qi, which is the source of congenital Qi. When these two points are joined, both congenital and postnatal Qi are strengthened, and the sinking of the middle Qi and ptosis of the internal organs is thereby corrected. S-36 *(zu san li)* is the lower uniting point of the Stomach. Lower uniting points are needled for disorders of the Yang Organs. This point also tonifies the middle Burner and replenishes Qi.

For points on the abdomen, the needles were inserted obliquely, and advanced about two units. Tonifying manipulation through twirling was then applied. There was local distention and soreness, followed by a sensation as if the stomach were pulling upward. At S-36 *(zu san li)*, the 'warm tonifying method' was used: after the arrival of Qi, the needle was twirled with forceful thrusting and gentle raising until a sensation of warmth was felt to course along the Stomach channel toward the stomach.

RESULTS

After eight treatments, the patient's appetite improved, and the sensation of distention and sinking (downward dragging) was substantially alleviated. A barium meal X-ray showed that the lower pole of her stomach was 4cm below the interiliac spinal line. After another two courses (a total of twenty-eight treatments), the patient's appetite was markedly improved, her facial color became rosy, and there was a gain of 3kg in body weight. Epigastric distention and pain completely disappeared. Another barium meal X-ray showed that the lower pole of her stomach was 2cm above the interiliac spinal line. Treatment was then discontinued. The patient was followed-up for six months and her condition remained stable. □

Fever from Internal Disharmonies
(Fever of Unknown Origin)

Nèi Shāng Fā Rè 内伤发热

Hua, female, 40 years old. The patient had a low grade fever for more than 3 months. It oc-
curred especially upon fatigue, and ranged from 37.5-38°C. Other symptoms included emacia-
tion, pallor, shortness of breath, general weakness and lack of spirit, dryness in the mouth with-
out desire to drink, sweating on exertion, poor appetite, and 2-3 bowel movements daily of soft
stools. The tongue was pale and the pulse was weak. No cause could be determined after inves-
tigations which included radiologic and clinical laboratory tests. The patient was therefore re-
ferred for acupuncture therapy.

SYNDROME DIFFERENTIATION

In Chinese medicine, fever is of two general patterns, exterior and interior. The exterior pattern is a reaction to an external pathogenic influence, such as Wind or Cold. Symptoms characteristic of this pattern are acute onset, chills, a thin, white tongue coating and a floating pulse. The fever is usually high because of the strong contention between the normal Qi and the pathogenic influence.

The interior pattern arises from internal Yin-Yang disharmonies, such as discord between the Yin and Yang Organs, or between Qi and Blood when either is deficient. The condition is usually one of gradual onset and protracted course, with changes in tongue appearance and pulse quality. The fever is generally low because it is caused by a relative imbalance between Yin and Yang, and not by contention between normal Qi and an external pathogenic influence.

The course of the illness in this case was over three months' duration and lacked the manifestations of an exterior pattern. The fever was thus of an interior pattern, due to internal Yin-Yang disharmonies.

Fevers from internal disharmonies may be further differentiated according to their pathogenesis. The three most frequently encountered syndromes are deficient Yin, deficient Qi, and stagnant Heat in the Liver channel.

Here, all of the signs and symptoms indicated deficiency of Spleen Qi. The Spleen is responsible for the transportation of nutrient matter throughout the body. Because of the deficiency of Spleen Qi, the nutrient matter, which brings color to the face, failed to ascend, hence the facial pallor. Similarly, because the limbs were undernourished, the patient was emaciated, short of breath, and lacked strength and spirit. Fever wastes the body fluids and causes thirst. In this case, however, the fever was low and was attributed to deficient Qi; the thirst was therefore not extreme, and the desire for drink was not too strong. Qi controls the sweat pores. Because Qi was deficient, the patient sweated upon slight exertion. Exertion consumes Qi; therefore the low grade fever occurred especially when the patient was fatigued. The pallor of the tongue and the weakness of the pulse were likewise expressions of deficient Qi.

The mechanism of fever here was that the deficiency of Spleen Qi led to sinking of the middle Qi and the non-ascent of clear Yang, which, when constrained, transformed into Heat.

TREATMENT

The principle of treatment was to tonify the Qi and invigorate the Spleen in order to eliminate the Heat.

Points selected:

CV-12 *(zhong wan)*, CV-6 *(qi hai)*, S-36 *(zu san li)*, B-20 *(pi shu)*, B-21 *(wei shu)*, LI-11 *(qu chi)*, GV-20 *(bai hui)*

Both acupuncture and moxibustion were administered at the first three points, and acupuncture alone at the latter four points. All of the points were tonified through raise-thrust and twirling manipulation of the needles. Moxibustion was administered with moxa stubs.

Discussion of points:

CV-12 *(zhong wan)* is the alarm point of the Stomach channel. CV-6 *(qi hai)*, the 'sea of Qi', regulates the Qi. S-36 *(zu san li)*, the lower uniting point of the Stomach, in-

vigorates the Spleen and Stomach, and tonifies weak and deficient conditions. These three points are indicated for protracted Qi deficiency. The use of moxibustion at these points augments the effect of needling in tonifying the Qi and strengthening the Spleen.

B-20 *(pi shu)* and B-21 *(wei shu)*, the associated points on the back for the Spleen and Stomach respectively, are the points through which the circulating Qi of the Spleen and the Stomach passes. Needling these two points regulates the Qi of the Spleen and the Stomach. LI-11 *(qu chi)* is a point on the Yang Brightness channel of the arm, while the Stomach channel is the Yang Brightness channel of the leg. These two channels are therefore closely related. Needling LI-11 *(qu chi)* cools the Heat and regulates the Qi in both of the Yang Brightness channels.

Needling GV-20 *(bai hui)*, located at the vertex of the head, causes the Qi of the Spleen and Stomach to rise. In this case, the elevation of the Yang Qi of the Spleen and Stomach was helpful in dispersing the sunken middle Qi, thereby eliminating the Heat.

B-20 *(pi shu)* and B-21 *(wei shu)* were needled first. Care was taken to insert the needles no more than 0.8 unit to avoid puncturing the kidneys and liver. After the arrival of Qi (signaled by a sensation of soreness and distention), the needles were retained for ten minutes. Only after the needles were withdrawn from these two points were the other points needled.

GV-20 *(bai hui)* was needled by oblique insertion from front to back. The needle sensation was one of local distention.

RESULTS

After two weeks of daily treatments, improvement was noted in the restoration of strength and appetite, and some diminishment in perspiration. However, the low grade fever persisted. This was thought to be a sign of continued Qi deficiency. The point prescription was therefore supplemented by administering moxibustion at CV-4 *(guan yuan)* to further tonify the Qi. Moxibustion was also increased to twice a day (needling remained at once a day). After daily treatment with the modified prescription for ten days, the low grade fever subsided, although some weakness remained. The frequency of treatment was then reduced to once every other day to consolidate the effect. After another two weeks of treatment, all symptoms disappeared and treatment was discontinued. During a follow-up of two months, there was no recurrence of fever. □

Goiter
(Hyperthyroidism)

Yǐng Bìng 瘿病

Zhang, female, 45 years old. The patient was diagnosed with hyperthyroidism over 3 years ago. The antithyroid drug propylthiouracil was discontinued because of adverse reactions. As a result, there was no amelioration of symptoms, which included palpitations, shortness of breath, fatigue, profuse sweating, irritability, thirst with a preference for cold beverages, hunger and excessive eating, insomnia and emaciation.

Physical examination showed a flushed complexion, diffuse grade 3 thyroid hypertrophy of soft consistency, no bruit, tremor of both hands, and exophthalmos. The pulse rate was 110/minute, blood pressure 110/60mm Hg, and body weight 43kg. Serum T_3 was 210ng/dL (normal 70-90ng/dL), serum T_4 was 5.2μg/dL (normal 4-12μg/dL), and the basal metabolic rate was +52%. The pulse was wiry and rapid, and the tongue was red.

SYNDROME DIFFERENTIATION

In Chinese medicine, hyperthyroidism falls under the category of 'goiter'. It is caused by emotional depression and stagnation of Liver Qi. Prolonged stagnation of Qi transforms into Fire, generates Phlegm, and induces Blood stasis. When Phlegm and Blood stasis combine and aggregate in the neck, goiter results. When Phlegm and Blood stasis combine and aggregate in the eyes, the eyeballs protrude. The presence of Fire damages the Yin.

In this case, the symptoms pointed to involvement of the Heart, Stomach and Liver. Insomnia, palpitations and profuse sweating are signs of Heart Fire and deficiency of Heart Yin. Irritability and hand tremors are signs of Liver Fire and deficiency of Liver Yin. Frequent hunger and excessive eating, emaciation, and thirst with a preference for cold beverages are signs of Stomach Fire and deficiency of Stomach Yin. Because Qi depends on the moistening and nourishing effects of the Yin Fluids, deficiency of Yin naturally results in deficiency of Qi. This accounts for the shortness of breath and fatigue, which are symptoms of Qi deficiency.

The pattern in this case was thus Fire from deficiency of Yin, stagnation of Phlegm and

Blood stasis, and deficiency of Qi. This is known as compounded deficiency-excess, since symptoms of both excess and deficiency were present.

TREATMENT

The principles of treatment were to nourish the Yin, drain the Fire, reduce the Phlegm, remove the stagnation and tonify the Qi.

Points selected:

Because of the complexity of the case, 16 points were selected according to the symptoms. In order to simultaneously treat the root and manifestations of this condition, the points were divided into 7 groups of 5 points each. Each of the groups was then used in rotation. The point groups were as follows:

1. K-3 *(tai xi)*, P-5 *(jian shi)*, S-10 *(shui tu)*, B-10 *(tian zhu)*, B-2 *(zan zhu)*

2. K-7 *(fu liu)*, S-36 *(zu san li)*, CV-22 *(tian tu)*, P-6 *(nei guan)*, G-1 *(tong zi liao)*

3. K-6 *(zhao hai)*, Sp-6 *(san yin jiao)*, LI-4 *(he gu)*, LI-11 *(qu chi)*, S-10 *(shui tu)*

4. K-3 *(tai xi)*, Liv-3 *(tai chong)*, S-40 *(feng long)*, S-10 *(shui tu)*, B-10 *(tian zhu)*

5. K-7 *(fu liu)*, S-36 *(zu san li)*, P-5 *(zan zhu)*, CV-22 *(tian tu)*

6. K-6 *(zhao hai)*, P-6 *(nei guan)*, Liv-3 *(tai chong)*, S-10 *(shui tu)*, B-10 *(tian zhu)*

7. K-3 *(tai xi)*, Sp-6 *(san yin jiao)*, LI-4 *(he gu)*, S-40 *(feng long)*, CV-22 *(tian tu)*

One group of points was needled each day (except Sunday), with seven treatments comprising one course of therapy. Three days' rest was allowed between courses. The points were needled bilaterally, except CV-22 *(tian tu)*, which is on the median line.

Discussion of points:

Since the underlying principles of treatment were to nourish the Yin and drain the Fire, the points that produce such effects, i.e., K-7 *(fu liu)*, K-6 *(zhao hai)*, K-3 *(tai xi)* and Sp-6 *(san yin jiao)*, were needled more often than the others. In addition, S-36 *(zu san li)*, the lower uniting point of the Stomach channel, was used as a supplementary point to replenish the Qi. These five points were tonified by combining twirling with forceful thrusting and slow raising of the needles.

P-6 *(nei guan)* and P-5 *(jian shi)* on the Pericardium channel are used to drain Fire from the Heart, and are especially effective for treating palpitations. Liv-3 *(tai chong)* on the Liver channel is used to drain Fire from the Liver, and is therefore useful for treating emotional irritability and tremor of the hands. LI-4 *(he gu)* on the Large Intestine channel is particularly effective in treating diseases of the head and eyes. S-40 *(feng long)* on the Stomach channel is effective in draining Fire from the Stomach and reducing Phlegm. LI-11 *(qu chi)* on the Large Intestine channel is also effective in draining Fire and clearing Heat. Since the Yang Brightness channels of the arm and leg (Large Intestine and Stomach) pass through the neck region, needling points on these channels promotes the flow of Qi through the Yang Brightness channels, and thereby reduces thyroid enlargement in the neck. Each of the aforementioned six points were drained by combining twirling with slow thrusting and forceful raising of the needles.

B-10 *(tian zhu)* was needled perpendicularly to a depth of 1 unit in order to transmit the needle sensation to the ocular region. Deep insertion upward and medially should be avoided. B-2 *(zan zhu)* and G-1 *(tong zi liao)* are local points situated in the vicinity of the eyes; these two points are effective in treating exophthalmos. B-2 *(zan zhu)* was needled obliquely downward for a distance of 0.5 unit through to B-1 *(jing ming)*. Painful distention in the orbital region was felt. G-1 *(tong zi liao)* was needled transversely toward M-HN-9 *(tai yang)* for a distance of 0.5 unit. This induced a local feeling of distention.

S-10 *(shui tu)* is located at the anterior margin of the sternocleidomastoid muscle. It is especially effective for treating thyroid enlargement. In this case, the needle was inserted into the substance of the thyroid gland to a depth of 1 unit. Another needle was then inserted obliquely (45° angle) at the lateral border of the gland at the same level of S-10 *(shui tu)* to a depth of 1 unit.

CV-22 *(tian tu)* is located in the center of the depression just above the suprasternal notch. Needling this point invigorates the Qi, and resolves the Phlegm and shortness of breath. Needle insertion was downward along the posterior aspect of the sternum to a depth of 1 unit. The needle was withdrawn immediately after needle sensation was obtained; manipulation of the needle was contraindicated.

The intensity of needle manipulation must be appropriate for the individual patient so that the stimulation can be tolerated without adverse reaction.

RESULTS

After four weeks of treatment, all symptoms began to show remission. Body weight increased from 43kg to 48kg. Heart rate was 80/minute, and blood pressure was 110/80mm Hg. The patient's emotions were stabilized, and she began eating less. The shortness of breath and fatigue disappeared. Enlargement of the thyroid was reduced to grade 2, but the protrusion of the eyeballs showed no improvement.

After another six weeks of treatment, all symptoms were further improved. Body weight increased to 52kg. Heart rate was 80/minute, blood pressure 110/80mm Hg, and thyroid enlargement remained at grade 2. Exophthalmos was still slight. Serum T_3 was 71ng/dL, serum T_3 was 1.3μg/dL, and the basal metabolic rate was+10%. Treatment was then discontinued.

Six months later, the patient reported some recurrence of symptoms. She was advised to resume antithyroid drug treatment at reduced levels. The symptoms were thus controlled with a much smaller dosage, and no adverse reaction was reported. □

Heart Pain
(Coronary Artery Disease)

Xīn Tòng 心痛

Lu, male, 68 years old. The patient had suffered from episodes of dull, precordial pain for 2 months. During this period, his office workload had become increasingly heavy. During the 2 weeks prior to his visit to the clinic, the episodes became more frequent when he was tired. Sometimes the attacks were accompanied by general weakness and palpitations. He was diagnosed at another hospital as having coronary artery disease, and was treated with western and traditional Chinese medicines, which provided some relief.

Examination found that the patient was mentally alert, but that his face was dull and his demeanor gloomy. He was obese. On auscultation, the first sound over the apex was diminished, and the second aortic sound was accentuated. The heart rate was 60 beats per minute. Breath sounds over the lungs were normal. The liver and spleen were not palpable. Blood pressure was 120/70mm Hg. The EKG showed a depression of the S-T segment. His tongue was dark red with a scanty coating, and the pulse was submerged and moderate.

SYNDROME DIFFERENTIATION

The patient was aged and weak, and the Qi of his Heart and Spleen was further weakened by mental fatigue. Qi and Blood are closely related. Qi is the 'commander' of Blood in that it impels the Blood's circulation. Blood serves as the 'mother' of Qi by providing its material basis. As long as Qi flows unimpeded, so too will Blood, but when Qi becomes stagnant, Blood stasis results. Deficiency of Heart Qi weakens its power in driving the Blood. Deficiency of Spleen Qi leads to disturbance in the transportation of nutrients and in the metabolism of water. This causes them to transform into Phlegm, which in turn obstructs the channels. The patient was obese, and such individuals are prone to suffer from Phlegm-Dampness.

In this case, Phlegm-Dampness combined with Blood stasis to produce an obstruction in the thorax which caused the pain. The palpitations were due to a lack of driving force in the Heart. The patient's general weakness was caused by deficiency of

Spleen Qi, since this Organ has the function of nourishing the muscles and limbs. The dull face and dark red tongue signified Blood stasis, and the submerged, moderate pulse indicated deficiency of Qi.

TREATMENT

The principle of treatment was to replenish the Qi and invigorate the Blood in order to resolve the Phlegm and alleviate the pain.

Points selected:

P-6 *(nei guan)*, Sp-4 *(gong sun)*, B-15 *(xin shu)*, CV-14 *(ju que)*, S-36 *(zu san li)*, Sp-6 *(san yin jiao)*

All points were needled with balanced tonifying-draining manipulation. Treatment was administered once daily, during which the needles were retained for 20 minutes. Ten treatments comprised one course of therapy, with 2-3 days' rest between courses.

Discussion of points:

P-6 *(nei guan)* is the confluent point of the Yin Linking channel, one of the eight miscellaneous channels. Conditions associated with this channel manifest primarily as pain in the Heart. P-6 *(nei guan)* was therefore selected in this case to treat the pain. Sp-4 *(gong sun)* is the confluent point of the Penetrating channel, another of the eight miscellaneous channels. Diseases associated with this channel manifest as contracting pains in the abdomen. Needling this point invigorates the Spleen and regulates the flow of Qi. The combination of these two points is often used in treating disorders of the Stomach, Heart and thoracic region in order to strengthen Spleen Qi, invigorate the

Blood, and alleviate pain.

B-15 *(xin shu)* is the associated point on the back for the Heart, and CV-14 *(ju que)* is the alarm point of the Heart. The combined use of these two points invigorates the Blood, alleviates pain, and replenishes Heart Qi, thus stopping the palpitations. Needling S-36 *(zu san li)* and Sp-6 *(san yin jiao)* replenishes Qi and Blood, and resolves Phlegm-Dampness.

P-6 *(nei guan)* was needled perpendicularly to a depth of 1 unit. Moderate raise-thrusting and twirling of the needle was utilized. The needle sensation was transmitted to the upper part of the forearm, or to the thorax. At Sp-4 *(gong sun)* the needle was inserted perpendicularly to a depth of 0.8 unit, producing a sensation of soreness and distention which was transmitted to the front of the medial malleolus. Needle insertion at B-15 *(xin shu)* was perpendicular to a depth of about 1 unit, producing local soreness and distention. At CV-14 *(ju que)* the needle was inserted perpendicularly to a depth of 1.2 units, producing local distention and pain.

RESULTS

After ten treatments, the precordial pain, palpitations and general weakness were all markedly improved. Two additional courses were administered for a total of thirty treatments, by which time all symptoms were alleviated. The patient's complexion was ruddy, his heart rate had increased to 75 beats per minute, and the EKG showed an S-T segment of normal level. The patient was followed-up for six months with no recurrence of symptoms. □

Hiccough

È Nì 呃逆

Zhang, female, 78 years old. Five days before admission, the patient had a heated argument with her family. Hiccough developed immediately afterward. The hiccough was continuous, clear and forceful. She had a feeling of uncontrollable upsurge of gas, with fullness in the epigastrium and hypochondria. Her appetite was diminished, and there was occasional acid regurgitation. She also had a bitter taste in her mouth, and suffered from restlessness and insomnia. Her tongue was slightly red with a thin, white coating, and her pulse was wiry.

SYNDROME DIFFERENTIATION

The immediate cause of hiccough is an abnormal movement of Stomach Qi upward. The condition may be one of either excess or deficiency, and can result from any of the following factors:

- Indigestion as a result of indulgence, or excessive intake of cold or uncooked foods.

- Invasion of external Cold, which accumulates in the middle Burner where it suppresses Stomach Yang and reverses the flow of Stomach Qi upward.

- Emotional disturbance causing stagnation of Liver Qi, which subjugates the Stomach and reverses the flow of its Qi upward.

- Stagnation of Phlegm, which causes obstruction and constraint and interferes with the normal descent of Stomach Qi, and eventually transforms into Heat.

- General debility due to old age, overwork and/or protracted disease, which reduces the Stomach and Spleen Yang such that the clear Yang does not rise and the turbid Yin does not descend.

The hiccough in this case was precipitated by a domestic argument. The symptoms associated with the epigastrium and hypochondria (fullness, occasional belching of sour fluid, poor appetite) were related to a disturbance of the Stomach. The slightly red tongue indicated the onset of Heat. The wiry pulse was characteristic of Liver disease. In sum, the pattern was one of stagnant Liver Qi subjugating the Stomach and causing its Qi to rebel upward.

TREATMENT

Treatment was directed at soothing the Liver to relieve its stagnant Qi, and pacifying the Stomach to suppress its rebellious Qi.

Points selected:

Liv-3 *(tai chong)*, B-18 *(gan shu)*, B-17 *(ge shu)*, CV-22 *(tian tu)*, CV-17 *(tan zhong)*, CV-12 *(zhong wan)*, P-6 *(nei guan)*

Draining manipulation was applied since the condition was one of excess.

Discussion of points:

B-18 *(gan shu)* is the associated point of the Liver on the back through which the circulating Qi of the Liver passes. The associated points on the back are used in connection with diseases of their associated Organs. Since this condition originated from stagnant Liver Qi, B-18 *(gan shu)* was of paramount importance in the prescription. Liv-3 *(tai chong)* is the source point of the Liver channel. The source points are those sites through which the source Qi of each of the 12 Organs flows, and is retained. The *Miraculous Pivot* (chapter 1) instructs: "For diseases of one of the five Yin Organs, needle its source [point]."

CV-12 *(zhong wan)* is the alarm point of the Stomach, and is the point at which the Qi of the Stomach converges. "When Yang is diseased, treat Yin." *(Simple Questions,* chapter 5) Since the Stomach is a Yang Organ and the abdomen is Yin, the alarm point of the Stomach was chosen to pacify the rebellious Stomach Qi. P-6 *(nei guan)* is one of the eight confluent points, connecting the Yin Linking channel with the Pericardium channel. Needling this point in combination with CV-12 *(zhong wan)* pacifies the Stomach.

CV-22 *(tian tu)* is a point of intersection of the Yin Linking channel on the Conception vessel. CV-17 *(tan zhong)*, one of the eight meeting points, is associated with Qi. Needling these two points restrains rebellious Stomach Qi. B-17 *(ge shu)* is associated with the diaphragm. Because hiccough is a disorder which affects the diaphragm, B-17 *(ge shu)* is traditionally used in its treatment.

RESULTS

After the arrival of Qi following insertion, the needles were retained in place. After 15 minutes, raise-thrust and twirling manipulation was administered for 1 minute. The hiccough was noticeably reduced. The needles were then retained for 50 minutes because prolonged needle retention is very useful for attack-type conditions such as this, or when pain is present.

Upon withdrawal of the needles, the hiccough stopped, and the distress in the epigastrium disappeared. The patient felt relaxed and left the clinic quite satisfied with the results. However, the next day she had a mild recurrence after lunch. Treatment was therefore resumed with the same points for two more sessions. The hiccough was then completely arrested, her appetite was restored and the other symptoms disappeared. Follow-up one week later found no relapse. ☐

Impotence
(Male Infertility)

Yáng Wěi 阳萎

Shi, male, 30 years old. About 1 year after marriage, the patient complained that his erection was weak and could not be sustained. His wife was examined and found to be normal. Examination of the patient showed a normal chest X-ray, the external genitalia were normally developed, cremasteric reflex was sluggish, and other neurological tests were negative. Microscopic examination of seminal fluid showed an absence of sperm. Bilateral biopsy of the testes showed moderate atrophy. The diagnosis was impotence and azoospermia (absence of sperm).

The four examinations of Chinese medicine found the patient to have a pale face. He experienced dizziness and blurred vision, lack of spirit, and disturbed sleep. He complained of soreness and weakness in the lower back and knees, weak and unsustainable erection during coitus, and occasional, involuntary nocturnal emissions. His tongue was pale. His pulse was thin and submerged, and weak at the rear position.

SYNDROME DIFFERENTIATION

In Chinese medicine, the Kidney stores the Essence, the physical manifestations of which include semen and sperm. This patient had a weak erection and absence of live sperm in the semen. The condition was attributed to deficient Kidney Qi.

The lower back houses the Kidney; thus, Kidney deficiency presents with soreness and weakness in the lower back and knees. The Kidney is also the source of energy and agility. When the Kidney is deficient, lassitude and general lack of spirit prevail, and the insufficiency of stored Essence gives rise to dizziness and blurred vision. Because the Kidney is responsible for the functions of the reproductive system, another symptom of Kidney deficiency is a weak erection. A pale tongue and a thin, submerged pulse are signs of deficient Yang. The rear position represents the Kidney, and a weak pulse at this position (especially on the right) points to a deficiency of Kidney Yang. In sum, the pattern was one of deficient Kidney Yang, with a resulting shortage of Essence.

It should be noted that deficient Kidney Yang is not the only cause of impotence. Other causes include:

- Injury to the Heart and Spleen. Constant worry and depression harm the Heart and Spleen, and thus the Stomach channel. The Spleen and Stomach are the source for the transformation of nutrients. When the Spleen and Stomach are deficient, Qi and Blood also become deficient; the sinews are thereby deprived of nourishment, thus causing impotence. Other symptoms include disturbed sleep, reduced appetite, a lackluster complexion, a pale tongue with a thin, greasy coating, and a thin pulse.

- Fright injures the Kidney and causes the sinking of Qi, thus affecting erection. Other symptoms include a thin, greasy tongue coating, and a wiry pulse.

- Downward pouring of Damp-Heat causes the penis to lose its rigidity. Other symptoms include dampness of the scrotum, weakness of the limbs, yellow urine, a yellow, greasy tongue coating, and a soggy, rapid pulse.

TREATMENT

The principle of treatment was to strengthen the Kidney Yang in order to replenish the Essence.

Points selected:
CV-4 *(guan yuan)* Sp-6 *(san yin jiao)*

Discussion of points:
The meaning of the point name CV-4 *(guan yuan)* is 'the passage for source [Qi]'. This is the point of intersection of the three Yin channels of the leg on the Conception vessel. Needling this point tonifies the Kidney Yang and replenishes the Essence. It is therefore effective in treating such manifestations of deficient Kidney Yang as impotence, nocturnal emissions, premature ejaculation and male infertility. Needling Sp-6 *(san*

yin jiao), the point of intersection of the three Yin channels of the leg on the Spleen channel, is also effective in treating disorders of the reproductive system resulting from Yang deficiency and insufficient Essence.

At CV-4 *(guan yuan)* the needle was inserted to a depth of 1 unit. 'Burning the mountain' tonification (see Introduction) was applied, and the needle was retained for 5 minutes. The sensation of warmth extended as far as the glans, testes and perineum. After withdrawal of the needle, direct moxibustion was administered using 5 cones, each the size of a grain of rice. A thin layer of vaseline was spread on the skin so that the cones would not fall off. The skin in the vicinity of the point was patted to reduce the pain from the smouldering cone. Moxibustion resulted in local erythema, but no actual burn, and was used to enhance the effect of the needling.

At Sp-6 *(san yin jiao)* raise-thrust and twirling manipulation was used to tonify the point. The needles were retained for 15 minutes, and manipulated once every 5 minutes. The sensation extended to the inner aspect of the thigh and the inguinal region, and down to the big toe and dorsum of the foot.

Treatment was administered once daily for the first five sessions, followed by once every other day. The patient was advised to abstain from intercourse during the first five treatments so that the Essence could be replenished. Fifteen treatments comprised one course of therapy, with a one week intermission between courses.

RESULTS

After five treatments, erection was somewhat strengthened, and by the end of the first course of therapy, it was distinctly stronger than before. After completion of the second course, erection and orgasm were essentially normal. Examination of semen showed a sperm count of about 10 million/ml, with poor motility and some aberrant forms. After the third course of treatment with the same points, the semen was found to be sticky, and milky white in color. Sperm count was approximately 40 million/ml. There were no aberrant forms, and sperm motility was also improved. By the end of the fourth course of treatment, sperm count and motility were normal. The other symptoms, including the general vitality of the patient, also showed marked improvement. The patient's wife became pregnant 7 months post-treatment. □

Impotence

Yáng Wěi 阳萎

Zou, male, 30 years old. The patient complained of impotence of 3 years' duration. His sexual life had been normal until sexual intercourse was interrupted one night when his wife fainted. From then on, he was unable to attain an erection. Herbal medications were ineffective. Three months ago he started intramuscular injections of testosterone propionate (25mg every other day), but this therapy was terminated when aching began in the right lower abdomen and testes. He then turned to acupuncture therapy.

The four examinations of Chinese medicine revealed a dark complexion, depression, palpitations, insomnia, intolerance of cold in the limbs, a pale tongue, and a wiry pulse which was thin and submerged in the rear position.

SYNDROME DIFFERENTIATION

Because the Kidney stores Essence, normal sexual function depends on a normal Kidney. When Kidney Qi is consolidated, erections can be sustained for normal intercourse. Deficiency of Kidney Qi, however, results in the inability to attain or sustain an erection. The impotence in this case appeared when sexual intercourse was interrupted by fright, when the patient discovered that his wife had fainted. According to Chinese medicine, fright impairs the Kidney Qi, thus the patient experienced impotence. Fright also affects the Heart and causes the Spirit to wander, which accounted for the palpitations and insomnia in this case.

Prolonged sexual dysfunction often leads to depression, which in turn causes constraint or stagnation of Liver Qi, expressed here by the wiry pulse. Other symptoms of deficient Kidney Qi in this case included the pale tongue, intolerance of cold in the limbs, and the thin, submerged pulse at the rear position.

TREATMENT

The primary focus of treatment was to replenish the Kidney Qi, and secondarily to relieve the stagnation of Liver Qi.

Points selected:

Principal points: CV-6 *(qi hai)*, CV-4 *(guan yuan)*, B-23 *(shen shu)*, GV-4 *(ming men)*, Sp-6 *(san yin jiao)*, S-29 *(gui lai)*, B-32 *(ci liao)*, Liv-3 *(tai chong)*

Supplemental points: B-15 *(xin shu)*, B-18 *(gan shu)*, B-19 *(dan shu)*, S-36 *(zu san li)*, K-3 *(tai xi)*

At each daily treatment, 2-3 principal points, and 1-2 supplemental points were needled.

Discussion of points:

CV-6 *(qi hai)* is the 'sea of Qi'. Needling this point regulates the lower Burner and tonifies the Kidney Qi. CV-4 *(guan yuan)* is the point at which the source Qi is stored; it functions to tonify the Kidney. B-23 *(shen shu)* is the associated point of the Kidney on the back. GV-4 *(ming men)* is located between the two kidneys, and is an important point for tonifying the Kidney. K-3 *(tai xi)* tonifies the Fire at the 'gate of vitality', and thus replenishes the Kidney. All of the aforementioned points were chosen for their common effect in tonifying Kidney Qi.

Liv-3 *(tai chong)* soothes the Liver and clears the Liver channel. S-29 *(gui lai)* regulates the lower Burner. B-18 *(gan shu)* is the associated point of the Liver on the back, and was needled to relieve the stagnant Liver Qi. B-19 *(dan shu)* is the associated point of the Gall Bladder on the back. Since the Gall Bladder and Liver are exterior-interiorly related, this point was also needled to relieve the stagnant Liver Qi.

Sp-6 *(san yin jiao)* is the point of intersection of the Liver, Spleen and Kidney channels, and functions to regulate and tonify the Qi in these channels. S-36 *(zu san li)* was cho-

sen as a general tonification point, and B-15 *(xin shu)* was chosen to nourish the Heart in order to relieve the insomnia and palpitations. B-32 *(ci liao)* is traditionally used for sexual dysfunction.

'Burning the mountain' tonifying manipulation (see Introduction) was utilized at all points to produce a comfortable feeling of warmth. To enhance the effect of acupuncture in replenishing the Kidney Qi, moxa stick moxibustion was applied after needling. Before needling the points on the lower abdomen, the patient was asked to urinate in order to prevent puncturing the bladder. These points were needled such that the needle sensation radiated to the penis, and even caused an erectile tendency.

RESULTS

After four treatments, the patient reported a slight erectile tendency in the morning and evening, and upon distention of the urinary bladder. He was advised to try sexual intercourse. At his fifth visit, he reported that he could perform intercourse, although the erection was not very firm, and ejaculation was premature. At his sixth visit, he was told to use moxibustion at CV-4 *(guan yuan)* and CV-6 *(qi hai)* with a moxa stick for 10-15 minutes every evening.

After 20 treatments, the patient was able to sustain a firm erection for about 5 minutes. After 30 treatments, all the symptoms disappeared and normal sexual function was restored. Treatment in the clinic was discontinued, but to consolidate the effect, he was advised to apply moxibustion periodically at CV-4 *(guan yuan)*, CV-6 *(qi hai)*, B-23 *(shen shu)* and GV-4 *(ming men)*. He was followed up for 8 months, and reported no further problems. □

Inhibited Orgasm

Yáng Qiáng 阳强

Lin, male, 34 years old. The patient was strong and healthy. He and his wife were childless, although they had been married for 2 years. He had frequent desire for intercourse, but never experienced ejaculation during coitus, which occasionally lasted for 30 minutes to an hour. Withdrawal was on account of fatigue, and his erection was maintained. Spontaneous emission often occurred later.

The patient complained of restlessness. He had a dry mouth, dark yellow urine, and red lips and tongue. His pulse was rapid and wiry. The external genitalia were normal.

SYNDROME DIFFERENTIATION

This case was characterized by the absence of intravaginal ejaculation and the maintenance of erection after the conclusion of intercourse, followed by spontaneous emission. These and other symptoms indicated a disorder of the Liver channel, and the presence of Liver Fire. Since the Liver channel encircles the external genitalia, dysfunction of this channel caused the erection to persist even after withdrawal. Liver Fire aroused sexual desire and caused the emissions after withdrawal. Other symptoms such as the restlessness, dry mouth, red lips

and tongue, dark urine, and the rapid, wiry pulse were all consequences of Liver Fire.

TREATMENT

The principles of treatment were to clear the Liver channel, soothe the Liver, and quell the Liver Fire.

Points selected:
CV-2 *(qu gu)*, Liv-11 *(yin lian)*, Liv-1 *(da dun)*
Acupuncture was administered once every other day. Ten treatments comprised one course of therapy, with 5-7 days' rest between courses. Moxibustion was self-administered once or twice daily at home, with twenty days comprising a course.

Discussion of points:
CV-2 *(qu gu)* is a point of intersection of the Liver channel on the Conception vessel

and is indicated for disorders of the genitalia. Liv-1 *(da dun)* is the well point of the Liver channel and is used to drain Liver Fire. Liv-11 *(yin lian)* relaxes the sinews and regulates the Conception vessel.

CV-2 *(qu gu)* was needled with the patient in a supine position; he was asked to empty his bladder beforehand. The needle was inserted to a depth of about 1.5 units, and the needle sensation spread to the root of the penis. Liv-11 *(yin lian)* was needled to a depth of 1-1.5 units. The sensation was one of local soreness, heaviness and distention. Liv-1 *(da dun)* was not needled because the sensation is not easily elicited at this point; sparrow-pecking moxibustion was used instead.

To obtain the needle sensation at the two points that were needled, draining through twirling manipulation was applied for one minute, and the needles were then retained for five minutes. If the needle sensation was too weak, it was strengthened by applying either the 'twisting' or 'flying' manipulation method.

'Twisting' involves twisting the needle like a thread, with wide amplitude. Care must be taken to avoid twisting too rapidly or too tightly, which causes the needle to catch. The 'flying' method is performed by rotating the needle in one direction until resistance is encountered, then suddenly releasing the needle, which creates a slight vibration. The sudden releasing action causes the fingers to resemble the spread wings of a bird, hence the term 'flying'. Generally, three releases or 'take-offs' are applied to achieve the best effect. These two methods have an excellent ability to propagate and prolong the needle sensation.

The patient was advised to refrain from sexual intercourse during the first course of therapy. This was done to allow the treatments to take effect, and also to avoid harming the Essence, which could lead to Fire from Yin deficiency and thus exacerbate the condition. (Overindulgence in intercourse leads to deficiency of Kidney Yang, and thus to deficiency of Essence.)

RESULTS

After the first course of treatment, the patient was permitted to have intercourse in order to judge how effective the treatment had been. There was still no intravaginal ejaculation. However, post-coital erection was reduced in duration, and spontaneous emissions disappeared. After the sixth day of the second course of treatment, post-coital erection was resolved, and the other symptoms were ameliorated. At the completion of the second course, intravaginal ejaculation and orgasm were experienced about ten minutes into intercourse. Treatment was then discontinued. Follow-up after three months found the patient to be enjoying a satisfactory sexual life. After another three months, the patient reported that his wife was pregnant.

Note: In treating male sexual dysfunction, the differences among three age groups should be taken into consideration. Among young men, i.e., those under 35 years of age, ascendant Yang is generally the cause of most cases of sexual dysfunction. Treatment should be directed at nourishing the Kidney Yin in order to subdue the ascendant Yang. Among middle aged men, Kidney Qi has begun to wane. Thus, both the Yin and Yang of the Kidney should be tonified in order to strengthen Kidney Qi. Among elderly men, the Kidney Qi, Yin and Yang have all waned, because the Fire at the 'gate of vitality' has declined. Treatment should therefore promote the latter. □

Insomnia

Bú Mèi 不寐

Liu, female, 62 years old. The patient complained of insomnia of 30 years' duration, and stated that she had been able to sleep for only about 3 hours each night. The condition had been diagnosed as neurasthenia. Various hypnotics had been used to induce sleep, but no cure was effected. The patient thereupon turned to acupuncture.

The four examinations of Chinese medicine found the patient to be emaciated. She lacked spirit and had malar flush. Inquiry revealed insomnia associated with palpitations, dizziness and tinnitus, and a sensation of heat in the lower back, buttocks, the posteriomedial aspect of the legs, and the soles. Palpation confirmed the presence of heat in those areas. Her tongue was red with a thin coating. The pulse was thin and rapid, and particularly frail at the rear position of the left wrist.

SYNDROME DIFFERENTIATION

The normal physiological process of sleep is related to the circulation of protective Qi. In the daytime, this Qi circulates in the Yang channels and wakefulness prevails; at night, it circulates in the Yin channels and sleep ensues. Normally, Yin regulates Yang, but when Yin is deficient, it cannot balance the Yang; as a result, there is an overabundance of Yang. Protective Qi pertains to Yang. When it encounters difficulty in entering the Yin channels, insomnia ensues.

There are several causes of insomnia, all of which ultimately result in an imbalance of Yin and Yang. Patterns of deficiency include the following:

- Deficiency of both the Spleen and Heart results in insufficient Blood, and thus restlessness of the Spirit, leading to insomnia and excessive dreaming. Other symptoms include a general lack of strength, loss of appetite, sallow complexion, a pale tongue with a thin coating, and a thin, frail pulse.

- Yin deficiency and blazing of Fire is caused by insufficient Kidney Yin, resulting in a lack of Yin to counterbalance the Heart Fire. The blazing of Heart Fire agitates the Spirit; restlessness and palpitations appear, causing insomnia. Symptoms of Kidney Yin deficiency include dizziness, tinnitus and soreness in the lower back. Symptoms of blazing Heart Fire are dryness in the mouth, a hot sensation in the chest, palms and soles, a red tongue, and a thin, rapid pulse.

- Qi deficiency of both the Heart and Gall Bladder induces restlessness of the Spirit, which causes insomnia. When the Spirit is restless, there is a propensity to become easily startled or frightened, leading to dream-disturbed sleep and wakefulness. Other symptoms of Qi Deficiency include shortness of breath, lassitude, clear and copious urine, a pale tongue, and a wiry, thin pulse.

Patterns of excess associated with insomnia include the following:

- Stagnant Liver Qi transforming into Fire results in insomnia. This often occurs when the Liver is affected by extreme anger. The Liver loses its function of spreading and regulating Qi, which then stagnates and transforms into Fire. Because the Spirit is disturbed by Fire, restlessness and insomnia ensue. Liver Fire may also induce Heat in the Stomach, which causes thirst. Other symptoms include red eyes, a bitter taste in the mouth, deep yellow urine, dry stools, a red tongue with a yellow coating, and a wiry, rapid pulse.

- Phlegm-Heat disturbing the interior is caused primarily by the stagnation of food leading to Dampness. Long-standing Dampness becomes Phlegm, which, if unresolved, transforms into Heat. Phlegm-Heat rises and disturbs the Heart; restlessness and insomnia follow. Other symptoms include heaviness of the head, fullness in the chest, nausea or vomiting. The tongue coating is greasy and yellow, and the pulse is slippery and rapid.

In this case, the patient suffered from dizziness, tinnitus, malar flush, and heat in the lower back, buttocks, the posteriomedial aspect of the legs, and the soles. The tongue was red with a thin coating. The pulse was thin and rapid, and was especially weak at the left rear position. All of these signs indicated Yin deficiency of the Kidney.

When Kidney Yin is deficient, there is not enough Water (Kidney Yin) to control Fire (Heart Yang). Heart Fire then blazes upward and disturbs the Spirit, causing insomnia and palpitations. Since the Kidney is one of the sources of nourishment for the brain (the 'sea of marrow'), Kidney Yin deficiency results in undernourishment of the brain, and thus dizziness. Tinnitus is also a sign of deficient Kidney Yin, as the ears are one of the exterior 'openings' of the Kidney.

TREATMENT

To ease the discord between the Kidney and Heart, the principles of treatment were to nourish the Yin in order to suppress the Fire, and to clear the Heart in order to calm the Spirit.

Points selected:
H-7 *(shen men)*, K-3 *(tai xi)*, B-14 *(jue yin shu)*, B-15 *(xin shu)*, B-23 *(shen shu)*, N-HN-54 *(an mian)*

All points were needled once daily with balanced tonifying-draining manipulation. Needles at points on the extremities were retained for 20 minutes, while those at the associated points of the back, and at N-HN-54 *(an mian)*, were retained for 10 minutes during each session.

Discussion of points:
Needling K-3 *(tai xi)* nourishes the Kidney Yin. H-7 *(shen men)* is the source and trans-

porting point of the Heart channel. Needling this point clears Fire from the Heart, and calms the Spirit. B-14 *(jue yin shu)* is the associated point of the Pericardium channel on the back. This point was chosen because of the close association between the Pericardium and Heart. B-15 *(xin shu)* and B-23 *(shen shu)* are the associated points on the back for the Heart and Kidney respectively. N-HN-54 *(an mian)* is especially effective for treating insomnia.

H-7 *(shen men)* was needled perpendicularly to a depth of 0.5 unit. The reaction to needling was one of soreness radiating to the little finger. K-3 *(tai xi)* was needled perpendicularly to a depth of about 0.5 unit. An electric shock-like sensation was felt radiating toward the sole. B-14 *(jue yin shu)* and B-15 *(xin shu)* were needled perpendicularly to a depth of 0.5 unit. Local soreness was experienced at these points. B-23 *(shen shu)* was needled perpendicularly to a depth of 1.2 units, and the needle sensation was one of soreness propagating downward along the Bladder channel toward the buttocks. N-HN-54 *(an mian)* was likewise needled perpendicularly to a depth of 1.2 units. The needle sensation was one of local soreness spreading to the side of the head.

RESULTS

Once acupuncture therapy was begun, all hypnotic drugs were discontinued in order to allow acupuncture to take its full effect. After five treatments, the patient's sleep increased to five hours at night. The heat in the thighs and soles disappeared, although some heat was still felt in the lower back and buttocks. The tongue became less red, and some white coating appeared. The pulse was still thin, but less rapid than before.

With the improvement in symptoms, needling was reduced to once every other day. After nine more treatments (for a total of fourteen), the patient was able to sleep for seven hours at night. All other symptoms basically disappeared, and treatment was terminated. The patient was followed-up for six months with no relapse. □

Pain in the Ribs
(Gallstone)

Xié Tòng 胁痛

Wang, female, 35 years old. The patient suffered from intermittent pain over the right abdomen for several months. Two years ago she was diagnosed as having gallstones, and underwent surgery to remove the stones. The symptoms recurred, however, and she had episodes of abdominal pain which radiated to the right scapula. Other symptoms included bitterness and dryness in the mouth, bloating, reduced appetite, aversion to greasy food, reduced urine, and difficult bowel movements with a burning sensation in the anus. She was irritable, and the abdominal pain was aggravated by her ill-temper.

Physical examination revealed an absence of jaundice. Her heart and lungs were normal, and her abdomen was soft. Murphy's sign was negative. The liver and spleen were not enlarged, but there was pain upon percussion over the gall bladder. The tongue was red with a yellowish-white coating, and the pulse was wiry, slippery and slightly rapid.

Ultrasound revealed several masses with strong reflection, the largest of which measured 0.9 x 0.5cm, suggesting the presence of stones.

Although the patient had taken herbal medicine for a prolonged period, and had also been treated with chenodeoxylic acid, no passage of stones was observed. Surgery was again recommended, but the patient refused. Instead, she decided to try acupuncture therapy.

SYNDROME DIFFERENTIATION

The Liver has the function of spreading and regulating the flow of Qi and Blood, while the Gall Bladder is the Organ in which the 'accumulated Essence' (bile) is stored *(Miraculous Pivot*, chapter 2). Emotional disturbance, intemperance in eating, and internal Damp-Heat interfere with the flow-regulating function of the Liver, and with the excretions of the Gall Bladder.

This was a case of recurrence of gallstones after temporary relief by surgical intervention. Such symptoms as the bitterness and dryness in the mouth pointed to the presence of internal Damp-Heat. The Liver and Gall Bladder are located in the costal region, and their channels are distributed over the sides of the ribcage; hence the upper abdominal pain and bloating. Since the normal digestive functions of the Spleen and Stomach depend on the Liver, the dysfunctioning of the Liver which resulted from the presence of Damp-Heat caused the reduced appetite and aversion to greasy food. Difficulty with urination and defecation was further evidence of the presence of internal Damp-Heat. When the Liver is affected by these pathogenic influences, irritability sets in. The resulting anger, in turn, worsens the condition of the Liver, thus aggravating the pain. Protracted Damp-Heat causes the bile to congeal into stones. The yellowish-white tongue coating, and the slippery, rapid pulse were consistent with this diagnosis. In sum, this was a case of Damp-Heat in the Liver and Gall Bladder.

TREATMENT

To eliminate the Damp-Heat from the body and restore normal function to the Liver, ear acupuncture was chosen as the mode of therapy. Recent clinical studies have shown that it is more effective than body acupuncture in expelling stones.[1]

Points selected:
Vaccaria seeds were applied at the ear points Gall Bladder, Pancreas, Liver, Sympathetic, Spleen, Stomach, Triple Burner and Shenmen.

Discussion of points:
The Gall Bladder, Pancreas and Liver points on the ear were chosen to normalize the function of the Liver, and to eliminate Damp-Heat. The Spleen and Stomach points were indicated for the reduced appetite and aversion to greasy food. The Sympathetic and Shenmen points were selected to relieve the pain and arrest the spasms, while the Triple Burner point also facilitated the elimination of Damp-Heat.

After disinfection of the skin, a vaccaria seed was applied to each point, bilaterally, and fixed in place with a small piece of adhesive tape, 5 x 5mm square. The seeds were pressed against the ear for five minutes until soreness was felt by the patient, and then left in place for seven days. Each course of treatment consisted of seven days, with three days' rest between courses. The seeds were removed at the end of each course.

The patient was asked to eat a stewed pig's foot (together with the broth) every day throughout the treatment in order to 'lubricate' the Gall Bladder, and to facilitate elimination of the gallstones.[2] In addition, the patient was advised to engage in physical exercise to the same end.

To evaluate the therapeutic effect, the stools were washed and sifted to search for stones, beginning with the first day of treatment.

RESULTS

After four days' treatment, the abdominal pain, bloating, and bitterness in the mouth began to subside. At the end of the second course, a stone 0.6 x 0.4cm in size was found in the stool. Altogether, three stones of various size were eliminated by the end of the fourth course. No other stones were found during two additional courses of treatment. The patient was then much more relaxed, her appetite returned, and the abdominal pain virtually disappeared. Ultrasound examination detected no other stones. The treatment was therefore discontinued, and there was no relapse during a follow-up of one year. □

---

[1]Zhang R, Ma SZ, Zhang TQ. The effect of auricular-plaster therapy on gallstone expulsion and on the expansion-contraction function of the biliary system: a clinical analysis of 57 cases. J Trad Chin Med 1986: 4;263.

[2]Any protein-rich liquid (e.g., chicken soup) can be used for this purpose.

Painful Obstruction of the Chest
(Angina Pectoris)

Xiōng Bì 胸痹

Li, female, 58 years old. The patient first experienced chest pain 3 years ago. The pain was rather dull, and often little more than a sensation of distention and constriction, usually precipitated by fatigue or emotional upset. During the past year, the pain worsened and became stabbing in nature. The episodes were relieved by nitroglycerin tablets. Other symptoms included palpitations, cough with expectoration of white, viscous sputum, and shortness of breath, all of which were aggravated by vigorous activity. Various remedies were tried, but were ineffective. Eventually, the patient was unable to manage daily household chores. She was then referred for acupuncture therapy.

Examination of the patient showed blood pressure of 170/110mm Hg, and weak cardiac sounds which were difficult to auscultate. The area of cardiac dullness to percussion was enlarged. Electrocardiogram revealed low T wave in V_3 and V_5 leads, and significant depression of the S-T segment.

The four examinations of traditional Chinese medicine found the patient to have a lackluster face, little spirit, and a rather stout figure. She complained of dizziness, and said that her head felt heavy, as if it were enclosed in a bag. She had a poor appetite, and she experienced epigastric and abdominal upset after eating. She also sweated spontaneously during the daytime. Her tongue was dark red with a white, greasy coating and purple spots. The pulse was thin, soggy and choppy.

SYNDROME DIFFERENTIATION

In traditional Chinese medicine, chest pain which is localized in the heart or substernal regions is attributed to Yang deficiency in the chest, which causes stagnation of Qi. This patient was rather obese, and her condition began with a sensation of distention and constriction, together with a productive cough. This was the result of the accumulation of Phlegm-Dampness, which interfered with the flow of Qi in the chest. (Obese individuals are prone to accumulation of Phlegm-Dampness.) The heavy sensation in the head, as if it were enclosed in a bag, was a sign of Dampness interfering with the ascent of clear Yang. This also accounted for the dizziness. The white, greasy tongue coating, and the soggy pulse, were likewise signs of Phlegm-Dampness.

Chronic disease injures Qi. Signs of deficient Qi were present in such symptoms as the palpitations, breathlessness, spontaneous sweating, lack of spirit, poor appetite and abdominal distention after eating. Qi is the 'commander' of Blood; when Qi is deficient, the movement of Blood is impeded. This impediment was aggravated by the lodging of Phlegm-Dampness in the Heart, and led to stasis of Blood, which was manifested in the episodes of chest pain, lackluster face, dark red tongue with purple spots, and choppy pulse. In sum, the pattern here was one of both excess (Phlegm-Dampness and stasis of Blood) as well as deficiency (deficient Qi).

TREATMENT

The principles of treatment were to resolve the Phlegm-Dampness, disperse the stasis of Blood, regulate the Qi and invigorate the Blood.

Points selected:

B-15 *(xin shu)*, B-14 *(jue yin shu)*, P-6 *(nei guan)*, H-5 *(tong li)*, S-40 *(feng long)*, S-36 *(zu san li)*, CV-17 *(tan zhong)*. Draining manipulation was applied at B-14 *(jue yin shu)* and S-40 *(feng long)*. S-36 *(zu san li)* was tonified.

Treatment was administered once daily. The needles were retained for 30 minutes. Ten treatments comprised 1 course of therapy, with 2-3 days' rest between courses.

Discussion of points:

B-15 *(xin shu)* is the associated point on the back for the Heart, and has the effect of clearing that channel, calming the Heart, regulating the Qi and invigorating the Blood. P-6 *(nei guan)* calms the Heart and suppresses pain. H-5 *(tong li)*, the connecting point of the Heart channel, regulates the Heart Qi and calms the Spirit. These were the three principal points in treating the

painful obstruction of the chest.

CV-17 *(tan zhong)* is the meeting point of Qi, and was used here to regulate the Qi in the chest. B-14 *(jue yin shu)*, the associated point on the back for the Pericardium, regulates Yang in the chest, and thereby resolves the Phlegm-Dampness lodged there. S-40 *(feng long)*, the connecting point of the Stomach channel, is traditionally indicated for Phlegm-Dampness. S-36 *(zu san li)* is one of the 'four dominant points' (see Introduction), and is an important point for promoting general health. Tonifying this point strengthens the Qi. It was used in this case to treat the deficiency of Qi.

When B-15 *(xin shu)* and B-14 *(jue yin shu)* were needled, care was taken not to insert the needles more than 0.5 unit deep to avoid puncturing the lung.

RESULTS

After five treatments, the distention and constriction in the chest diminished, the palpitations disappeared, and all other symptoms showed improvement. By the completion of the first course of therapy, the distention and constriction were completely alleviated. An increase in strength and spirit was noted, and other symptoms such as the shortness of breath, spontaneous sweating, dizziness and poor appetite continued to improve. The patient was able to walk at a leisurely pace for two miles without any discomfort in the chest. By the end of the second course of treatment with the same set of points, the patient could walk three miles at a rapid pace without any discomfort. Her appetite was improved, as was her complexion, which appeared healthier-looking. All other symptoms subsided. Electrocardiogram showed normal T waves, without any depression of the S-T segment.

To consolidate the therapeutic effect, a third course of treatment was administered. By the end of this course, the patient was able to perform ordinary household chores with ease. Treatment was therefore discontinued. Throughout her therapy, the patient had no attacks of angina. A follow-up one year later showed normal electrocardiogram, although the patient did complain of occasional mild and short-lived sensations of distention and constriction in the chest. □

Painful Urinary Dysfunction
(Renal Calculus)

Lín Zhèng 淋症

Wu, male, 45 years old. The left kidney of the patient was removed 5 years ago because of renal calculi that could not be effectively treated by more conservative measures. Several months ago, the patient suffered sudden, severe, colicky pain in the right lumbar region. X-ray revealed a pea-sized oval stone in the right kidney. The patient experienced constant, heavy and painful distention in the lower abdomen, and was fatigued. Urination was dribbling, and colic attack often recurred after hard work. His appetite was poor, and his stools were unformed. His tongue was light in color, and his pulse was frail.

SYNDROME DIFFERENTIATION

In Chinese medicine, symptoms associated with urinary infections and stones, such as painful, dribbling urination and pain in the lower abdomen and lumbar region, fall in the category of painful urinary dysfunction. This syndrome is attributed to the accumulation of Damp-Heat in the lower Burner, which affects the normal Bladder functions of water circulation and urination. If not effectively treated, the Kidney and Spleen will be injured in turn.

Clinically, there are three common types of painful urinary dysfunction:

• Accumulation of Damp-Heat. Due to excessive intake of pungent, hot, greasy foods, or of alcohol, Damp-Heat is generated and pours into the lower Burner, where it interferes with the urinary functions. When the Blood vessels are damaged by Heat, hematuria results. The tongue coating is greasy and yellow, and the pulse is slippery and rapid.

• Liver Qi stagnation. When the Liver is injured by anger, Liver Qi stagnates and transforms into Fire, which accumulates in the lower Burner along the course of the Liver channel and disrupts the normal function of the Bladder. The tongue is bluish, and the pulse is wiry and submerged.

• Deficiency of Spleen and Kidney Qi. When old age and overexertion, or prolonged accumulation of Damp-Heat, overcome the body's resistance (true Qi),

70

the result is deficiency of Spleen and Kidney Qi. Bladder function is disrupted, causing dribbling urination, which is exacerbated by fatigue. Other manifestations of Spleen and Kidney Qi deficiency are soreness in the lower back, lassitude and diminished appetite. The reported case pertained to this type of painful urinary dysfunction.

TREATMENT

The principles of treatment were to warm the Kidney, invigorate the Spleen, relieve the painful urinary dysfunction and eliminate the stone.

Points selected:

B-23 *(shen shu)*, B-28 *(pang guang shu)*, B-20 *(pi shu)*, CV-4 *(guan yuan)*, CV-3 *(zhong ji)*, Sp-6 *(san yin jiao)*, K-8 *(jiao xin)*, Sp-15 *(da heng)*

Treatment was administered once daily. Ten treatments comprised one course of therapy, with 3-5 days' rest between courses.

Discussion of points:

B-23 *(shen shu)*, B-28 *(pang guang shu)* and B-20 *(pi shu)* are the associated points on the back for the Kidney, Bladder and Spleen respectively. Needling these points regulates the functions of the Spleen and Kidney, and all of these points work in concert to aid the urinary function of the Bladder.

CV-4 *(guan yuan)* is where true Qi is stored. Needling and moxibustion at this point warms the Kidney and invigorates Kidney Yang. CV-3 *(zhong ji)* is the alarm point of the Bladder. Treating this point relieves

painful urinary dysfunction and eliminates urinary stones.

Sp-6 *(san yin jiao)* is the point of intersection of the three Yin channels of the leg. Combined with Sp-15 *(da heng)* and K-8 *(jiao xin)*, these three points have the effect of relieving painful urinary dysfunction and eliminating stones. K-3 *(jiao xin)* is the accumulating point of the Yin Heel channel. Accumulating points are used for emergency symptoms, hence K-8 *(jiao xin)* was specifically used here for treating the acute renal colic induced by the urinary stone.

Following the principle of tonifying deficiency and draining excess, the Spleen and Kidney deficiency was tonified by raise-thrust and twirling manipulation. At CV-4 *(guan yuan)* and CV-3 *(zhong ji)* the needle sensation was induced to spread into the bladder. Warm needle moxibustion (two stubs per point) was then applied at these two points while the needles were in place.

RESULTS

After the first course of therapy, there was little improvement in the symptoms. In order to strengthen the therapeutic effect, warm needle moxibustion (two stubs per point) was added at B-20 *(pi shu)* and B-23 *(shen shu)*. The patient was advised to drink a lot of water to facilitate expulsion of the stone.

After the third course of treatment, X-ray showed that the stone had dropped to the lower part of the ureter. After one more week of treatment, the pea-sized stone was expelled, and the other symptoms were relieved. Treatment was then terminated. During a follow-up of one year there was no recurrence of stones. □

Palpitations
(Paroxysmal Supraventricular Tachycardia)

Xīn Jì 心悸

Wang, male, 28 years old. About 5 years ago, the patient suffered an attack of palpitations, dizziness and loss of strength without any apparent precipitating cause. He counted his own pulse rate and found it to be 150 beats per minute. Such episodes recurred about 1-3 times per month, each of which lasted 3-5 days, and followed periods of overwork or anxiety. The patient took Chinese and western medicines, but with no appreciable effect. He then turned to acupuncture.

The four examinations of Chinese medicine revealed that the patient was pale, and appeared listless and weak. He suffered from dizziness, insomnia and excessive dreaming during sleep. The episodes were especially severe when he was tired. His memory was failing, and just one hour of mental work or reading would bring on the dizziness and palpitations. His appetite was fair, and urination and bowel movements were normal. The tongue was pale with a thin, white coating, and the pulse was submerged, thin and frail.

SYNDROME DIFFERENTIATION

Chinese medicine considers palpitations to be a common disorder of the Heart. They can be brought on by deficiency of Qi and Blood of the Heart, or by lack of nourishment to the Heart and the Spirit.

The patient was a composer who regularly overtaxed his mental faculties. Over the course of time, this led to consumption of Qi and impairment of Blood.

Deficient Qi caused the listlessness and lack of strength, while deficient Blood deprived the Spirit of its nutritional support, thus giving rise to insomnia, dream-disturbed sleep, and failing memory. Deficiency of Qi and Blood deprived the head of adequate nourishment, which caused the dizziness. Since overtaxation of the mental faculties impairs Qi and Blood, the sudden onset of symptoms was generally precipitated by mental fatigue. The pale tongue, and the thin, frail and submerged pulse likewise indicated deficiency of Qi and Blood. This case was therefore diagnosed as deficiency of Qi and Blood.

TREATMENT

Treatment was directed at replenishing the Qi and Blood, pacifying the Heart and relieving the mental strain.

Points selected:

P-6 *(nei guan)*, H-7 *(shen men)*, Sp-6 *(san yin jiao)*

Tonifying manipulation was applied at all points.

Discussion of points:

P-6 *(nei guan)* is the connecting point of the Pericardium channel, and H-7 *(shen men)* is the source point of the Heart channel. The selection of these two points illustrates the treatment principle of combining source and connecting points. These two points are commonly used together in treating diseases of the Heart. In this case, they served to pacify the Heart, and to relieve the mental strain.

Sp-6 *(san yin jiao)* is the point of intersection of the Liver, Spleen and Kidney channels. The Liver has the function of storing Blood, and the Spleen has the functions of producing Blood and maintaining its circulation within the vessels. This point was therefore selected to regulate the Liver and Spleen, and thereby replenish the Qi and Blood.

RESULTS

The first treatment was by chance administered during an attack of palpitations, when the heart rate was 148/minute. After tonifying manipulation was applied for 3 minutes at the prescribed points, the heart rate slowed to 110/minute. The needles were retained for 30 minutes and then removed, by which time the heart rate was 100/minute. At the next treatment on the following day, the patient did not experience any palpitations, and his heart rate was 92/minute.

Treatment was continued once daily for a total of ten sessions, which comprised one course of therapy. By the end of the first course, the patient had no further episodes of palpitations. He could also sleep better, but his other symptoms remained essentially unchanged.

The patient had been suffering from deficiency of both Qi and Blood, and the disease was focused in the Heart. The selection of points primarily on the Heart and Pericardium channels was therefore suited only for the chief symptoms. Theoretically, for deficiency of both Qi and Blood, treatment should be directed mainly at tonifying the former. This is because Qi produces Blood, and when Qi thrives, Blood will follow. Unlike herbal therapy which can directly tonify Blood, acupuncture indirectly tonifies Blood by regulating the Qi in order to open up the source of Blood. Since the Spleen and Stomach are the source of nutrients for the development of Qi and Blood, tonifying these Organs is very important in treating Qi and Blood deficiency.

Based upon this analysis, a new point prescription was formulated: P-6 *(nei guan)*, H-7 *(shen men)*, CV-6 *(qi hai)*, S-36 *(zu san li)*, Sp-6 *(san yin jiao)*. Moxibustion was also administered at CV-6 *(qi hai)* and S-36 *(zu san li)*.

CV-6 *(qi hai)*, the 'sea of Qi', is often used for strengthening the Qi. S-36 *(zu san li)* is an important point for invigoration in general. Its use strengthens the Spleen and Stomach. Moreover, when combined with CV-6 *(qi hai)*, its action in tonifying Qi is enhanced.

Treatment was resumed every other day using the modified prescription, and the needles were retained for 30 minutes. After 5 sessions, all symptoms gradually abated. The dizziness was alleviated, and the patient no longer experienced insomnia. After 20 treatments, the patient reported that he felt excellent. He was energetic, his memory was improved, and he was able to perform mental work and read for extended periods of time. No recurrence of palpitations occurred during the period of treatment. Another 5 treatments were administered to consolidate the therapeutic effect.

The patient was followed up for six months. He was found to have recovered completely, and in fact was preparing to travel abroad for further studies. Since the patient's illness originated from overwork and anxiety, he was advised to avoid undue mental strain. □

Palpitations
(Ventricular Septal Defect)

Xīn Jì 心悸

Zhang, female, 23 years old. The patient suffered from frequent colds since childhood, and had pneumonia when she was 10 years old. She had palpitations and shortness of breath, which were especially severe after exertion. Sometimes cyanosis of the lips was noted. An examination 1 year ago revealed a regular heartbeat with a rate of 74 beats per minute. Both lungs were clear; a systolic murmur was heard in the 3rd and 4th intercostal spaces along the sternum. The second heart sound was accentuated. No thrill was palpable. EKG showed hypertrophy of the right ventricle. Right heart catheterization revealed a ventricular septal defect with bidirectional shunt, and a pulmonic pressure of 90mm Hg. The diagnosis was congenital heart disease with ventricular septal defect and severe pulmonary hypertension. The cardiologist felt that the patient was not suited for surgery at the time, and suggested acupuncture.

The four examinations of Chinese medicine revealed that the patient's face was lackluster. She complained of an oppressive sensation in the chest, palpitations, shortness of breath and general weakness. The palpitations and shortness of breath were aggravated by mild exertion. She had a dry sensation and a bitter taste in her mouth, but did not drink much. She suffered from frequent night sweats, a sensation of heat in the soles of her feet, and soreness and weakness in her legs. She slept little and dreamed excessively. Her appetite was normal. She was constipated, and her urine was scanty. The menses were light in color and reduced in amount. The tip of her tongue was red, and there were cracks over the front; the tongue coating was scanty. Her pulse was thin and weak.

SYNDROME DIFFERENTIATION

According to Chinese medicine, the Heart controls the Blood circulation and mental activities, which are closely related. When Qi and Blood are abundant, the individual is full of vigor, with ruddy cheeks and a moderate, strong pulse. When Qi and Blood are deficient, the heartbeat is feeble and there is not enough Blood to nourish the Heart, resulting in such symptoms as palpitations, an oppressive sensation in the chest, shortness of breath, weakness and a lackluster demeanor. When the Heart lacks nourishment, it is unable to restrain the Spirit, thus causing disturbed sleep and excessive dreaming. Deficiency of Heart Yin leads to loss of control of the Yang and to the generation of internal Heat, manifested in night sweats and a hot sensation in the soles. Deficiency of Yin causes constipation and scantiness of urine. Deficiency of Qi and Blood may also be manifested in light-colored, scanty menses, and a thin, weak pulse.

The diagnosis here was accordingly deficiency of Heart Qi and Blood.

TREATMENT

The principles of treatment were to tonify the Heart Qi, nourish the Heart Yin and replenish the Heart Blood.

Points selected:

P-6 *(nei guan)*, H-7 *(shen men)*, CV-17 *(tan zhong)*, S-36 *(zu san li)*, CV-6 *(qi hai)*, Sp-6 *(san yin jiao)*, K-6 *(zhao hai)*, B-14 *(jue yin shu)*, B-15 *(xin shu)*, B-17 *(ge shu)*

Discussion of points:

P-6 *(nei guan)* is the connecting point of the Pericardium channel. It is also one of the confluent points of the eight miscellaneous channels, intersecting with the Yin Linking channel. It is the principal point for treating diseases of the Heart. B-15 *(xin shu)* is the associated point on the back for the Heart; its combination with P-6 *(nei guan)* acts to tonify the functional activities of the Heart, and to nourish its Yin.

B-14 *(jue yin shu)* is the associated point on the back for the Pericardium, and CV-17 *(tan zhong)* is the alarm point of that Organ. Using these two points together is an example of combining an associated point on the back of the body with an alarm point on the front. In this case, the two points were used to regulate cardiac function and tonify the

Qi and Yin of the Heart. CV-17 *(tan zhong)* is also the meeting point of Qi, and was therefore used to regulate the circulation of Qi in treating the oppressive sensation in the chest, and the shortness of breath.

CV-6 *(qi hai)* is the 'sea of Qi'. B-17 *(ge shu)* is the meeting point of Blood, and is the site where Blood converges; it is used primarily in treating Blood-related disorders. S-36 *(zu san li)* is an important point for tonifying Qi and promoting the production of Blood. CV-6 *(qi hai)* and S-36 *(zu san li)* are general tonification points, used in this case with B-17 *(ge shu)* to tonify Heart Qi and Blood.

K-6 *(zhao hai)* on the Kidney channel is another of the confluent points of the eight miscellaneous channels, intersecting with the Yin Heel channel. The Kidney channel has a branch which connects with the Heart via the Lung. Needling K-6 *(zhao hai)* in combination with H-7 *(shen men)*, the source point of the Heart channel, has the effect of nourishing the Heart Yin, calming the Heart and relieving anxiety.

Because the condition was one of deficiency, the points were tonified using raise-thrust and twirling manipulation.

B-14 *(jue yin shu)*, B-15 *(xin shu)* and B-17 *(ge shu)* were needled first, with the patient in a sitting position. One-unit needles were inserted 0.8 unit deep. When a local sensation of soreness and distention was obtained, tonification was applied. The needles were retained for 10 minutes. The other points were needled with the patient lying supine.

At CV-17 *(tan zhong)* a 1.5-unit needle was inserted obliquely downward under the skin. The needle sensation radiated to the region around the xiphoid process.

There are two ways of locating K-6 *(zhao hai)*: either 1 unit below the tip of the medial malleolus, or in the depression immediately below the tip. In this case, a distinct needle sensation was obtained 1 unit below the tip of the bone.

All other points were needled in the conventional manner.

RESULTS

After daily acupuncture treatments for two weeks, the patient felt relaxed and was able to sleep for longer periods of time. The palpitations and shortness of breath were also alleviated. After two more weeks of treatment, the night sweats were significantly improved. Six weeks into treatment, her face began to show a ruddy tinge, and she became more energetic. She no longer experienced palpitations or shortness of breath while walking; however, climbing the stairs of a three-story building still left her breath-less. In order to consolidate the therapeutic effect, treatment was continued every other day for another month with the same points. Acupuncture was then discontinued, and the patient was advised to recuperate at home. During a follow-up of three months, there was no recurrence of symptoms.

Note: For this type of disorder, amelioration of the symptoms is the goal of treatment. Recurrence of symptoms is probable without continuous treatment, or surgical intervention. □

Pulseless Syndrome
(Takayasu's Syndrome)

Wú Mài Zhèng 无脉症

Tan, female, 27 years old. One year ago, the patient suddenly fainted while at work. She was revived with oxygen at a hospital. Two similar episodes occurred during the next 6 months. She then began to suffer intense pain in her left arm, especially around the elbow, and the pain was aggravated by pressure. The affected limb was pale and cold, and the pulses at the radial and brachial arteries were not palpable. Her condition was diagnosed as pulseless syndrome (Takayasu's syndrome). In the past month the pain increased, the fingers became numb, and the patient was unable to grasp chopsticks. She was then referred for acupuncture therapy.

The four examinations of Chinese medicine revealed that the patient was emaciated, depressed, dizzy, weak, and had frequent fainting spells. She also suffered from palpitations and insomnia. Her tongue was pale. The pulse, which was not palpable on the left wrist, was choppy and thin on the right. Blood pressure could not be taken on the left arm, but was 110/170mm Hg on the right.

SYNDROME DIFFERENTIATION

In Chinese medicine, the absence of pulse signifies the complete obliteration of the channel. This implies Yang deficiency and internal Cold, resulting in stagnation of Qi and stasis of Blood. This patient presented with no pulse on the left wrist. Her skin was pale, her left arm was cold, and her tongue was pale. These were all signs of Yang deficiency and internal Cold. Pain completed the picture of stagnation of Qi and stasis of Blood, as pain usually occurs when the flow of Qi and Blood is impeded.

The Heart controls the Blood vessels. When the vessels are affected by long-standing disease, the Heart is affected. Here, the deficiency of Heart Yang resulted in palpitations, insomnia, dizziness, lack of strength and frequent episodes of fainting.

TREATMENT

The principles of treatment were to strengthen the Yang and dissipate the Cold, regulate the Qi and invigorate the Blood.

78

Points selected:

H-3 *(shao hai)*, H-5 *(tong li)*, H-7 *(shen men)*, P-3 *(qu ze)*, P-6 *(nei guan)*, P-7 *(da ling)*

All points were needled on the left arm only, in accordance with the method of local point selection. Treatment was administered once every other day, and the needles were retained for 30 minutes during each session.

Discussion of points:

H-3 *(shao hai)* calms the Spirit and clears the Heart channel. It was used here for the numbness of the forearm, and the elbow pain. H-5 *(tong li)* is the connecting point of the Heart channel. Its effect is to calm the Spirit and regulate the Heart Qi. H-7 *(shen men)*, the source point of the Heart channel, likewise calms the Spirit and clears the Heart channel. It was selected for treating the palpitations and insomnia. Needling P-3 *(qu ze)* invigorates the Heart Qi. P-6 *(nei guan)*, the connecting point of the Pericardium channel, calms the Spirit, pacifies the Heart, and alleviates pain. In this case, it was selected for treating the palpitations, insomnia and pain. P-7 *(da ling)* is the source point of the Pericardium channel. It too calms the Spirit and regulates the Heart.

When combined, these six points can achieve the therapeutic effect of regulating the Qi, invigorating the Blood, restoring flow in the channel and arresting the pain. At the same time, the Spirit will be calmed and the Heart pacified. Furthermore, the combined use of the source and connecting points links the interior and exterior channels, regulates the Yin and Yang, and enhances the needling effect.

All six points were tonified. At H-3 *(shao hai)*, P-3 *(qu zi)* and P-6 *(nei guan)*, the technique of 'burning the mountain' (see Introduction) was used to elicit warmth under the needle until the skin began to sweat. The other three points were tonified through raise-thrust and twirling manipulation.

RESULTS

After three treatments, the pain in the left elbow diminished. After seven treatments, the pulses at the brachial and radial arteries were faintly palpable, and the patient was able to grasp chopsticks. After an additional ten treatments, the pain was completely alleviated, and there was further improvement in the strength of the pulses.

'Burning the mountain' technique was then replaced with raise-thrust and twirling manipulation, because the symptoms had improved, and it was no longer necessary to use such strong manipulation. After the needle sensation was obtained, the needles were retained in place for 30 minutes, and manipulated once every 10 minutes. Needling was also commenced at H-3 *(shao hai)*, H-5 *(tong li)* and P-7 *(da ling)* on the *right* arm, using tonifying manipulation. These points were added to regulate the flow of Qi and Blood in the bilateral channels, and thereby to enhance the therapeutic effect.

After ten treatments with the modified point prescription, marked improvement was seen, although the left radial pulse was still weak and easily lost on pressure. Because most of the symptoms had disappeared, acupuncture therapy was discontinued. Follow-up eight months later found that the patient's condition had remained stable.

Note: Acupuncture for Takayasu's syndrome is only a palliative therapy. There is no cure for this condition, although some success has been obtained through surgery. □

Rectal Prolapse

Tuō Gāng 脱肛

Zhao, female, 56 years old. The patient complained of rectal prolapse of 3 years' duration. She had a history of constipation for 30 years, but only in the past 3 years had she experienced prolapse of the rectum after bowel movements. The prolapsed rectum was reduced manually. Minor prolapses also occurred when she was fatigued. The prolapse was about 3cm maximum. She had always suffered from poor health, and had symptoms such as dizziness, forgetfulness, soreness in the lower back, weakness of the limbs, aversion to cold, and frequent urination. She had also suffered from a duodenal ulcer, now much improved, but at times her appetite was still poor, and she had abdominal distention. Fifteen years ago, she had chronic pyelonephritis, which was treated successfully.

On examination, the patient appeared emaciated and listless. Her face and lips were pale. The prolapsed rectum was light in color, without congestion, swelling or pain. The tongue was pale with a thin, white and moist coating. The pulse was submerged, thin and frail.

SYNDROME DIFFERENTIATION

The patient's history indicated that she was past middle age, and had suffered chronic illness for more than ten years. Old age and prolonged illness are apt to lead to deficiency syndromes. In old age, the Kidney Qi becomes deficient. When the Kidney Qi is deficient, two of the Kidney's 'openings'—the urethra and anus—lack control. This was manifested here by frequent urination and rectal prolapse. Other symptoms of Kidney deficiency included dizziness, soreness in the lower back and weakness of the limbs, sensitivity to cold, and forgetfulness.

Chronic illness consumes Qi. The functioning of an Organ depends on the adequacy of its Qi. The symptoms of this patient indicated deficiency of Spleen Qi; the Spleen's Blood-producing function was thus disturbed, resulting in the pale face and tongue. Deficient Spleen Qi was also marked by emaciation and lassitude, because the Spleen's function of transporting nutrients was impaired. Spleen Qi is known as the 'middle Qi', and is responsible for holding the Organs in place. Deficient middle Qi causes the Organs to sink, which in this case resulted in the sinking (prolapse) of the rectum.

In sum, the patient's condition was due to deficiency of the Kidney and Spleen.

TREATMENT

Treatment was directed at tonifying the Kidney to improve its function, and strengthening the Spleen to replenish the Blood and to raise the sinking Qi.

Points selected:

GV-20 (bai hui), GV-1 (chang qiang), B-23 (shen shu), B-20 (pi shu), B-25 (da chang shu)

Discussion of points:

GV-20 (bai hui) is the point at which the Qi of the Yang channels accumulates. Needling this point replenishes Qi, and raises the sinking Qi of the Spleen. GV-1 (chang qiang) is a local point. Tonifying this point strengthens the restraining function of the anus. B-23 (shen shu) is the associated point on the back for the Kidney, and helps tonify Kidney Qi. B-25 (da chang shu) is the associated point on the back for the Large Intestine. Needling this point tonifies and warms the Qi of the Large Intestine, thus restoring its restraining function. B-20 (pi shu) is the associated point on the back for the Spleen. This point replenishes Qi and Blood, thus treating deficiency of the middle Burner.

GV-20 (bai hui) was needled with a 1.5-unit needle inserted forward, forming an angle of 15^0 to the scalp. The depth of insertion was about 1 unit. GV-1 (chang qiang) was needled with a 2-unit needle inserted in the direction of the rectum to a depth of about 1.5 units, producing a sensation of soreness and distention, and sometimes retraction. B-20 (pi shu), B-23 (shen shu) and B-25 (da chang shu) were needled with 1.5-unit needles inserted perpendicularly to a depth of about 1.2 units, producing soreness and distention which was transmitted downward along the Bladder channel to the buttocks, and upward to the back.

Treatment was administered once every other day, and the needles were retained for 20 minutes. During this time, a moxibustion box measuring about 20 x 15cm was placed over B-25 (da chang shu) and B-23 (shen shu). Two 5cm moxa sticks were burned on the wire mesh inside the box.

RESULTS

When the needles were removed after the first treatment, the patient had a feeling of warmth in the anus, accompanied by a sensation of retraction. After three more treatments, the rectum prolapsed only after bowel movements, and the extent of the prolapse was reduced to about 1cm. Treatment was continued for a total of eleven sessions. By this time, prolapse no longer occurred, even after bowel movements. The patient was livelier, felt stronger in her back and limbs, and had a better appetite. Her face assumed a ruddy complexion, and the dizziness was substantially improved. Treatment was then discontinued. The patient was advised not to tire herself, and to eat more nourishing foods. She was followed up for three months, with no recurrence of symptoms. □

Stomachache
(Peptic Ulcer)

Wèi Tòng 胃痛

Jian, female, 45 years old. The patient suffered from frequent, dull pains in the epigastrium for over 20 years. Two years ago, after barium meal examination and gastroscopy, she was diagnosed as having a peptic ulcer in the duodenal bulb, and chronic superficial gastritis. She took cimetidine and various Chinese medicinal preparations, but with little effect; the stomachache recurred frequently. During the 2 weeks prior to her visit to the clinic, the condition worsened. The pain radiated to the back, and was accompanied by nausea and regurgitation of clear fluid. Other symptoms included reduced appetite, a dulling of the sense of taste, a preference for hot beverages, alleviation of pain when the stomach was pressed, aggravation of pain during cold weather, sticky, loose stools (not black), a pale tongue with a thin, white coating, and a frail pulse.

SYNDROME DIFFERENTIATION

Stomach pain is a condition commonly seen in the clinic. In Chinese medicine, it may be attributed to a variety of factors, the most common of which are externally-contracted Cold, or over-indulgence in raw or cold food, which gives rise to Cold in the Stomach; stagnation of Liver Qi, which rebels transversely and encroaches upon the Stomach; or to overwork or protracted illness, which leads to deficiency of Yang, and the presence of Cold in the Spleen and Stomach.

Cases associated with externally-contracted Cold generally present with an acute onset of pain, an aversion to Cold and a desire for warmth, a white tongue coating, and a tight pulse. Symptoms associated with adverse flow of Liver Qi encroaching upon the Stomach include a feeling of fullness in the stomach that extends to the hypochondria, frequent hiccoughs, and a wiry pulse. Deficiency of Yang and the presence of Cold in the Spleen and Stomach manifests as dull epigastric pain and a desire for warmth. The patient will tend to press the stomach when it hurts, and will have cold hands and feet.

According to the above analysis, the present case was one of deficiency of Yang and the presence of Cold in the Spleen and Stomach. The dull pain resulted from deficiency of Yang, which deprived the channels of vigor and nourishment. Deficiency of Yang also led to disturbance in the transportation of water, which gave rise to nausea and regurgitation of clear fluid. Because of the deficiency of Yang, internal Cold was generated, and the related pain was aggravated by cold temperatures. Other symptoms such as the preference for hot beverages, the sticky, loose stools, and the tongue and pulse signs confirmed the diagnosis of Yang deficiency and the presence of Cold in the Spleen and Stomach.

TREATMENT

Treatment was directed at warming the Spleen and Stomach (the middle Burner) to dispel the Cold, and to regulate the functions of these two Organs.

Points selected:

CV-12 *(zhong wan)*, S-36 *(zu san li)*, P-6 *(nei guan)*, Sp-4 *(gong sun)*, B-20 *(pi shu)*, B-21 *(wei shu)*

Two moxa sticks, 7cm in length, were burned in a moxibustion box over CV-12 *(zhong wan)*. After the first two sticks were consumed, two more sticks were burned. Tonifying manipulation was applied at the remaining points, utilizing raise-thrust and twirling techniques. Treatment was administered once daily.

Discussion of points:

CV-12 *(zhong wan)* is the alarm point of the Stomach and the meeting point of the Yang Organs. It is used primarily in treating diseases of the Stomach. Strong moxibustion at this point warms the middle Burner and dispels the Cold.

P-6 *(nei guan)* and Sp-4 *(gong sun)* are two of the confluent points of the eight miscellaneous channels, and are useful in treating diseases of the Heart, chest and Stomach. P-6 *(nei guan)* pacifies the Stomach and al-leviates epigastric pain, while Sp-4 *(gong sun)* strengthens the Spleen and Stomach. The two points work synergistically. S-36 *(zu san li)* is the uniting point of the Stomach channel and is one of the 'four dominant points'. S-36 *(zu san li)* is especially effective in regulating the Spleen and Stomach.

B-20 *(pi shu)* and B-21 *(wei shu)* are the associated points on the back for the Spleen and Stomach respectively. They are situated where the Qi of the Spleen and Stomach are conveyed and spread over the back. These points were selected to help regulate the functions of those Organs. Generally, when the Spleen and Stomach are affected by disease, a stiff, cord-like structure can be palpated in the vicinity of B-20 *(pi shu)* or B-21 *(wei shu)*. When needling these points, the best results are obtained when the needles are directed toward the cord, or are inserted at the spot where the tenderness is most distinct.

B-20 *(pi shu)* and B-21 *(wei shu)* were treated first, with the patient in a sitting position. One-unit needles were inserted 0.8 unit deep. After the needle sensation was obtained, the handles of the needles were flicked lightly. This caused the needles to gently vibrate, and enhanced the needle sensation. Needle flicking was applied at both points for five minutes; the two needles were flicked at the same time, using both hands. The needles were then removed, and the patient was asked to lie down so that the other points could be needled.

RESULTS

After three treatments, the stomach pain improved slightly, and the regurgitation of clear fluid was also somewhat ameliorated. However, canker sores appeared in the mouth and on the tongue, and there was a sensation of dryness in the mouth. The stools also turned dry. These symptoms were attributed to the excessive use of moxibustion. Although moxibustion at CV-12 *(zhong wan)* was appropriate for this condition, the dosage of moxibustion might have been too large for the patient's tolerance in light of her protracted and debilitating illness. As a result, excessive warmth dissipated the body Fluids, which caused a flaring-up of Fire from deficiency, manifested by the ulcers in the mouth.

Therefore, from the fourth day onward, CV-12 *(zhong wan)* was treated only with acupuncture. CV-23 *(lian quan)* was added to help regenerate the body Fluids, and P-8 *(lao gong)* was added to suppress the Fire from deficiency. All other points remained the same. Treatment with these points continued for five days, and the ulcers in the mouth healed.

Treatment was then suspended for three days. Upon resumption, the use of CV-23 *(lian quan)* and P-8 *(lao gong)* was discontinued, and moxibustion at CV-12 *(zhong wan)* was restored. This time, however, only one moxa stick, about 3cm in length, was used at each session. After ten treatments, the patient's appetite improved, and her stomachache was much better. Treatment was then reduced to every other day for another two weeks. When all of the symptoms had subsided, therapy was terminated. The patient was followed up for one year, and there was no recurrence of symptoms. □

Sweating of the Hands and Feet

Shǒu Zú Duō Hàn Zhèng 手足多汗症

Fang, female, 23 years old. Since childhood, the patient's hands and feet had a tendency to sweat profusely, especially during menstrual periods and when she was excited. Sweat would drip from her palms, and the sweat from the soles of her feet would soak through her socks and shoes. The western medical diagnosis was functional disturbance of the autonomic nervous system. Various vitamins and other medicines were prescribed, but with little effect. She also took Chinese herbs which were astringent or sedative in nature, as well as preparations for replenishing Yin and clearing Heat. These too were of no avail. She therefore turned to acupuncture therapy.

The patient was lively and healthy-looking. Examination of the heart and lungs was negative. The liver and spleen were not palpable. The spinal column and extremities were normal. Body temperature, blood pressure and other laboratory findings were all within normal limits. Her palms and soles were normal in color and temperature, but were so sweaty that perspiration streamed down her skin. She complained of thirst, preferred cold beverages, and was irritable. The tongue was red without coating, and the pulse was thin and rapid.

SYNDROME DIFFERENTIATION

Except for the chronic sweating of the palms and soles, no other abnormalities were noted. Together with the thirst and desire for cold beverages, irritability, red tongue and thin, rapid pulse, this condition was attributed to the presence of Fire and Heat.

Although Chinese medicine holds that deficiency of Yin leads to night sweats, and deficiency of Yang to spontaneous sweating, the true nature of sweating in a particular case must be determined by consideration of both the general constitution of the patient as well as the accompanying symptoms. This patient appeared to be healthy and lively, and showed no signs of deficiency; therefore, deficiency was ruled out as the cause of the condition. Sweat is regarded as the Fluid of the Heart because it originates from Blood, which is regulated by the Heart. Excessive sweating can thus be caused by Fire in the Heart, which is a

85

condition of excess. The symptoms in the present case corresponded with this diagnosis. This was an excellent example of a chronic disorder (originating in childhood) which was excessive in nature.

TREATMENT

The principle of treatment was to dispel the Heat and quell the Fire in the Heart.

Points selected:

H-6 *(yin xi)*, H-7 *(shen men)*

Treatment was administered once daily. Draining manipulation was used at both points.

Discussion of points:

H-6 *(yin xi)* is the accumulating point of the Heart channel. Draining manipulation at this point acts to dispel the Heat and quell the Fire in the Heart. This point is often used in treating excessive sweating. H-7 *(shen men)*, the source point of the Heart channel, was added to enhance the therapeutic effect. There is another way of understanding the use of this second point. In the five phases scheme, H-7 *(shen men)* is the earth point on the Heart channel. Earth is the 'son' of fire in the generation cycle of the five phases. Draining the 'son' drains the 'mother'; therefore, draining this point quells the Fire in the Heart.

After five treatments, the sweating was reduced. However, the effect was unstable

for the symptoms recurred after a three-day interruption in treatment. Because the patient had suffered from this disorder since childhood, it was a very deep-rooted condition. Clearly, other points were needed.

In the *Great Compendium of Acupuncture and Moxibustion,* Yang Jizhou noted that excessive sweating should be treated by first draining LI-4 *(he gu),* and then tonifying K-7 *(fu liu).* This has long been an effective method for treating this condition. When applied to the present case, draining at LI-4 *(he gu)* was performed first, using a method of strong draining manipulation known as 'cooling the sky' (see Introduction). Vigorous tonification at K-7 *(fu liu)* was then performed, using a method called 'burning the mountain' (see Introduction). H-6 *(yin xi)* and H-7 *(shen men)* were drained in the conventional manner.

RESULTS

After two treatments with the new combination of points, the sweating of the palms and soles was markedly reduced, and the thirst and preference for cold beverages was less pronounced. After seven treatments, the excessive sweating disappeared entirely. Seven more treatments were administered to consolidate the effect. Altogether, twenty-one treatments were administered, including those before the change in prescription. The patient was followed up six months later and the symptoms had not recurred. □

Urinary Retention
(Benign Prostatic Hypertrophy)

Lóng Bì 癃闭

Zhang, male, 68 years old. Five years ago, the patient began experiencing increased frequency of urination, especially at night. There was no urgency or pain during urination, or hematuria. However, after urinating he had a feeling that some urine remained. Over time, increasing effort was needed to urinate, and the stream of urine became thin. Enuresis occurred at times. Three days ago, after becoming tired, he was unable to pass water, which resulted in marked distention of the lower abdomen and extreme discomfort. After consulting with western medical doctors, his condition was diagnosed as retention of urine due to benign prostatic hypertrophy. The abdominal distention was relieved by catheterization, and oral administration of both diethyl stilbestrol and traditional Chinese medicinal preparations were instituted simultaneously. Two days later, voluntary micturition was still impossible, and catheterization was repeated. Surgery was recommended, but the patient refused. He turned instead to acupuncture therapy.

The four examinations of Chinese medicine revealed that the patient was dejected and apathetic. His inability to urinate had caused marked distention of the lower abdomen. His ears were slightly dark and dull. He felt weak and was debilitated. His breathing was shallow, and he experienced an aversion to cold.

In addition to the history of enuresis, the patient stated that his lower back was weak, and was frequently sore. He also experienced tinnitus. His tongue was pale, and tooth-marked along the edges; the coating was white and slippery. The pulse was submerged and wiry, and both rear positions were thin and weak.

SYNDROME DIFFERENTIATION

The Bladder's functions of storing and releasing urine are facilitated by the Qi of the Kidney. In Chinese medicine, the Kidney is said to 'open' through the urethra and anus; urination and defecation are thus influenced by this Organ. Most abnormalities in passing water are therefore related to the Kidney and Bladder.

The patient was over 60 years old. By this age, the Kidney Qi has declined, and its vital functions have become deficient. Its control over the Bladder is thus diminished. This was manifested by an increase in the frequency of urination in the early stages. Progressive dysfunction of the Kidney and Bladder disturbed water circulation and distribution, and resulted in such symptoms as the feeling of incomplete urination, straining during urination, and reduced volume of urine. Overwork (the patient continued to engage in farm work) further weakened the Kidney Qi, leading to even greater dysfunction in water circulation, and ultimately to retention of urine. Other symptoms such as the tinnitus, aversion to cold, dejection, and soreness in the lower back were all manifestations of deficiency of Kidney Qi. The weakness and shallow breathing, and the pale, tooth-marked tongue are common symptoms of Qi deficiency. The submerged pulse indicated a condition of the interior. The wiry pulse, and the white, slippery tongue coating indicated stagnation of Fluids. The thin, weak rear pulses on both wrists (the Kidney position) reflected Kidney deficiency. In summary, the condition was one of deficiency of Kidney Qi.

TREATMENT

The principle of treatment was to strengthen the Kidney Qi in order to facilitate urination.

Points selected:
CV-4 *(guan yuan)*, B-23 *(shen shu)*, K-7 *(fu liu)*, Sp-6 *(san yin jiao)*

Tonification of all points was accomplished through raise-thrust and twirling manipulation of the needles, which were retained for 30 minutes during each session. Warm needle moxibustion was applied at CV-4 *(guan yuan)*.

Discussion of points:
CV-4 *(guan yuan)* has the action of tonifying source Qi and is an important point used for systemic invigoration. When combined with K-7 *(fu liu)* and B-23 *(shen shu)*, the as-

sociated point on the back for the Kidney, the Kidney Qi is tonified, and the source Qi is invigorated. K-7 *(fu liu)* was chosen in accordance with the 'mother-son', tonifying-draining method. The Kidney corresponds to water in the five phases system. Because the Kidney was deficient, the Kidney channel's 'mother' point, K-7 *(fu liu)*, was selected for tonification. Sp-6 *(san yin jiao)* is the point of intersection of the three Yin channels of the leg. This point regulates the Qi in these channels (all of which traverse the lower abdomen), thus facilitating urination.

RESULTS

Two hours after the first treatment, voluntary micturition occurred. The volume of urine was very small, however, and the patient had to make strenuous efforts to expel it. After 200ml of urine had been forced out, the patient was so tired that the process was stopped. Eight hours later, bladder distention became worse, and catheterization was again administered.

Although the underlying condition of the patient was deficiency of Kidney Qi, it was clear that tonification of Kidney Qi was of little value in this case. Upon review, it was determined that we had overlooked the principle in Chinese medicine of treating diseases by considering *both* the symptoms and the root cause.

Signs and symptoms are the outward manifestations, and the root cause is the essence of a disease. While it is true that Chinese medicine stresses that resolving the root cause of a disease should be the ultimate goal of therapy, under certain circumstances the symptoms can be so severe that they must be treated first. Otherwise, they may hinder treatment of the root cause, or even endanger the life of the patient. In such cases, it is only after the acute symptoms are alleviated that the physician deals with the root cause.

In *Simple Questions* (chapter 65), it is noted that in cases of constipation or retention of urine, treatment should be directed at these symptoms. Thus, although deficiency of Kidney Qi was the root of the disorder in this case, the retention of urine was so severe that it should have been given priority in treatment. Based upon this analysis, the point prescription was modified.

Points selected:

CV-3 *(zhong ji)*, B-28 *(pang guang shu)*, Sp-9 *(yin ling quan)*, Sp-6 *(san yin jiao)*

The points were drained using twirling manipulation. The needles were retained for one hour, during which time the needles were manipulated once.

Discussion of points:

CV-3 *(zhong ji)* is the alarm point of the Bladder, and B-28 *(pang guang shu)* is the associated point on the back for this Organ. The use of both points is an example of combining the alarm point with the associated point of the same Organ. This point combination was used here to help regulate the Qi of the Bladder, and thus facilitate urination.

Sp-9 *(yin ling quan)* promotes urination, the effect of which is enhanced when combined with Sp-6 *(san yin jiao)*, which regulates the Qi of the three Yin channels of the Leg.

One and one-half hours after the first treatment with the modified point prescription, micturition occurred. About 700ml of urine was expelled with less effort than before, and the distention was eased. However, the stream of urine was still thin, and the act of urinating somewhat strained. The next day, another treatment was administered with the same points. Following the second treatment, the patient could urinate more freely, and had no further retention of urine, or abdominal distention.

With the alleviation of symptoms, attention was again directed at the root cause of the disorder, deficient Kidney Qi. The use of the original set of points was resumed to strengthen the Kidney Qi. Tonifying manipulation was used by applying warm needle moxibustion at CV-4 *(guan yuan)*. After four daily treatments, the patient was in much better spirits, and could urinate without difficulty. Following one week's rest, he was reexamined and found to have no retention of urine. Urination remained effortless, although the stream was thin, and there was still a feeling of incomplete urination. Regrettably, the patient failed to return to the clinic for a follow-up. □

Wasting and Thirsting Syndrome
(Diabetes Mellitus)

Xiāo Kě 消渴

Zhang, male, 52 years old. During the past 3 years, the patient often felt hungry and thirsty. He experienced frequent urination and loss of weight. He reported that he had always enjoyed rich foods and alcohol. Laboratory tests found his fasting blood sugar to be 150mg%, and blood sugar 2 hours post-prandial to be 180mg%. Fasting urine sugar was (+), and 2 hours post-prandial was (+++). The diagnosis was diabetes mellitus, and he was started on tolbutamide. His symptoms improved with the drug, but recurred when use of the drug was suspended. The patient therefore decided to try acupuncture therapy.

The four examinations of Chinese medicine found a tired-looking patient with a dull complexion and a low, weak voice. He stated that he was always thirsty and drank several quarts of water every day. Urination was frequent, five to six times during the day, and two to three times at night. The tongue coating was thin, yellow and greasy, and his pulse was wiry and deficient. Laboratory tests conducted a few days prior to his visit revealed that blood sugar was 142mg%, and urine sugar (+).

SYNDROME DIFFERENTIATION

Wasting and thirsting syndrome is generally characterized by thirst, hunger, frequent urination, and wasting. These symptoms may also be accompanied by cloudy urine and sugar in the urine. The condition may be caused by three factors: improper diet, emotional disturbance, and a constitution that is Yin-deficient.

Improper diet refers to excessive intake of rich, fatty foods, as well as alcohol. This impairs the transportive and digestive functions of the Spleen and Stomach. The accumulated food thereupon transforms into Heat. Heat consumes the Fluids, thus bringing on wasting and thirsting.

Prolonged emotional disturbance may contribute to wasting and thirsting by hindering the flow of Qi. Stagnant Qi transforms into Fire, which then consumes the Yin of the Lung and Stomach.

When an individual is constitutionally Yin-deficient, factors such as overwork or excessive sexual activity can consume the

Essence. The result is deficient Yin and blazing Fire, which impairs the Lung and Stomach, thus giving rise to wasting and thirsting.

In this case, the patient was fond of rich foods and alcohol. The Heat generated in the Stomach and Intestines impaired the Kidney and Lung Yin. Long-term deficiency of Kidney Yin led to deficiency of Kidney Qi, which caused the Kidney to lose its ability to hold the urine; this resulted in frequent urination. The patient had been ill for over three years. His tired appearance, dull complexion, low, weak voice and frequent urination reflected deficiency of Kidney Yin and Kidney Qi. Thirst and hunger with excessive water and food intake, and the thin, yellow coating on the tongue indicated Heat in the Stomach, combined with deficiency of Lung Yin. The chief problems of this patient were therefore deficiency of Kidney Yin and Kidney Qi, combined with deficiency of Lung Yin, and Heat in the Stomach.

TREATMENT

Treatment was directed at tonifying the Yin of the Lung and Kidney, and at regulating the Spleen and Stomach.

Points selected:

B-23 *(shen shu)*, the 'pancreas points' *(yi dian)*, Sp-6 *(san yin jiao)*, L-10 *(yu ji)*

The points were needled once daily, and the needles retained for 30 minutes during each session. Balanced tonifying-draining manipulation was utilized.

Discussion of points:

B-23 *(shen shu)* was selected to tonify the Kidney Yin and Qi, and L-10 *(yu ji)* to clear the Heat from the Lung, and thereby replenish the Lung Yin. Sp-6 *(san yin jiao)* was chosen to regulate the functions of the Spleen and Stomach, and the 'pancreas points' to regulate the function of the pancreas. The 'pancreas points' are tender points located

about 0.5 unit on both sides of the spinous processes at the level of the sixth through eighth thoracic vertebrae.

B-23 *(shen shu)* was needled to a depth of 1.2 units. This produced a sensation of local soreness and distention that traveled up and down. The 'pancreas points' *(yi dian)* were needled at a slightly oblique angle in the direction of the spine, to a depth of about 1 unit. This produced a sensation of soreness and distention that was transmitted to the ribs. Sp-6 *(san yin jiao)* was needled to a depth of 0.8 unit, which produced a sensation of electric tingling that traveled up and down along the Spleen channel. L-10 *(yu ji)* was punctured to a depth of 0.8 unit. A sensation of distention reached the medial side of the thumb.

RESULTS

During the course of treatment, the patient was asked to suspend all hypoglycemic agents, and to abstain from rich foods and alcohol. After five treatments, the feeling of thirst abated, and water intake was reduced by one-half. The excessive hunger was also somewhat alleviated. Urination was reduced to three or four times during the day, and only once at night.

To further strengthen the tonification of the Lung and Kidney Yin, K-3 *(tai xi)* and B-13 *(fei shu)* were added to the prescription. These two points were tonified. After five more treatments with the modified prescription, the excessive hunger, thirst and urination continued to show improvement. The tongue coating became white and moist, and the pulse turned wiry and moderate, indicating restoration of the Kidney Yin and Qi.

Two more points were then added: CV-6 *(qi hai)* and S-36 *(zu san li)*. These points were needled with balanced tonifying-draining manipulation to clear Heat from the Stomach, and thus promote that Organ's digestive function. After needling, the plum-blossom needle was used to tap the M-BW-35 *(jia ji)* vertebral points from the eleventh thoracic to the fifth lumbar vertebrae. This was done to tonify the Kidney and Spleen, and to regulate the Qi of those Organs. After fifteen treatments with this second modified prescription, the patient was in better spirits, and the symptoms of thirst, hunger and frequent urination were completely relieved. Laboratory tests showed that fasting blood sugar was 130mg%, blood sugar two hours post-prandial was 170mg%, and urine sugar (−).

By this time, although the Yin and Yang of the Organs had gradually become balanced, the patient was still weak from the long illness and needed further strengthening for full restoration of health. Additional treatment was therefore directed at tonifying the Kidney to strengthen the body resistance, and at regulating the Spleen and Stomach. The points selected for consolida-tion were B-23 *(shen shu),* the 'pancreas points' *(yi dian),* B-20 *(pi shu),* CV-3 *(zhong ji),* S-36 *(zu san li),* Sp-6 *(san yin jiao)* and G-34 *(yang ling quan).*

Three to four points were used during each session, and tonifying manipulation was applied. Needling was administered every other day, and the needles were retained for thirty minutes. At the end of each session after the needles had been withdrawn, plum-blossom needling was applied at the M-BW-35 *(jia ji)* vertebral points.

After two more months of treatment (for a total of fifty-five sessions), the patient felt energetic and free of all symptoms associated with this disease. The fasting blood sugar was then 100mg%, and urine sugar (−). Acupuncture therapy was therefore terminated. The patient was advised to refrain from excessive intake of food and alcohol. During a follow-up period of six months, the symptoms did not recur. □

Wind Edema
(Acute Nephritis)

Fēng Shuǐ 风水

Chen, female, 34 years old. The patient began to suffer from general malaise with poor appetite 5 days prior to her first visit. She soon had chills, fever (39.5°C) and a headache. Acetaminophen was prescribed to reduce the fever. Two days later, she lost her appetite completely; any attempt at eating led to vomiting, and she could not even drink water. The vomit was sometimes bitter, and yellow-green in color. The left lumbar region was painful. Her stools were dry. Her urine was yellow, scanty, painful and frequent (about 20 times per day). She also sweated profusely.

Upon examination, the patient's body temperature was found to be 38⁰C. The white blood cell count was 19,600/mm³. Neutrophils were 88%, lymphocytes 9%, and monocytes 3%. Urine was yellowish and clear, reaction acidic, specific gravity 1.04, protein (+++), glucose (−), RBC 5-6/hpf, WBC 10-15/hpf, epithelial cells 10-20/hpf. The diagnosis was acute nephritis.

The tonsils were red and swollen. Her complexion was pale, and there was slight edema of the eyelids. The tongue was light red, with a thin, yellow coating. The pulse was rapid and slippery.

SYNDROME DIFFERENTIATION

This patient was affected by external Wind-Heat, which was manifested in the symptoms of chills, fever, headache, general malaise and sore throat. When the Wind-Heat reached the middle Burner, the functions of the Spleen and Stomach were disturbed. This led to impaired appetite and vomiting after eating. In the control cycle of the five phases, wood controls earth. Deficiency of the Spleen and Stomach (earth) led to hyperfunction of the Liver (wood) by 'inviting' overcontrol. This in turn led to adverse or rebellious flow of the Liver Qi, manifested in the vomiting of bitter, yellow-green fluid. Because it was unchecked in the middle Burner, the Heat proceeded to the lower Burner, where it affected the functions of the Kidney and Bladder. The Kidney is in charge of water, and is the Yin Organ that is paired with the Yang Bladder. Consequently, symptoms such as edema of the eyelids, urgent and frequent urination, and pain in the lumbar region appeared. The thin, yellow tongue coating, and the rapid, slippery pulse reflected the presence of Heat.

TREATMENT

Although the middle and lower Burners were simultaneously affected, the symptoms of the middle Burner were more acute. In such cases, the acute symptoms should be treated first. This patient was therefore treated first by clearing the Heat from the middle Burner to regulate the Spleen and Stomach, and then by resolving the Heat in the lower Burner.

Points selected:

GV-14 *(da zhui)*, CV-12 *(zhong wan)*, CV-4 *(guan yuan)*, P-6 *(nei guan)*, Sp-4 *(gong sun)*

Needling was administered once daily. Draining manipulation was applied through raise-thrust and twirling techniques, and the needles were retained for 30 minutes.

Discussion of points:

GV-14 *(da zhui)* is the point at which the six Yang channels of the arm and leg intersect. Its use has a fever-reducing effect. CV-12 *(zhong wan)* is the alarm point of the Stomach. Draining this point clears Heat from the Stomach, and thus arrests vomiting. P-6 *(nei guan)* and Sp-4 *(gong sun)* are two of the confluent points of the eight miscellaneous channels. Needling these points regulates the ascending and descending functions of the Spleen and Stomach, facilitates the flow of Qi, and arrests vomiting. CV-4 *(guan yuan)* is the alarm point of the Small Intestine. Draining this point clears Heat from the lower Burner, and promotes diuresis.

GV-14 *(da zhui)* was needled to a depth of 1.2 units in a slightly upward direction. The sensation was one of soreness and distention that traveled up and down the Governing vessel. CV-12 *(zhong wan)* was needled perpendicularly to a depth of 1.2 units. The sen-

sation was one of distention in the vicinity of the point. CV-4 *(guan yuan)* was needled perpendicularly to a depth of 1.3 units. The sensation was one of sore numbness that radiated to the genitals. P-6 *(nei guan)* was needled to a depth of 0.8 unit. The sensation of soreness and distention was transmitted to the middle finger, and to the middle of the forearm. Sp-4 *(gong sun)* was needled to a depth of 0.8 unit. This produced a sensation of soreness and distention that reached the medial side of the big toe.

RESULTS

After one treatment, the vomiting was arrested, and the body temperature dropped to 37°C. With improvement in the symptoms of the middle Burner, treatment was then directed to the lower Burner. Since the patient presented with signs of deficiency after coping with the disease for one week, and going without food for three days, the clearing of the Heat was accompanied by strengthening the patient's constitution. A modified prescription was formulated for this purpose.

Points selected:

CV-12 *(zhong wan)*, CV-4 *(guan yuan)*, S-36 *(zu san li)*, K-7 *(fu liu)*

The points were needled once daily, and the needles retained for 30 minutes.

Discussion of points:

Tonifying manipulation was applied at S-36 *(zu san li)* to replenish the Qi, invigorate the Stomach, and strengthen the constitution. Draining manipulation was applied at the other three points. K-7 *(fu liu)* was needled perpendicularly to a depth of 0.5 unit, which produced a sensation of soreness and numbness that radiated to the middle of the sole. This point was chosen in order to clear Heat and promote diuresis, thus reducing the edema.

The four points in the modified prescription were needled for eight days. The patient's temperature remained normal during this time. By the eighth treatment, edema of the eyelids, frequent urination, urinary pain and left lumbar pain were completely alleviated. Laboratory tests showed the following: WBC 9800/mm^3, neutrophils 58%, lymphocytes 37%, monocytes 3%; the urine was clear and slightly yellow, specific gravity 1.0, protein (−), glucose (−), epithelial cells 2-4/hpf, WBC 3-5/hpf. The patient was discharged, and there was no recurrence of symptoms on follow-up one month later. □

CHAPTER TWO
Neurological Disorders

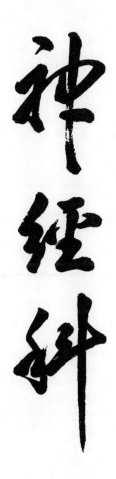

Aphasia

Shī Yǔ 失语

Chi, male, 23 years old. Two months ago, while working in a coal mine, the patient suffered a blow to his head and became unconscious. He regained consciousness at a hospital about 1 hour later, but was unable to speak. He was diagnosed as having contusions of the brain and neck, fracture of the 2nd and 3rd left ribs, compressed fracture of the 12th thoracic and 1st lumbar vertebrae, and motor aphasia. He remained hospitalized for about 1 month. On discharge, the contusions and fractures were resolved, but the aphasia remained.

The four examinations of Chinese medicine revealed that the patient was unable to speak, but could understand others. He had impaired hearing of the left ear. His complexion was lackluster. His appetite and bowel movements were normal. The tongue was dull red, and the pulse was choppy.

SYNDROME DIFFERENTIATION

Aphasia is a frequent sequela of Wind-stroke, however in this case it resulted from trauma. The brain is the center for mental activities. When the head suffers external trauma, the Blood and Qi in the head are disturbed. This may cause stagnation of Qi and stasis of Blood, with subsequent obstruction of the orifice of speech, or aphasia.

The dull, red tongue, and the choppy pulse

were further evidence of Blood stasis.

TREATMENT

Treatment was directed at clearing the channels by invigorating the Blood and moving the Qi.

Points selected:
GV-20 *(bai hui)*, CV-23 *(lian quan)*, L-7 *(lie que)* and K-6 *(zhao hai)* bilaterally; G-20 *(feng chi)* and SI-19 *(ting gong)* on the left side only

The points were needled once daily with balanced tonifying-draining manipulation, and the needles were retained for 30 minutes during each session.

Discussion of points:
GV-20 *(bai hui)* regulates the Blood and Qi in the head. In the *Great Compendium of*

Acupuncture and Moxibustion, Yang Jizhou noted that this point can be used in treating speech disorders. CV-23 *(lian quan)* is an important point in treating aphasia because it facilitates the movement of the tongue.

L-7 *(lie que)* and K-6 *(zhao hai)* are two of the confluent points of the eight miscellaneous channels. L-7 *(lie que)* on the Lung channel is linked with the Conception vessel, both of which traverse the throat region. K-6 *(zhao hai)* on the Kidney channel is linked with the Yin Heel channel. The Kidney channel has a branch that enters the root of the tongue, while the Yin Heel channel passes through the throat before emerging in front of S-9 *(ren ying)*. L-7 *(lie que)* and K-6 *(zhao hai)* are thus effective in treating aphasia.

G-20 *(feng chi)* and SI-19 *(ting gong)* were needled only on the left side in order to regulate the Blood and Qi in the left ear, where the hearing was impaired.

GV-20 *(bai hui)* was punctured by transverse insertion toward the front for about 1.2 units. Twirling manipulation was applied, which produced a feeling of local distention. CV-23 *(lian quan)* was punctured by a slanted insertion toward the base of tongue to a depth of 1.3 units. The sensation produced was one of itching and distention in the throat. L-7 *(lie que)* was needled by oblique insertion upward to a depth of 0.5 unit, producing local soreness and distention which extended toward the elbow. K-6 *(zhao hai)* was needled perpendicularly to a depth of 0.5 unit. This produced an electric shock-like sensation which extended toward the sole of the foot. G-20 *(feng chi)* was needled obliquely to a depth of 1.3 units in the direction of the opposite orbit. Soreness and distention extended to the temple and eye region of the same side. SI-19 *(ting gong)* was needled, with the mouth open, to a depth of 1.2 units. Soreness and distention was felt in the ear.

RESULTS

After ten treatments, the patient was able to recite numbers, but his voice was so low that it was inaudible beyond a foot or so. After an additional eight treatments, his voice was much louder, and he was able to clearly enunciate short and simple sentences. Treatment was continued with the same points for another ten sessions. After a total of twenty-eight treatments, examination by a neurologist verified complete restoration of speech, normal cognitive and motor functions, and normal hearing in the left ear. □

Atrophy Syndrome
(Guillain-Barré Syndrome)

Wěi Zhèng 痿症

Yi, female, 21 years old. The patient complained of pain and weakness in the limbs of over 1 week's duration. Two weeks ago, sudden onset of high fever, chills and general discomfort marked the beginning of the disorder. Her temperature rose to 39.2°C, and she began to cough and had a sore throat. She took aspirin and erythromycin, and the symptoms subsided after 3 days. However, muscle pain developed, which interfered with walking. Shortly thereafter, she found herself too weak to stand, walk or raise her arms. Her hands became clumsy, and could not bear any weight.

Upon admission to the hospital, examination revealed an alert person with normal temperature, a supple neck, pupils of equal size and normal light reflexes. No abnormality of the heart or lungs was found. The abdomen was soft, and the liver and spleen were not palpable. Muscular strength in the limbs was diminished, and the extremities were cold to the touch. Tendon reflexes were markedly depressed, but no pathological reflexes were elicited. A red tongue, and a thin, weak and rapid pulse were noted. The cerebrospinal fluid was clear and colorless, with normal pressure. The Queckenstedt test showed no sign of blockage. The protein content was 50mg/100ml, but no coagulate formed on standing. Cerebrospinal fluid glucose and chlorides were within normal range. She was diagnosed as having acute polyneuropathy (Guillain-Barré syndrome).

Treatment with neostigmine, vitamin B_1 and physical therapy stabilized the condition. The weakness and pain of the limbs did not improve, nor did the difficulty in movement. The acupuncture department was thereupon consulted for help.

SYNDROME DIFFERENTIATION

This case was characterized by weakness of the muscles of the limbs such that movement was impaired. The condition resembles atrophy syndrome in Chinese medicine, which is marked by weakness of the limbs and difficulty in voluntary movement. Weakness confined to the lower limbs is more common, although involvement of all four limbs is not rare.

Since this case presented with high fever, chills, cough and sore throat caused by an external pathogenic influence (Heat), the Lung was regarded as the primary focus. Despite the subsidence of fever, the external Heat persisted and consumed the Fluids, leading to malnutrition of the muscles and tendons. This resulted in weakness of the muscles of the limbs, and difficulty in body movement. In addition, the persistence of the external pathogenic influence blocked the circulation of Qi and Blood in the muscles of the limbs, giving rise to pain. Because the Fluids correspond to Yin, deficiency of Fluids is a form of Yin deficiency. Internal Heat arises as a result of Yin deficiency, hence the red tongue, and the thin, weak and rapid pulse.

TREATMENT

The principles of treatment were to clear the Heat, nourish the Yin, promote the generation of Fluids, and invigorate circulation in the channels of the limbs.

Points selected:

Principal points: L-7 *(lie que)*, L-5 *(chi ze)*, LI-4 *(he gu)*, LI-11 *(qu chi)*, S-36 *(zu san li)*, Sp-6 *(san yin jiao)*, Sp-10 *(xue hai)*, K-7 *(fu liu)*, K-3 *(tai xi)*, Liv-3 *(tai chong)*, Liv-5 *(li gou)*

Supplemental points: LI-15 *(jian yu)*, G-30 *(huan tiao)*, B-54 *(zhi bian)*, G-34 *(yang ling quan)*, M-LE-8 *(ba feng)*, M-UE-22 *(ba xie)*

Treatment was administered once daily, and the needles were retained for 30 minutes. Seven sessions comprised 1 course of therapy, with 3 days' rest between courses.

Discussion of points:

Among the principal points, L-7 *(lie que)*, L-5 *(chi ze)*, LI-4 *(he gu)*, LI-11 *(qu chi)* and Liv-5 *(li gou)* were chosen to clear the Heat. K-7 *(fu liu)*, K-3 *(tai xi)*, S-36 *(zu san li)* and S-6 *(san yin jiao)* were used to nourish the Yin, and to promote the generation of Fluids.

Liv-3 *(tai chong)* and Sp-10 *(xue hai)* were needled to regulate the Qi and Blood. The supplemental points were chosen to enhance the effects of the principal points in invigorating the circulation of Qi and Blood in the channels of the limbs.

During each treatment, four or five principal points, and three or four supplemental points were used. Points on the upper limbs were combined with those on the lower. In this case, it should be noted that the principal points were intended to deal with the root cause of the condition, and the supplemental points to relieve the manifestations or symptoms.

At the principal points, the needles were inserted perpendicularly to a depth of 1-1.5 units, except at L-7 *(lie que)*, where the needle was inserted obliquely to a depth of 0.5-1.0 unit. Balanced tonifying-draining manipulation was applied to induce a mild needle sensation.

The supplemental points were needled in the following manner. At LI-15 *(jian yu)* the arm was raised by a nurse, and the needle was directed toward H-1 *(ji quan)* at the center of the armpit to a depth of 2-3 units. This induced an intense sensation which radiated to the forearm. At G-30 *(huan tiao)* and B-54 *(zhi bian)* the needles were inserted perpendicularly to a depth of 3 units, with the needle sensation radiating through the lower limbs. At G-34 *(yang ling quan)* the needle was inserted perpendicularly to a depth of 1.5 units.

The M-UE-22 *(ba xie)* points were punctured perpendicularly, with the needles oriented toward the metacarpal bones, to a depth of about 1 unit. At the M-LE-8 *(ba feng)* points the needles were inserted perpendicularly to a depth of 1 unit. The needle sensation radiated to the tips of the fingers and toes respectively.

Draining manipulation was applied at all supplemental points in order to enhance the effect of the principal points in invigorating the circulation of Qi and Blood.

RESULTS

After 14 treatments, the patient was able to extend and flex her elbows and knees. She could raise her arms, and could also elevate her legs 3 inches above the ground. The muscle pain had disappeared. After another 7 treatments, she was able to stand and walk with the aid of a cane, and could grasp objects.

After a total of 30 treatments, the symptoms disappeared completely, and normal muscle function was restored. She could walk without assistance for 5-10 minutes; she could also move her arms freely, and carry objects weighing 3-5kg. Treatment was then terminated. The patient was discharged from the hospital and advised to continue with strengthening exercises at home. Follow-up 6 months later found that she could run and jump, and could walk as far as 5km. □

Atrophy Syndrome
(Median Nerve Palsy)

Wěi Zhèng 痿症

Guang, male, 30 years old. Forty days ago, the patient's left hand was caught in a machine at work. The hand was crushed, with a bleeding wound 1cm in length on the dorsum of the hand over the 2nd metacarpal bone. Because of the heavy bleeding, tourniquets were applied at two points: the left wrist and the upper part of the left arm. The tourniquets were left in place, without any attempt to loosen them, for over 2 hours. The day after the tourniquets were removed, the left arm could be raised, but wrist-drop had set in. The diagnosis was injury of the left brachial plexus and traumatic median nerve palsy. The patient was referred for acupuncture therapy.

Examination showed muscular atrophy of the forearm, and of the thenar and hypothenar regions. The skin of the left hand was bluish. The left elbow could be extended, but flexion was impossible. The wrist was movable, but the hand was unable to grasp. Biceps reflex and Hoffmann reflex were absent. Subjective numbness and weakness were felt in the left hand. The tongue was lusterless, with red spots. The pulse was deep and thin.

SYNDROME DIFFERENTIATION

The muscular atrophy, disability in flexion, and wrist-drop are all characteristic of atrophy syndrome. This syndrome can be sub-divided into flesh, sinew, vascular, skin and bone types. Here the presence of muscular atrophy, and the absence of flexion, made this case a combination of flesh and sinew atrophy. The cause was evidently the loss of blood, and the subsequent overuse of tourniquets. This resulted in insufficiency of Qi and Blood, and interfered with their movement in the channels, thereby depriving the flesh and sinews of necessary nutrients.

TREATMENT

Since the condition resulted from interference with the flow of Qi and Blood to the flesh and sinews, treatment was aimed at warming the channels to promote the flow of Qi and Blood.

Points selected:

Points on the three Yang channels of the arm were selected: SI-10 *(nao shu)*, SI-3 *(hou xi)*, LI-11 *(qu chi)*, TB-13 *(nao hui)*, TB-12 *(xiao luo)* and TB-5 *(wai guan)*. These points were supplemented by B-11 *(da zhu)*.

Treatment was administered once daily for two weeks, and then once every three or four days for six weeks.

Discussion of points:

SI-10 *(nao shu)* is traditionally used for treating weakness of the arm. SI-3 *(hou xi)* is one of the points of confluence of the eight miscellaneous channels and communicates with the Governing vessel, which controls all of the Yang channels. LI-11 *(qu chi)* is a point on the Yang Brightness (Large Intestine) channel of the arm, a channel rich in both Qi and Blood. TB-13 *(nao hui)* and TB-12 *(xiao luo)* are used to promote the flow of Qi and Blood in the channels to relieve pain in the arm and numbness of the hand. TB-5 *(wai guan)*, another of the points of confluence of the eight miscellaneous channels, which communicates with the Yang Linking channel, is traditionally used to promote circulation of stagnant Qi in the channels. B-11 *(da zhu)* is a point of intersection of the Bladder and Small Intestine channels. Its use promotes movement of Qi and Blood in the channels, and strengthens the sinews.

The sequence of needling in a case such as this is rather important. Needling should begin with B-11 *(da zhu)*, followed in order by SI-10 *(nao shu)*, TB-13 *(nao hui)*, TB-12 *(xiao luo)*, LI-11 *(qu chi)*, TB-5 *(wai guan)* and SI-3 *(hou xi)*. In other words, the order of insertion is one-by-one from proximal to distal, so that the needle sensation may propagate sequentially from one locus to the next.

To obtain maximum effect, the 'burning the mountain' technique was used, which induces a warm sensation. The technique is performed in the following manner. The needle is inserted during exhalation to a depth one-third the distance between the surface of the skin and the site of the acupuncture point. The 'flying' method is then applied, either three or nine times, to hasten the arrival of Qi. If Qi arrives quickly, 'fly' the needle three times; if slowly, 'fly' it nine times. The needle is then advanced to two-thirds depth, and finally to the point itself. At each of the latter depths, the needle is 'flown' again. After the induction of Qi at each depth, the needle is thrust forcefully and raised gently three times within a range of 0.1 unit to elicit a warm sensation.

When the warmth is perceived by the patient, the needle may be 'pushed' to help spread the warm sensation. 'Pushing' involves a very slight twirling of the needle in a forward direction until resistance is felt. The needle is then 'pushed' against the resistance to maintain its tautness, but without actually moving the needle. If warmth is not felt, the needle is withdrawn to the first depth, and the procedure is repeated. 'Flying' and 'pushing' induce the propagation and prolongation of the warm sensation. At the completion of the procedure, the needle is withdrawn during inhalation, and the opening is quickly pressed to prevent the release of Qi.

Supplementary moxibustion with a moxa stick was administered for 15-20 minutes after needling at LI-11 *(qu chi)*, TB-5 *(wai guan)* and SI-3 *(hou xi)*, as these were points selected specifically to aid wrist and finger movement.

RESULTS

After two months of treatment, the range of motion of the left shoulder, elbow, wrist and fingers was normal. However, active movement of the wrist and finger joints was still awkward. Palmar flexion of all fingers was possible. Muscular strength and tone were weak when compared to the right arm. The circumference of the arm and forearm was about 1cm smaller than that of the unaffected side. Thenar, hypothenar and interosseous muscular atrophy was still evident. Tremor was not detected. There was slight sensitivity to pain in the upper arm and forearm to a distance 2cm proximal to the wrist. But from this point down to the fingertips, the sense of pain, touch and temperature were all diminished. Proprioceptive sense was intact. All reflexes—biceps, radial and ulnar—were absent on the left side; the triceps was occasionally positive. Hoffmann reflex was negative on both sides.

Because the condition had improved, the point prescription was modified by eliminating some of the back and shoulder points. The modified prescription included LI-15 *(jian yu)*, TB-12 *(xiao luo)*, LI-11 *(qu chi)*, TB-5 *(wai guan)* and TB-3 *(zhong zhu)*. The method of manipulation and the sequence of needling were unchanged. This small variation in the point prescription gave the patient a psychological boost. He realized that the acupuncturists were doing their best to help him.

After another month of treatment, most of the symptoms were alleviated. Normal color tone of the hand returned, and movement of all joints was normal. The senses of touch, pain and temperature were restored. The strength in the left arm returned and the patient was able to carry a load of 15kg. However, muscle atrophy showed no significant improvement.

With the course of treatment completed, the patient was told to return to his job as a manual laborer after another month of rest. He was also encouraged to exercise his left arm. Follow-up two months later found the patient to be well, with no evidence of muscular atrophy or any other disability. □

Atrophy Syndrome
(Multiple Sclerosis)

Wěi Zhèng 痿症

Li, female, 46 years old. The patient complained of failing vision, together with numbness and weakness of the lower limbs. About 10 months ago, she began to experience rapidly failing vision of both eyes, which dropped from 20/20 to 20/200 in the left eye, and from 20/16 to 20/25 in the right eye, in just a few days. Eight months ago, she noted numbness in the left toes and marked pain over the back which prevented her from sleeping for 3 days. A few days later, she felt numbness below the 5th thoracic vertebra on the back, and below the xiphoid process on the front, and was unable to urinate and defecate. She was taken to a hospital and diagnosed as having multiple sclerosis. Supportive measures were given, including enema and catheterization. When she was discharged 40 days later, she could urinate and defecate by herself, but experienced weakness during voiding. The numbness remained unchanged. She received acupuncture and massage therapy for 3 months at another hospital, but with only slight improvement.

Upon examination at this clinic, the patient's symptoms included numbness extending from the level of the 5th thoracic vertebra down to the hips on the back, and from the xiphoid process down to the pubic symphysis on the front; numbness of both legs, which was more pronounced on the right; weakness of the right leg, which was most noticeable when walking; fullness in the abdomen; bowel movements every three days, and frequent urination, both of which actions were weak. The patient was corpulent. Her tongue was pale with a greasy, white coating, and her pulse was slippery and rapid.

SYNDROME DIFFERENTIATION

This condition was caused by Damp-Heat, which affected the Governing vessel and disrupted the circulation of Qi. The Governing vessel controls the Yang of the entire body. Since the Yang Organs are connected by the Yang channels, all of which converge at the Governing vessel, dysfunction of the Governing vessel is characterized by impairment of the functions of the Yang Organs. In this case, disturbance of the Large Intestine led to difficulty in defecation, dysfunction of the Bladder to difficulty in urination, and disturbance of the digestive system as a whole led to abdominal distention. In addition, because the Yang and Yin channels are interconnected by the sequential circulation of Qi through the primary and connecting channels, the impaired circulation of Qi gave rise to numbness of the abdomen and back, and weakness of the lower limbs. With impaired circulation, moreover, the diminished supply of Qi and Blood resulted in atrophy of the muscles. The abdominal distention, the greasy, white tongue coating, and the slippery, rapid pulse were all manifestations of Damp-Heat.

TREATMENT

Points were chosen primarily from the Governing and Conception vessels, and from the Bladder, Spleen and Stomach channels. Draining manipulation was utilized to dispel the Damp-Heat, and to invigorate the circulation of Qi and Blood in the channels.

Treatment was administered once daily, and the needles were retained for 20 minutes during each session. Ten treatments comprised a course of therapy, with 3 days' rest between courses.

Points selected:

One of the following groups of points was used each day in rotation:

Group 1: GV-11 *(shen dao)*, GV-9 *(ling tai)*, M-BW-35 *(jia ji)* from the 5th to the 7th thoracic vertebrae, B-23 *(shen shu)*, B-25 *(da chang shu)*, G-30 *(huan tiao)*, B-40 *(wei zhong)*, B-57 *(cheng shan)*

Group 2: CV-12 *(zhong wan)*, S-21 *(liang men)*, S-25 *(tian shu)*, CV-6 *(qi hai)*, CV-3 *(zhong ji)*, S-36 *(zu san li)*, Sp-9 *(ying ling quan)*, Sp-6 *(san yin jiao)*, M-LE-8 *(ba feng)*

Discussion of points:

In the first group of points, GV-11 *(shen*

dao), GV-10 *(ling tai)* and M-BW-35 *(jia ji)* were chosen as local points in the vicinity of the numbness on the back. They function to invigorate the circulation of Qi and Blood. As the associated point on the back for the Kidney, B-23 *(shen shu)* was selected to normalize urination and bowel function; the Kidney controls these two functions. B-25 *(da chang shu)*, the associated point on the back for the Large Intestine, was also selected to regulate the bowels. G-30 *(huan tiao)*, B-40 *(wei zhong)* and B-57 *(cheng shan)* were chosen to regulate the flow of Qi in the channels in order to alleviate the numbness and weakness of the lower limbs.

Among the points listed in the second group, CV-12 *(zhong wan)* and S-25 *(tian shu)* are the alarm points of the Stomach and the Large Intestine respectively, and CV-6 *(qi hai)* is the point at which the circulating Qi converges. The combined use of CV-12 *(zhong wan)*, S-21 *(liang men)*, S-25 *(tian shu)* and CV-6 *(qi hai)* was aimed at normalizing the flow of Qi in the digestive system to resolve the fullness and numbness in the abdomen. As the alarm point of the Bladder, CV-3 *(zhong ji)* was selected to facilitate urination. Sp-9 *(yin ling quan)* and Sp-6 *(san yin jiao)* were needled to dispel Damp-Heat, and S-36 *(zu san li)* to relieve abdominal distention. These three points were also used to alleviate numbness and weakness of the lower limbs by regulating the flow of Qi.

In the first group, all of the points are located on the back of the body, and were needled with the patient lying prone. In the second group, all of the points are on the front of the body, and were needled with the patient lying supine. The functions of the various points in both groups are similar. Since both the front and back of the body were affected, these particular groups of points were selected both for the sake of convenience (to avoid the necessity of needling both sides of the body during a single treatment), as well as to enhance the therapeutic effect.

RESULTS

After ten treatments, the upper boundary of the numbness on the front moved downward from the level of the xiphoid process to the level of CV-12 *(zhong wan)*. The numbness in the back and lower limbs was significantly reduced in intensity, abdominal distention was diminished, bowel movement occurred daily and with more force, and urination became less frequent and with more force. After another twenty treatments, the upper boundary of numbness on the front moved further downward to the level of the umbilicus, the abdominal distention disappeared, bowel movement and urination returned to normal, sensation in the lower limbs recovered, and locomotion was much improved.

After more than four months' treatment, most of the symptoms were alleviated, except for slight numbness in the umbilical region, back, and the lateral aspect of the right leg. No improvement, however, was noted in the muscular atrophy of the right leg. Vision in the left eye improved to 20/25, and in the right eye to 20/16. During the next six months, treatment was continued once or twice a month to consolidate the effect. Follow-up during this time found that the atrophy of the right leg was slightly improved, and that there was no recurrence of the other symptoms. □

Deaf-Mutism
(Sequelae of Drug Ototoxicity)

Lóng Yǎ 聋哑

Sun, male, 10 years old. The patient began to pronounce syllables at 1 year of age, and simple words at 2. At 3, the child suffered pneumonia with fever and convulsions, which was treated successfully with penicillin and streptomycin injections. Afterward, however, the child no longer responded to voices or other sounds, and was also less inclined to speak. At 4 years of age, the child was diagnosed as being completely deaf due to streptomycin ototoxicity. He was prescribed vitamin B_{12} and traditional Chinese herbs for 6 months, but without apparent effect. His parents were advised that the case was hopeless. The child was then brought to the acupuncturist as a last resort.

Upon examination, the child was found to be totally deaf and unable to speak. He was otherwise healthy, with a good appetite, and showed no signs of mental retardation. His tongue was light red with a thin, white coating, and the pulse was slightly wiry.

SYNDROME DIFFERENTIATION

The deaf-mutism in this case occurred after a high fever and injections of streptomycin. The child was completely normal in other respects. According to Chinese medicine, high fever and convulsions are signs of invasion by external Heat, which can travel upward to attack the channels of the ears. Deaf-mutism results from diminished circulation of Qi in the region of the ears. Streptomycin is known to be toxic to the auditory nerve. In this case, therefore, it was the ototoxicity of this drug that attacked the channels of the ears (which were vulnerable due to the invasion of external Heat) and caused dimished circulation of Qi in the ear region.

The principal channels in the region of the ear are those of the arm Lesser Yang (Triple Burner), which passes behind and then enters the ears, and the leg Lesser Yang (Gall Bladder), which travels from the sides of the head to the back of the ears where it enters. The deafness thus arose from diminished circulation of Qi in the Lesser Yang channels; the mutism resulted from the deafness.

The Kidney is usually involved in diseases of the ears because the Kidney 'opens' through the ears. However, in this case, the child had no underlying disorder of the Kidney.

TREATMENT

The principle of treatment was to promote the circulation of Qi in the ear region.

Points selected:

G-20 *(feng chi)*, SI-19 *(ting gong)*, G-2 *(ting hui)*, TB-5 *(wai guan)*, G-41 *(zu lin qi)*, Sp-6 *(san yin jiao)*, Liv-3 *(tai chong)*

Treatment was administered once daily, and the needles were retained for 15-20 minutes during each session. Six sessions comprised a course of therapy, with 3 days' rest between courses.

Discussion of points:

G-20 *(feng chi)* and G-2 *(ting hui)* belong to the Gall Bladder channel, and SI-19 *(ting gong)* to the Small Intestine channel; both channels enter the ears. These three proximal points were used to promote local circulation of Qi. TB-5 *(wai guan)* belongs to the Triple Burner channel, and G-41 *(zu lin qi)* to the Gall Bladder channel. These two distal points were chosen to promote circulation of Qi in the Lesser Yang channels.

Liv-3 *(tai chong)* belongs to the Liver channel. Although this point is generally used to spread Liver Qi, because the Liver and Gall Bladder channels are interior-exteriorly related, needling Liv-3 *(tai chong)* also promotes the flow of Gall Bladder Qi. Similarly, Sp-6 *(san yin jiao)* is the point of intersection of the three leg Yin channels; by regulating the Liver channel, this point promotes the circulation of Qi in the Gall Bladder channel as well. The combination of these two points thus regulates Liver Qi so that it rises to support and promote the circulation of Gall Bladder Qi in the ear region.

Balanced tonifying-draining needle manipulation was used at all points because no definite signs of excess or deficiency were apparent.

RESULTS

After two courses of treatment, the child began to respond to the honking of cars. After the fourth course, he could hear his parents' voices. By the end of the fifth course (still with the same set of points), the child began to utter syllables, indicating that he could speak. CV-23 *(lian quan)* was then added, since this point stimulates the root of the tongue and aids speech. Two additional courses of treatment were administered with this modified prescription. The patient was then discharged and the parents were advised to give their child language training. Follow-up six months later found the child's hearing to be stable, and his speech intelligible.

Note: Deaf-mutism from drug ototoxicity is not uncommon in China. As with any condition, the earlier it is treated, the better the outcome. Before treatment begins, patients and their families are told that they must be persistent, since quite often it is a long process. As soon as hearing is restored, language training should begin. □

Depression

Yù Zhèng 郁症

Wang, female, 28 years old. Ten day ago, the patient had a quarrel after which she was unable to calm down. That evening she experienced fullness in the chest, felt sick, and vomited. She went immediately to an emergency clinic. Examination showed her blood pressure and cardiac rhythm to be normal; the laboratory findings were also within normal limits. She was admitted for overnight observation. After taking valium and vitamin B complex, the patient slept peacefully. The next morning she still experienced fullness in the chest, and complained of dull pain in the ribs. The nausea and vomiting became worse; she threw up immediately after eating, drinking or taking medicine. Fluid was given by intravenous drip. The condition, however, did not improve, and the patient was transferred to the acupuncture department.

The four examinations of Chinese medicine revealed that the patient was slightly pale, with a pained and gloomy expression. She had vomited clear fluid, and there was no desire for food or drink. Bowel movement and urination were essentially normal. The tongue was pink with a white coating, and the pulse was wiry. Blood pressure was 130/80mm Hg. Neurological examination showed no abnormalities, and the patient had no prior history of significant psychopathology.

SYNDROME DIFFERENTIATION

This condition appeared as a result of pent-up anger. When anger and other strong emotions affect the Liver, its function of spreading and regulating Qi is disturbed, and stagnation of Liver Qi results. Since the Liver channel traverses the costal region and chest, stagnation of Qi in the Liver channel here caused the fullness in the chest and pain in the ribs.

Stagnant Liver Qi can also affect the Stomach and Spleen. Stomach Qi normally flows downward, but when its function is disturbed, vomiting occurs, as it did in this case. The Spleen controls the transportation of water and nutrients. Here this action was lost, hence the lack of desire for food and drink.

Because the disorder was of recent occurrence, and was primarily due to stagnation of Qi, the tongue was normal. The wiry pulse was associated with the Liver trouble and severe pain.

TREATMENT

Treatment was aimed at regulating the flow of Liver Qi, and suppressing the rebellious flow of Stomach Qi.

Points selected:

GV-20 *(bai hui)*, S-36 *(zu san li)*, Liv-3 *(tai chong)*

GV-20 *(bai hui)* and Liv-3 *(tai chong)* were drained, and balanced tonifying-draining manipulation was applied at S-36 *(zu san li)*. Treatment was administered once daily, and the needles were retained for 30 minutes during each session. Each of the needles was manipulated once while in place.

Discussion of points:

GV-20 *(bai hui)* is located at the vertex and meets the Liver channel. Needling this point has the effect of calming the Liver. Liv-3 *(tai chong)* is the source and transporting point of the Liver channel. Its use promotes the flow of Liver Qi, and in this case is an example of using a point on the lower part of the body to treat a disorder affecting the upper part of the body. S-36 *(zu san li)* is the lower uniting point of the Stomach channel. Needling this point regulates the functions of the Spleen and Stomach, and was chosen here to arrest the vomiting.

RESULTS

After two treatments, there was no improvement. This was attributed to an inadequate number of points in the prescription. P-6 *(nei guan)* and Sp-6 *(san yin jiao)* were

therefore added. P-6 *(nei guan)* is the point of confluence of the Yin Linking channel, one of the eight miscellaneous channels. It is commonly used for disorders of the chest, Heart and Stomach. When used in combination with S-36 (zu san li), the function of the Stomach is regulated such that the proper downward flow of its Qi is restored. P-6 *(nei guan)* is thus often used in the treatment of vomiting. Sp-6 *(san yin jiao)* is the point at which the three Yin channels of the leg intersect, and is therefore used for regulating the Qi of the Liver, Spleen and Kidney. In this case it was used in combination with Liv-3 *(tai chong)* to strengthen the action of regulating Liver Qi.

After the first treatment with the modified point prescription, the nausea and vomiting were resolved. The patient could eat, and the fullness in the chest and pain in the costal regions were substantially alleviated. All of the symptoms of stagnant Liver Qi were now subdued, and the patient complained only of lack of strength.

Since she had been unable to eat or drink for over three days, causing insufficiency of Qi and Blood of the Spleen and Stomach, the emphasis then shifted to invigorating the Spleen and replenishing Qi. Only GV-20 *(bai hui)*, S-36 *(zu san li)* and Liv-3 *(tai chong)* were used for this purpose. The first two points were tonified, and balanced tonifying-draining manipulation was applied at the latter point. After one more treatment, the patient did not return to the clinic. A follow-up two weeks later found that she had recovered completely and had returned to work.

Note: In China this type of condition is rather common in rural areas, where it is considered to be an isolated occurrence, and not a precursor of a chronic psychiatric disorder. □

Depression

Yù Zhèng 郁症

Lu, male, 48 years old. Two years ago, the patient fell from a bicycle and suffered a Colles' fracture of his right arm. The injury healed after orthopedic treatment. However, the patient complained of weakness in his right arm ever since, and became depressed from worrying about being unable to continue his work as a driver. During the past year, he developed insomnia and his memory became bad. He often laughed or wept for no apparent reason. Neurological and EEG examinations revealed no abnormalities, nor was there a history of hypertension. Anti-anxiety drugs such as diazepam were not helpful, and the patient decided to try acupuncture.

The four examinations of Chinese medicine revealed that the patient had a dull and pale complexion. He was gloomy and responded slowly. He laughed and wept for no apparent reason, but exhibited no manic behavior. His appetite was poor, and he complained of a feeling of fullness in the chest. He had difficulty falling asleep, and when he did sleep, he had nightmares. The tongue was pale with a greasy, white coating. The pulse was wiry and thin.

SYNDROME DIFFERENTIATION

This condition was induced by emotional depression and excessive worry. In Chinese medicine, excessive worry is thought to impair the Heart and Spleen. The Heart controls the Blood, and the Spleen generates the Blood. When the Heart is not properly nourished by Blood, the result is insomnia, excessive dreaming and impaired memory.

Deficiency of Blood adversely affects the Liver. The Liver not only regulates the flow of Qi and Blood, but also the distribution of Fluids. Excessive worry induces stagnation of Liver Qi, which in turn hinders the proper distribution of Fluids. Fluids which are stagnant transform into Phlegm. The Phlegm may then combine with stagnant Qi to disturb the Heart, which controls the emotions. This accounts for the gloominess and the uncontrollable laughter and weeping of the patient. The Liver is associated with dreaming and nightmares. The stagnation of Liver Qi and deficiency of Blood in the Liver caused the patient's sleep to be disturbed by nightmares.

The patient's dull and pale complexion, and pale tongue, indicated deficiency of Qi and Blood. The greasy, white tongue coating was a sign of Phlegm. The wiry pulse indicated Liver disease.

In summary, the patient was suffering from depression due to stagnation of Phlegm and Qi, with impaired nutrition of the Heart and Liver.

TREATMENT

The principles of treatment were to regulate the Liver and invigorate the Spleen, soothe the Heart and thus calm the mind.

Points selected:

P-6 *(nei guan)*, H-7 *(shen men)*, CV-17 *(tan zhong)*, S-36 *(zu san li)*, Sp-6 *(san yin jiao)*, Liv-3 *(tai chong)*

H-7 *(shen men)* and S-36 *(zu san li)* were tonified, and the other points were needled with balanced tonifying-draining manipulation. Treatment was administered once daily, and the needles were retained for 30 minutes during each session. Six sessions comprised one course of therapy, with one day of rest between courses.

Discussion of points:

Needling H-7 *(shen men)* has the effect of soothing the Heart and calming the mind. CV-17 *(tan zhong)* is the meeting point at which Qi assembles; it is used for regulating the functional activities of Qi. P-6 *(nei guan)* is the point of confluence of the Yin Linking channel, one of the eight miscellaneous channels, and is used for diseases of the Heart, chest and Stomach. Together with H-7 *(shen men)*, it soothes the Heart and calms the mind; and together with CV-17 *(tan zhong)*, it clears the chest and regulates the Qi. Needling S-36 *(zu san li)* invigorates the Stomach and Spleen, which are the source for the generation of Qi and Blood; it also clears Dampness and reduces Phlegm.

Sp-6 *(san yin jiao)* is the point on the leg where the Liver, Spleen and Stomach channels intersect. Together with S-36 *(zu san li)*, it invigorates the Spleen. Liv-3 *(tai chong)* is the source point of the Liver channel. This point regulates the Liver and dispels stagnation. This effect is enhanced when used in combination with Sp-6 *(san yin jiao)*. Combining H-7 *(shen men)*, P-6 *(nei guan)* and Sp-6 *(san yin jiao)* is a common and very effective prescription for the treatment of insomnia.

RESULTS

After two courses of treatment, the patient was able to fall asleep more readily, and his appetite was markedly improved. His memory also improved. Weeping became less frequent, but uncontrollable laughter still occurred. The nightmares also persisted, indicating that the stagnation of Phlegm and Qi still remained.

To promote the transformation of Phlegm, H-5 *(tong li)* and S-40 *(feng long)* were added. H-5 *(tong li)* was chosen to regulate the Heart and clear its channel in order to treat the uncontrollable laughter. S-40 *(feng long)* is an important point for transforming Phlegm. Both points were needled with balanced tonifying-draining manipulation. The use of P-6 *(nei guan)*, which had been chosen to enhance the calming effect of H-7 *(shen men)*, was discontinued because the insomnia had improved.

After three sessions with the modified point prescription, the uncontrollable laughter ceased, and the nightmares decreased in frequency. The use of H-5 *(tong li)* was therefore discontinued. During three more courses of treatment, all the symptoms gradually subsided, and there was an increase in body weight. The patient's complexion improved. The tongue turned pink, and had a thin, white coating. The pulse was only slightly wiry.

Treatment was then terminated, and the patient returned to work as a driver. Follow-up six months later found him to be in good spirits, with no signs of his previous depression. ☐

Deviation of the Mouth and Eye
(Facial Paralysis)

Kǒu Yǎn Wāi Xié 口眼喎斜

Liu, male, 48 years old. One morning 6 months ago, the patient awoke to find signs of facial paralysis: numbness and stiffness of his right cheek, deviation of the mouth to the left, inability to close his right eye and raise his right eyebrow, and pain behind and below his right ear. He recalled that the night before he had slept with the door and window open. He was diagnosed at a hospital as having facial paralysis, and was given traditional massage therapy (tuī nà) along with vitamins. The pain behind the ear disappeared 2 weeks later, but the paralysis remained. He received 10 acupuncture treatments at another hospital, but without apparent effect. Afterward, he was too busy to continue therapy. However, because the condition persisted, he decided to come to our clinic for treatment.

Examination revealed numbness of the right cheek, deviation of the mouth to the left, and leakage of air from the mouth when the patient puffed out his cheeks. There was constant drooling from the right corner of the mouth, and a tendency for food to escape. The right nasolabial groove was shallow. The patient could not close his right eye completely, leaving an opening 5mm wide. There was constant tearing in the right eye, and he was unable to raise the eyebrow on that side. The wrinkles on the right side of the forehead had flattened out. When the patient smiled, only two upper and three lower teeth on the right, and four upper and five lower teeth on the left, were visible. The tongue was pale with a thin, white coating, and the pulse was floating and weak. Be-

cause this condition was a case of channel pathology, other systemic aspects of the patient's conditions were not considered important.

SYNDROME DIFFERENTIATION

Deviation of the mouth and eye is caused by invasion of the channels of the face by Wind-Cold. In this case, the patient had probably been exposed to a draft. The channels involved were the Yang Brightness and Lesser Yang channels of the arm and leg. When Wind-Cold invaded these channels, stagnation of Qi and Blood resulted, leading to a lack of nourishment in the muscles and other tissues of the face. This lack of nourishment caused the numbness and flaccidity. Because the flaccid muscles were unable to contract, there was paralysis.

TREATMENT

Points were chosen primarily from the Yang Brightness channels of the arm and leg, supplemented by local points. Balanced tonifying-draining manipulation was applied to facilitate the circulation of Qi in the face, and to dispel, and strengthen the body's resistance to, the pathogenic influence of Wind-Cold.

Points selected:

LI-4 *(he gu)*, G-14 *(yang bai)*, B-2 *(zan zhu)*, B-1 *(jing ming)*, TB-23 *(si zhu kong)*, point of pain on the upper eyelid, S-1 *(cheng qi)*, LI-20 *(ying xiang)*, SI-18 *(quan liao)*, N-HN-20 *(qian zheng)*, S-4 *(di cang)*, S-6 *(jia che)*

LI-4 *(he gu)* was needled bilaterally, and the other points on the right side only. Treatment was administered once daily, with ten sessions comprising one course of therapy. Three days' rest was allowed between courses.

Discussion of points:

B-2 *(zan zhu)*, B-1 *(jing ming)*, TB-23 *(si zhu kong)*, S-1 *(cheng qi)* and the point of pain on the upper eyelid are all located near the eye. Needling these points helped to normalize the flow of Qi to the eye, thus improving the strength of the eye muscles. LI-20 *(ying xiang)*, SI-18 *(quan liao)*, S-4 *(di cang)*, S-6 *(jia che)* and N-HN-20 *(qian zheng)* were chosen to normalize the flow of Qi to the cheek, thus strengthening the cheek muscles. G-14 *(yang bai)* was needled to normalize the flow of Qi in the channels of the forehead, thus improving the strength of local muscles.

G-14 *(yang bai)* was needled with a 1-unit needle inserted transversely toward the eyebrow 0.8 unit. B-2 *(zan zhu)* was needled

transversely toward B-1 *(jing ming)* about 0.8 unit. At B-1 *(jing ming)*, with the eyeball pushed to the side, the needle was inserted slowly along the medial orbital wall 1.2 units; no manipulation was attempted. At TB-23 *(si zhu kong)* the needle was directed transversely toward G-1 *(tong zi liao)* about 1 unit. The 'point of pain' was located at the center of the upper eyelid. With the eyelid pinched horizontally to avoid puncturing through the eyelid, a 34-gauge needle was inserted in the direction of B-1 *(jing ming)* about 0.3 unit. At S-1 *(cheng qi)* the needle was inserted perpendicularly, and very slowly, about 1 unit. At LI-20 *(ying xiang)* the needle was inserted perpendicularly to a depth of 0.4 unit, and at SI-18 *(quan liao)* perpendicularly to a depth of 1.2 units. At all of the above points, the needling produced a sensation of local soreness and distention.

N-HN-20 *(qian zheng)* was needled perpendicularly to a depth of about 1 unit, which produced a feeling of soreness and distention that radiated to the zygomatic arch and upper teeth. S-4 *(di cang)* was joined to S-6 *(jia che)*, and the soreness and distention produced thereby spread throughout the cheek.

RESULTS

After one course of therapy, the opening left when the patient attempted to close his right eye had diminished to 3mm, and he was able to slightly raise his right eyebrow. Leftward deviation of the mouth was reduced, as was the tendency for food to escape. When the patient smiled, more teeth (three upper and four lower) were visible on the right side than before. Treatment was therefore continued with the same points.

After a total of 42 treatments, the patient was able to close his right eye. The number of teeth showing when he smiled was the same on both sides. There was no deviation of the mouth, and food no longer fell out.

Wrinkles on the right side of the forehead reappeared. Treatment was then terminated. The patient was followed-up for six months, with no evidence of relapse.

Note: In treating facial paralysis, the best results are obtained if treatment is begun immediately after the onset of symptoms. The more protracted the condition, the more resistant it becomes to acupuncture. In this case, more than four courses were necessary to effect a cure, compared to less than three courses in the case which follows. □

Deviation of the Mouth and Eye
(Facial Paralysis)

Kǒu Yǎn Wāi Xié 口眼喎斜

Bi, female, 40 years old. Two nights ago, the patient slept facing an open window. The next morning numbness was felt over the right side of the face, and there was deviation of the mouth to the left side. There was also some salivation. When the patient ate, food collected in the right cheek, with some leakage from the mouth. Blurred vision and tearing was experienced in the right eye.

Examination showed deviation of the mouth to the left, and an inability to close the mouth securely. The wrinkles on the right side of the forehead had disappeared. The ability to frown and puff out the right cheek was absent, and the right nasolabial groove had disappeared. The right eye could not be closed completely, leaving an opening 4mm wide. The pulse was floating, and the tongue had a thin, white coating.

SYNDROME DIFFERENTIATION

Various names are ascribed to this condition in Chinese medical literature, including 'deviation of the mouth from Wind' *(wāi zuǐ fēng)* and 'deviation of the mouth and eyes' *(kǒu yǎn wāi xié)*. Its pathogenesis is attributed to local disturbance in the flow of Qi and Blood in the Yang Brightness and Lesser Yang channels, rendering the face vulnerable to invasion by external Wind-Cold. This results in further disruption, depriving the sinews of nutrients. The diagnosis is supported by the exposure to a draft during sleep, the sudden onset of the condition, the floating nature of the pulse, and the thin, white coating on the tongue.

TREATMENT

Treatment was directed at dispersing the Wind, clearing the channels and regulating Yin and Yang.

Points selected:

L-7 *(lie que)*, K-6 *(zhao hai)*, SI-3 *(hou xi)*, B-62 *(shen mai)*, G-20 *(feng chi)*, SI-18 *(quan liao)*, GV-26 *(ren zhong)*, CV-24 *(cheng jiang)*, S-6 *(jia che)*, S-4 *(di cang)*, G-14 *(yang bai)*, B-2 *(zan zhu)*

Needling was administered once daily, with ten treatments comprising one course of therapy.

Discussion of points:

L-7 *(lie que)* and SI-3 *(hou xi)* are two of the points of confluence of the eight miscellaneous channels. The former communicates with the Conception vessel, and the latter with the Governing vessel. The Governing vessel functions to unite all of the Yang channels. It is thus known as the 'sea of the Yang channels', and controls the exterior of the body. The Conception vessel unites all of the Yin channels. It is called the 'sea of the Yin channels', and controls the interior of the body. Needling L-7 *(lie que)* and SI-3 *(hou xi)* therefore serves to regulate Yin and Yang.

B-62 *(shen mai)* and K-6 *(zhao hai)* are also points of confluence of the eight miscellaneous channels. B-62 *(shen mai)* communicates with the Yang Heel channel, and K-6 *(zhao hai)* communicates with the Yin Heel channel. These two channels traverse the face and meet at the inner canthus. They function to regulate Yin and Yang. These two points are therefore effective in treating diseases of the face, and were used here for dysfunction in the movement of the eyelid.

G-20 *(feng chi)* acts to disperse Wind and is therefore frequently used in the treatment of facial paralysis. SI-18 *(quan liao)*, S-6 *(jia che)*, S-4 *(di cang)*, B-2 *(zan zhu)* and G-14 *(yang bai)* are local points which were selected to regulate Qi in the channels of the face. GV-26 *(ren zhong)* is the point of intersection of the Governing vessel with the Stomach and Large Intestine channels, while CV-24 *(cheng jiang)* is a point of intersection of the Conception vessel with the Stomach channel. Needling GV-26 *(ren zhong)* and CV-24 *(cheng jiang)* clears the channels and facilitates the flow of Qi, primarily in the Stomach channel.

In treating the facial paralysis, the points on the face were needled superficially with balanced tonifying-draining manipulation. The point penetration method (joining points) was utilized: S-4 *(di cang)* to S-6 *(jia che)*, G-14 *(yang bai)* to TB-23 *(si zhu kong)*, and B-2 *(zan zhu)* to B-1 *(jing ming)*. Facial points on the affected side were needled one day, and points on the healthy side the following day. The points on the extremities were needled on the affected side only.

RESULTS

After the first course of treatment, there was a marked reduction in tearing. Eye closure was almost complete when lying down, but not while sitting. No change was noted in the deviation of the mouth. The patient was then allowed to rest for three days.

Upon commencement of the second course, moxibustion of the right cheek was administered on a daily basis. Moxibustion warms the channels to dispel Cold. In this case, moxibustion was added to enhance the effect of acupuncture because the disease was due to invasion of Wind-Cold. In general, for cases of facial paralysis, only needling is used at the outset since it is usually effective. In this case, however, it was not, and moxibustion was therefore added.

The same points were needled in the second course, and treatment was continued on a daily basis. By the end of the second course, some wrinkles could be seen upon raising the brow. There was also substantial improvement in the deviation of the mouth, and the forming of words was easier.

Beginning with the third course of therapy, needling and moxibustion were administered together every other day. After seven treatments, the deviation of the mouth was resolved. Measurements from the bottom of the earlobe to the corner of mouth, and from the outer canthus to the corner of the mouth, were the same on both sides. Eye closure was complete, and the nasolabial grooves were symmetrical. Wrinkling of the forehead upon raising the brow, and protrusion of the cheek upon puffing, were the same on both sides. Treatment was therefore terminated. □

Excessive Sleeping
(Narcolepsy)

Duō Mèi Zhèng 多寐症

Wang, male, 51, years old. Unusual drowsiness was first experienced 3 months ago, with sleep sometimes continuing for 24 hours. Upon awakening, the patient still felt tired. The symptoms worsened and eventually became so uncontrollable that the patient would fall into a deep sleep while attending a meeting, or while reading or writing, and even while eating. He slept well at night. He was diagnosed as having narcolepsy at another hospital, and was prescribed stimulants such as caffeine. Relief, however, was not long-lasting, and he was referred for acupuncture therapy.

The four examinations of Chinese medicine found an overweight man with a tired and drowsy expression. His appetite was poor, and he complained of distention in the abdomen and loose stools. The tongue was pale with a white, greasy coating. His pulse was deep and moderate.

SYNDROME DIFFERENTIATION

The patient complained of uncontrollable drowsiness during the day. In Chinese medicine, the daytime belongs to Yang; during the day, people are spirited because of the predominance of Yang. Conversely, the nighttime belongs to Yin; during the night, people sleep because of the predominance of Yin. When the body is deficient in Yang, the balance is tipped toward a relative predominance of Yin. This is why the patient fell asleep during the day.

Besides narcolepsy, the patient also suffered from loss of appetite, abdominal distention and loose stools, and had a pale tongue. All of these symptoms pointed to deficiency of Spleen Yang, which is responsible for the transportation of nutrients. The Spleen is also associated with the health of the limbs. When the Spleen is weak, the limbs become flabby and lack strength. In addition, the Spleen regulates the movement of Fluids. When the Spleen is deficient, Fluids are not moved properly, but instead accumulate as Dampness. The patient's overweight appearance was thus attributed to an accumulation of Dampness, proving the adage that overweight people are prone to suffer from Dampness.

An inverted sleep rhythm is also a reflection of the dysfunction of the Yin and Yang Heel channels. In the *Miraculous Pivot* (chapter 21), a close relationship is noted between the Qi in both Heel channels. When the Qi of the Yang Heel channel travels inward, the Qi of the Yin Heel channel travels outward, balancing each other. When Yang Heel Qi is relatively excessive, and Yin Heel Qi relatively deficient, the mind becomes excited and insomnia ensues. Conversely, if Yin Heel Qi is relatively excessive, drowsiness and fatigue occur in the daytime. The daytime sleepiness in this patient indicated that the pattern was one of deficiency of Yang Heel Qi, and excess of Yin Heel Qi. This is an example of syndrome differentiation in accordance with the theory of the channels.

To summarize, this case was one of Yang deficiency and Yin excess. There was a deficiency of Spleen Yang, which resulted in an accumulation of Dampness, and there was a deficiency of Yang Heel channel Qi, and an excess of Yin Heel channel Qi.

TREATMENT

Treatment was directed at tonifying the deficient Yang and draining the excessive Yin.

Points selected:
S-36 *(zu san li)*, Sp-6 *(san yin jiao)*, B-62 *(shen mai)*, K-6 *(zhao hai)*, GV-20 *(bai hui)*
Needling was administered once daily.

Discussion of points:
S-36 *(zu san li)* is an important point for tonifying the Spleen and warming the Yang. Sp-6 *(san yin jiao)* was used to strengthen the Spleen and resolve the Dampness. B-62 *(shen mai)* and K-6 *(zhao hai)* are the confluent points of the Yang Heel and Yin Heel miscellaneous channels, which communicate with the Bladder and Kidney channels respectively. These two points were needled to regulate the flow of Qi in the two channels; they are specifically indicated for the treatment of both excessive sleeping and insomnia. GV-20 *(bai hui)* was needled to tonify the Yang and invigorate the Qi.

Each of the five points in the prescription belongs to a different Yin or Yang channel. The method of manipulation, and the sequence of treatment, are therefore noteworthy. The Yang channel points, S-36 *(zu san li)*, B-62 *(shen mai)* and GV-20 *(bai hui)*, were needled first, with tonifying manipulation. The Yin channel points, K-6 *(zhao hai)* and Sp-6 *(san yin jiao)*, were needled next, with draining manipulation. This is in accord with a principle first enunciated in the *Classic of Difficulties* (chapter 64): "When the Yang is deficient and the Yin is excessive, tonify the Yang first, and then drain the Yin."

When needling K-6 *(zhao hai)*, twirling manipulation with large amplitude should be applied so that the draining stimulation is strong. This causes propagation of the needle sensation upward. When the needle sensation reaches the vicinity of Sp-6 *(san yin jiao)*, the needle at K-6 *(zhao hai)* should be withdrawn at once, and Sp-6 *(san yin jiao)* needled with raise-thrust manipulation, also of large amplitude. When Qi is obtained at this point, the needle is withdrawn. This method enhances the therapeutic effect, and reduces the time needed to treat each of the points.

RESULTS

After two treatments, the patient felt that his mind was clearer. After five treatments, he was more spirited during the day, and his drowsiness could be overcome with conscious effort. After ten treatments, all of the symptoms had substantially improved. Acupuncture therapy was therefore terminated.

Follow-up after three months found that there had been no relapse of narcolepsy, and that the patient had returned to work.

Note: Other etiologies of excessive sleeping include the following:

- Insufficiency of Spleen Qi: This may be caused either by mental fatigue or improper diet, resulting in disturbance of the Spleen's functions of transportation and transformation. The clear Yang is unable to rise, leading to lassitude and a desire to sleep. Other symptoms include drowsiness especially after meals, weakness of the limbs, a pasty complexion, reduced appetite, watery stools, a deficient and frail pulse, and a thin, white tongue coating.

- Deficient Yang Qi: This pattern generally occurs in the elderly after a protracted illness. Such patients have a deficiency of Kidney Qi and a diminishing Fire at the 'gate of vitality', as well as a deficiency of Yang Qi. They therefore lack energy, and become drowsy. Other symptoms include an aversion to cold, coldness of the limbs, forgetfulness, a submerged, thin and weak pulse, and a pale tongue with a thin coating.

- Stagnant Blood blocking the senses: This condition may result either from external head injury, or from fright which causes stagnation of Qi and disturbance in the flow of Qi and Blood, or from Phlegm which blocks the vessels and channels. Any of these factors may impede the flow of Qi and Blood, such that the Yang Qi is obstructed, and a desire for sleep ensues. Other symptoms include dizziness, headache, mental fatigue, a choppy pulse, and a purple tongue, or one with purple eruptions along the edges. □

Facial Tic

Miàn Jī Jìng Luán 面肌痉挛

Li, male, 67 years old. Over 2 years ago, the patient suddenly suffered deviation of the mouth to the left, drooling from the right corner of the mouth, and incomplete closure of the right eye. The diagnosis was facial paralysis due to exposure to a draft. Acupuncture was administered for 2 years at another clinic, and there was moderate improvement in the paralysis. However, sudden, involuntary spasms developed, localized in the right lower submaxillary region. Acupuncture was continued for more than 2 months using facial points on the right side. No appreciable result was obtained, and the patient was referred to our clinic.

Examination showed a slight deviation of the mouth to the left, rigidity of the right facial muscles, and diminished wrinkles on the right side of the forehead upon raising the eyebrows. The patient experienced dizziness, and dryness of the mouth with no desire to drink. His pulse was slippery and wiry, and his tongue was red with a thick, white coating.

SYNDROME DIFFERENTIATION

The underlying cause of this condition was an invasion of Wind, which lodged in the facial portion of the Stomach channel. This hindered the flow of Blood and Qi, and deprived this part of the face of nutrients. Because of ineffective treatment, the primary condition persisted. The persistence of Wind, compounded by the patient's obesity, impaired the metabolism of Fluids and gave rise to Phlegm. This further interfered with the function of the channels, and resulted in spasmodic contractions. The dizziness was due to an upsurge of Wind-Phlegm, which was also reflected in the slippery, wiry pulse, and in the thick, white tongue coating. When Phlegm is protracted, it tends to transform into Heat, which in this case was manifested in the red tongue and dryness of the mouth. Because of the stagnation of Fluids (Phlegm), there was no desire to drink. The diminution of forehead wrinkles was evidence of the incomplete resolution of the initial paralysis.

In summary, this syndrome was one of obstruction of the channels by Wind-Phlegm, which had transformed into Heat.

TREATMENT

Treatment was directed at eliminating the Wind-Phlegm and removing the Heat in order to clear the channels.

Points selected:

Left side: S-2 *(si bai)*, S-4 *(di cang)*, S-6 *(jia che)*, M-HN-18 *(jia cheng jiang)*

Right side: G-14 *(yang bai)*

Bilateral: SI-18 *(quan liao)*, LI-4 *(he gu)*, S-40 *(feng long)*, S-44 *(nei ting)*, Liv-3 *(tai chong)*

Treatment was administered once daily.

Discussion of points:

The spasms were the primary focus of therapy. Because the prolonged use of points on the affected (right) side of the face had led to the development of spasms, we intentionally used those on the left side as the principal points of therapy. The rationale was that since the bilateral aspects of the Stomach channel intersect, treating the healthy (left) side would be just as effective as treating the diseased side. This is particularly true with points on the Stomach channel, which encircles the mouth.

SI-18 *(quan liao)* is a point on the Small Intestine channel, which intersects the Stomach channel on the face. M-HN-18 *(jia cheng jiang)* is especially useful for treating facial paralysis or tic. G-14 *(yang bai)* and SI-18 *(quan liao)* on the affected side were used to supplement the points on the left in order to regulate the Yin and Yang on both sides.

LI-4 *(he gu)* is a point on the Large Intestine channel, which travels around the lip. LI-4 *(he gu)* is commonly used for spasms of the masseter muscle. S-44 *(nei ting)* is the gushing point of the Stomach channel, and was chosen in accordance with the principle of using points on the lower body for diseases of the upper body. Furthermore, the gushing points are particularly effective in treating Heat syndromes. S-40 *(feng long)* is traditionally used for resolving Phlegm.

Liv-3 *(tai chong)* is the source point of the Liver channel, and is often used for dispersing Wind.

Points on the healthy side were strongly stimulated. After the needle sensation was obtained, raise-thrust manipulation of small amplitude was applied continuously for two minutes. Points on the affected side were only mildly stimulated. M-HN-18 *(jia cheng jiang)* was needled obliquely inward and downward to a depth of 0.5 unit.

RESULTS

After five sessions, the facial spasms were substantially alleviated. However, the patient had loose stools for two days. Since he previously had regular bowel movements, and no cause such as exposure to wind, eating of contaminated food, or overindulgence could be found, it was suspected that the needling of S-44 *(nei ting)*, which drains Heat, might be the reason. This hypothesis was supported by a change in the color of the tongue from red to pink. Accordingly, on the sixth day the use of S-44 *(nei ting)* was discontinued. On the following day, bowel movements were normal.

After ten treatments, the rigidity of the facial muscles was relieved, the spasmodic contractions stopped, the nasolabial grooves became symmetrical, and the deviation of the mouth was no longer apparent. Some slight dizziness remained, and the wrinkles on the right side of the forehead were still incomplete. Treatment was suspended for four days.

Upon resumption of treatment, only G-14 *(yang bai)*, B-2 *(zan zhu)* and G-34 *(yang ling quan)*, all on the right side, were needled once every other day. After ten treatments with these points, the wrinkles on the forehead upon raising the brow appeared to be normal. Treatment was therefore discontinued. The patient was followed-up for three months, during which time he remained in good health, and experienced no recurrence of symptoms.

Note: A comparison of this case with the one that follows is instructive. In this case, the condition was caused by three factors — Wind, Phlegm and Heat — whereas in the following case, the condition was caused solely by Wind. Here, the condition had become refractory, thus more local points, as well as those for resolving Phlegm and Heat, were used to clear the channels. In the following case, distal points alone proved to be effective. It should also be noted that in both cases the principle of needling one side to treat the opposite side was effectively utilized. □

Facial Tic

Miàn Jī Jìng Luán 面肌痉挛

Wang, male, 45 years old. One year ago, the patient suddenly began to feel twitching in his left eyelid. The twitching gradually spread to the entire left cheek, and was more frequent when he became excited. No apparent cause for the disorder could be found.

Examination revealed a facial tic on the left side, spasmodic contractions of the left eyelid, and a narrowing of the left palpebral fissure. The patient had a wiry pulse, and a thin, white tongue coating.

SYNDROME DIFFERENTIATION

This condition was manifested by spasms of the facial muscles and eyelid. In Chinese medicine, spasms are considered to be caused by an invasion of Wind, the characteristics of which include motion and variation: "Prevailing of Wind produces movement" (Simple Questions, chapter 5). Therefore, an invasion of Wind can lead to such symptoms as convulsions of the extremities, muscular spasms, rigidity of the neck and back, and tremors of the head.

With facial tic, the spasms are in the cheek and eyelid. Since the cheek and inner canthus are traversed by the Yang Brightness and Greater Yang channels of the arm and leg, the diagnosis of the condition was therefore made with reference to these channels. Thus, the condition was attributed to an invasion of external Wind, resulting in obstruction to the flow of Qi in the Yang Brightness and Greater Yang channels.

TREATMENT

Treatment was directed at dispersing the Wind, checking the spasms, and removing the obstruction from the channels.

Points selected:
SI-3 (hou xi) and B-62 (shen mai) on the right, LI-4 (he gu) and G-20 (feng chi) on the left, and S-36 (zu san li) bilaterally
Treatment was administered once daily.

Discussion of points:
LI-4 (he gu) is an important point for treating diseases of the head and face. It is said

in the classics that LI-4 *(he gu)* governs the face and mouth, indicating that this is an important point for treating headache, toothache and other conditions affecting the face. SI-3 *(hou xi)* and B-62 *(shen mai)* are the confluent points for the Governing vessel and Yang Heel channel respectively. They are often used together as supplemental points for relieving spasms, and are especially effective in the treatment of convulsions of the extremities, muscular spasms, and rigidity of the neck and back due to various causes. S-36 *(zu san li)* is commonly used for general invigoration. It is also used to remove obstruction to the flow of Qi in the leg Yang Brightness (Stomach) channel, in order to relax spasms of the facial muscles. G-20 *(feng chi)* is frequently used for treating conditions caused by Wind.

LI-4 *(he gu)* and G-20 *(feng chi)* on the left were selected in order to produce a strong needle sensation at the site of the disorder, since the Large Intestine and Gall Bladder channels on which these points are located traverse the affected area. While the same points on the right side could have been chosen instead, their effect would not have been as pronounced as those on the left. Thus, in this case, only the points on the left side were chosen. Strong manipulation was applied.

SI-3 *(hou xi)* and B-62 *(shen mai)* were needled on the right, conforming to the principle of selecting points on the right side to treat diseases on the left. Although this principle of point selection was applied here, the left points could also have been needled together with those on the right.

SI-3 *(hou xi)* was needled perpendicularly to a depth of 1.5 units; deep needling was utilized to enhance the point's Wind-dispersing action. Strong draining manipulation was applied by twirling the needle through a wide angle two or three times. At LI-4 *(he gu)* the needle was inserted close to the radial surface of the second metacarpal bone to induce a strong needle sensation, which was transmitted up the arm. G-20 *(feng chi)* was needled with the 'burning the mountain' technique (see Introduction), causing a hot sensation to be transmitted to the cheek. This technique was used because the elicited sensation is stronger, and is better transmitted along the channel. At B-62 *(shen mai)* the needle was inserted 1 unit, penetrating through to K-6 *(zhao hai)*. S-36 *(zu san li)* was drained, using raise-thrust and twirling manipulation, in order to clear the Stomach channel which courses through the face.

RESULTS

After four treatments, the facial spasms had improved, but the twitching of the eyelid was still unresolved. After an additional fourteen treatments with the same set of points, the symptoms were under control, and the palpebral fissure resumed its normal width, but mild relapses still occurred from time to time when the patient became excited. Treatment was discontinued after ten more treatments. The patient was followed up for six months, and no recurrence was reported. □

Spasms of the Hands and Feet
(Hypocalcemia)

Shǒu Zú Chì Zhòng 手足瘈疭

> *Nie, female, 7 years old. This child had suffered from involuntary spasms, which occurred more than 20 times per day for a week. Each episode lasted 3-5 seconds, during which time either the hands clenched, or all the fingers were extended, with the thumb approximating the palm; the feet and toes were plantar flexed; the head trembled, the eyelids fluttered, and the teeth clenched. The episodes were more frequent during the day than at night. Her parents could not recall any precipitating factor or condition which led to the onset of the spasms.*

Physical examination found the child to be of average development. Her complexion was pale, and she was listless. The heart, lungs and abdomen were normal. The liver and spleen were not palpable. The tongue was pale with a thin coating, and the pulse was wiry and thin.

Laboratory tests showed serum calcium of 8mg/100ml, and serum phosphorus of 5.05mg/100ml. The child was diagnosed as having hypocalcemia.

SYNDROME DIFFERENTIATION

The chief symptoms of the patient were spasms of the hands and feet. Spasms are associated with Wind in Chinese medicine, since Wind is characterized by incessant movement. In this case, the Wind was inter-nally generated because of deficiency of Liver Blood. This was manifested by the pale complexion, listlessness, and the wiry, thin pulse.

In differentiating the syndrome according to the theory of the channels and collaterals, this was a condition of the Governing vessel, which is the confluence of all the Yang channels. Its function is to regulate the Yang Qi of the body. Abnormalities of the Govern-ing vessel can cause the body to lose balance, hence the spasms.

The root of this condition was therefore deficiency of Liver Blood, manifested as dys-function of the Governing vessel.

TREATMENT

The principles of treatment were to extin-guish the Wind and resolve the spasms,

131

regulate the Governing vessel, and replenish the Blood.

Points selected:

GV-26 *(ren zhong)*, GV-14 *(da zhui)*, SI-3 *(hou xi)*, Liv-3 *(tai chong)*, Sp-6 *(san yin jiao)*

Treatment was administered once every other day. Balanced tonifying-draining manipulation was applied through raise-thrust and twirling techniques. The needles were retained for ten minutes during each session, except at GV-26 *(ren zhong)*, where the needle was removed immediately after obtaining the needle sensation. This is because the needle sensation at this point is rather strong.

Discussion of points:

GV-26 *(ren zhong)* functions to extinguish Wind and to calm the Spirit. GV-14 *(da zhui)* is the point of intersection of all the Yang channels, and is thus capable of regulating both the Governing vessel as well as the body as a whole. SI-3 *(hou xi)* is the confluent point of the Governing vessel. These three points were chosen to resolve the 'branch' or manifestation of the condition — dysfunction of the Governing vessel.

Liv-3 *(tai chong)* was used to extinguish the Liver Wind, and to tonify the Liver Blood. Sp-6 *(san yin jiao)* was used to tonify the Spleen and Stomach, and to regulate the Liver. These two points were chosen to treat the root of the condition — deficiency of Liver Blood.

RESULTS

By the third treatment, the frequency of spasms was reduced by about one-half, according to the parents. After three more treatments, the child experienced only one or two transient spasms over a period of two days. Six more treatments were administered to consolidate the therapeutic effect. Laboratory tests revealed that the serum calcium had increased to 9.5mg/100ml. The child remained healthy during a follow-up of one year. □

Traumatic Paraplegia

Jié Tān 截瘫

Li, 48 years old. Six months ago, the back of the patient's neck was severely injured in an accident involving a coal-cart; he was unconscious for 40 minutes. When he revived, it was found that he had completely lost the ability to move his extremities, and suffered incontinence of urine and stool. X-ray revealed that the 3rd, 4th and 5th cervical vertebrae were severely out of alignment. Traction was immediately applied, and the patient was hospitalized for 6 months, during which time partial function was restored to the limbs.

When the patient was brought to the acupuncture clinic, myodynamia of both arms near the shoulders reached grade 3 or 4 (out of 5), as he was able to raise them at will. But both wrists had dropped, and his fingers had slight muscular atrophy, which made their movement clumsy. Myodynamia of both legs was about grade 2, and the patient could not walk, even with the aid of a cane. Muscular atrophy was not observed. There was slight hypertonicity of the muscles. Bowel movements were continent, but overflow incontinence of urine occurred frequently. The pulse was tight, and the tongue was pink with a thin, white coating.

SYNDROME DIFFERENTIATION

Traumatic paraplegia is attributed in Chinese medicine to severe injury of the Governing vessel. This channel travels up from the coccyx along the midline of the back and enters the Brain. Because it is the confluence of all the Yang channels, it governs the Yang Qi of the entire body. By virtue of its pathway along the spine, the Governing vessel affects the function of the spinal cord.

The injury to the cervical vertebrae in this case had a direct and catastrophic effect on the Yang Qi in the Governing vessel. Because one of the principal functions of the Yang Qi is to invigorate the channels and promote the flow of Qi and Blood, the injury to the Yang Qi impeded the flow of Qi in the channels. This in turn deprived the sinews, bones and muscles of replenishment of Qi and Blood, thus rendering the limbs weak and unable to perform their normal functions.

TREATMENT

Treatment was directed primarily at removing the stagnation from the Governing vessel, and regulating the flow of Qi and Blood.

Points selected:

Two groups of points were used in rotation on alternating days:

Group 1: GV-14 *(da zhui)*, M-BW-35 *(jia ji)* from the 2nd to the 6th cervical vertebrae, GV-4 *(ming men)*, B-32 *(ci liao)*, B-36 *(cheng fu)*, B-40 *(wei zhong)*, B-57 *(cheng shan)*, B-60 *(kun lun)*

Group 2: CV-4 *(guan yuan)*, CV-3 *(zhong ji)*, TB-5 *(wai guan)*, LI-4 *(he gu)*, M-UE-50 *(shang ba xie)*, S-31 *(bi guan)*, S-36 *(zu san li)*, G-34 *(yang ling quan)*, G-39 *(xuan zhong)*, K-3 *(tai xi)*

Discussion of points:

G-14 *(da zhui)* is the point of intersection of the six Yang channels of the arm and leg, and is regarded as the site at which the Yang of the entire body converges. Needling this point helped to remove the stagnation from the Governing vessel, and to regulate the flow of its Qi. The vertebral points M-BW-35 *(jia ji)* from the 2nd to the 6th cervical vertebrae corresponded to the injured area in this case. Needling these points promoted the flow of Qi and Blood in this region. Treating GV-4 *(ming men)* and CV-4 *(guan yuan)* helped warm and replenish the Yang Qi.

CV-3 *(zhong ji)* is the alarm point of the Bladder. Needling this point improved the function of that Organ. TB-5 *(wai guan)*, LI-4 *(he gu)* and M-UE-50 *(shang ba xie)* were used primarily for opening the channels in the wrists and fingers. S-36 *(zu san li)* is an important point on the Stomach channel, which is exterior-interiorly related to the Spleen channel. The Stomach is the reservoir of water and food, and the Spleen serves as the source of nutrients for the development of Qi and Blood. When these two Organs were regulated by needling S-36 *(zu san li)*, Qi and Blood were replenished.

B-32 *(ci liao)*, B-36 *(cheng fu)*, B-40 *(wei zhong)*, B-57 *(cheng shan)*, B-60 *(kun lun)*, S-31 *(bi guan)*, G-34 *(yang ling quan)*, G-39 *(xuan zhong)* and K-3 *(tai xi)* were used primarily for clearing the channels in the lower extremities, and regulating their Qi and Blood.

Balanced tonifying-draining manipulation of the needles through raise-thrust and twirling techniques with strong stimulation was used to obtain a distinct needle sensation. Points in the first group were needled with the patient lying prone, and those in the second group with the patient lying supine.

At GV-14 *(da zhui)* a 1.5-unit needle was inserted to a depth of 1 unit. The needle sensation was transmitted downward along the spinal column. The vertebral points M-BW-35 *(jia ji)* from the 2nd to the 6th cervical vertebrae were treated with 1-unit needles, inserted perpendicularly to a depth of 0.8 unit. This produced a sensation of local soreness, distention and numbness. At CV-14 *(guan yuan)* and CV-3 *(zhong ji)*, 2-unit needles were used. The needle tips were directed slightly toward the external genitalia in order to induce a sensation that was transmitted to the perineum. The M-UE-50 *(shang ba xie)* points were treated with 1-unit needles, which produced a sensation of local soreness and distention. Needling of the other points was performed in the conventional manner.

RESULTS

Treatment was administered once daily for three months. The incontinence of urine was basically brought under control. Myodynamia of both legs was markedly improved, and the patient was able to walk, with help, about twenty meters, and to stand on his own for about thirty minutes. However, my-odynamia of the lower arms and hands did not show much improvement.

Treatment was suspended for two weeks, and was then resumed. To improve the my-odynamia in the lower part of the arms, the local points SI-3 *(hou xi)*, TB-4 *(yang chi)* and LI-5 *(yang xi)* were added. Treatment was continued on a daily basis, using the two groups of points in rotation on alternating days as before. After two months, the patient could move the fingers of both hands to a limited extent, but still lacked gripping

power. He could stand on both legs for about one hour. In order to consolidate the therapeutic effect, treatment was continued every other day for another four months.

By the end of this extended period of treatment, the patient was able to hold an empty cup with either hand, myodynamia of both legs had reached about grade 4, and he could walk slowly with the aid of a cane. Treatment continued for four more months, but because no further improvement was observed, acupuncture treatment was then discontinued. □

Tremors
(Parkinson's Disease)

Zhèn Chàn 震颤

Li, male, 17 years old. The patient complained of hand tremors since childhood. Involuntary tremors of both hands first appeared with no obvious cause when he was 3 years old. The tremors were rhythmic and occurred at rest. They were accentuated when he reached for an object, but decreased during active movement, and disappeared during sleep. His daily life and study were severely affected. Repeated symptomatic treatment during the past 10 years, using both traditional herbs and modern drugs, had no effect upon the condition. Neurological tests revealed no abnormalities. No Kayser-Fleischer ring was found. The diagnosis was Parkinson's disease (primary paralysis agitans).

The four examinations of Chinese medicine revealed a sallow complexion and mask-like demeanor, lassitude, a feeble voice, dizziness, spontaneous sweating and a poor appetite. His pulse was weak, and his tongue was pale and swollen with a thin, white coating.

SYNDROME DIFFERENTIATION

This case was characterized by involuntary tremors of both hands. In Chinese medicine, shaking movements are attributed to Wind: "Prevalence of Wind produces involuntary movement" (*Simple Questions,* chapter 5).

Diseases caused by Wind are of two types: those induced by external Wind, and those induced by internal Wind. The former are among the class of conditions caused by external pathogenic influences, with such symptoms as simultaneous chills and fever, and coughing. Conditions caused by internal Wind from the Liver are related to disturbances in the Liver functions of storing Blood, nourishing the sinews and sustaining normal eyesight. Common manifestations include shaking, dizziness and convulsions. "Internal Wind symptoms of dizziness and tremors always indicate involvement of the Liver" (*Simple Questions,* chapter 74).

In this case, the condition was present since childhood, and there were no symptoms suggestive of external Wind, such as fever and chills. Rather, this was a typical case of internal Wind.

Diseases associated with internal Wind are further divided into three subtypes. The first arises from the transformation of Liver Yang into Wind. It is caused by deficiency of Liver Yin and/or ascendant Liver Yang. The second is caused by extreme Heat, which harms the nutritive and Blood levels and damages the Liver channel, thus giving rise to internal Wind of the Liver. The third subtype of internal Wind is caused by deficiency of Blood that is stored in the Liver, resulting in undernourishment of the sinews, and eventually in tremors, dizziness and convulsions.

Based upon the four examinations of Chinese medicine, no signs of deficient Yin, ascendant Liver Yang, or transformation of Liver Yang into Wind were found. Nor was there a history of such symptoms as high fever, thirst and red tongue, which would have indicated Wind due to extreme Heat. Instead, all of the positive findings (sallow complexion, lassitude, feeble voice, weak pulse, and pale, swollen tongue) were related to deficiency of Blood.

Proper functioning of the body's motor activities depends on adequate nourishment of the sinews, which in turn depends on sufficient Blood stored in the Liver. In this case, the deficient Liver Blood did not provide adequate nourishment to the sinews, thus giving rise to internal Wind, leading to tremors. Because only the hands were involved, the internal Wind was mild. In severe cases, tremors may appear in other parts of the body, such as the arms and head.

TREATMENT

In this case, the tremors arising from internal Wind were a manifestation of deficiency of Blood, which was the root cause. Treatment was therefore directed at nourishing the Blood in order to subdue the internal Wind.

Points selected:

G-20 *(feng chi)*, Liv-3 *(tai chong)*, B-17 *(ge shu)*, B-20 *(pi shu)*, B-18 *(gan shu)*

Deficiency of Blood requires tonification, while the tremors from internal Wind require draining. Therefore, both tonifying and draining manipulation was applied through raise-thrust and twirling techniques.

Treatment was administered once daily, and the needles were retained for 20 minutes during each session. Six treatments comprised a course of therapy, with 3 days' rest between courses.

Discussion of points:

G-20 *(feng chi)* and Liv-3 *(tai chong)* were drained to subdue the internal Wind. The head and neck are common targets of Wind, and the point name *fēng chí* means the 'pool where wind gathers'. Thus, G-20 *(feng chi)* is one of the chief points for dispelling Wind. Liv-3 *(tai chong)*, the source point of the Liver channel, is where Blood and Qi of that channel flourish. According to the *Miraculous Pivot* (chapter 1), the 12 source points are indicated for diseases involving the Yin and Yang Organs. Liv-3 *(tai chong)* is therefore often selected for internal Wind arising from the Liver.

B-20 *(pi shu)* is the associated point on the back for the Spleen. It is an important point for regulating the transportation and distribution of nutrients and Fluids. The Spleen regulates the flow of Blood. The Spleen and Stomach are the source of nutrients for Blood and Qi. Tonification of B-20 *(pi shu)* regulates the Spleen and Stomach, thus facilitating the production of Blood and Qi.

B-18 *(gan shu)* is the associated point on the back for the Liver. It is an important point for promoting the circulation of Liver Qi. Tonifying the Liver strengthens the functioning of the Liver, so that the Blood stored in the Liver is replenished, and the deficiency of Blood is corrected.

B-17 *(ge shu)* is the point associated with Blood among the eight meeting points. It is indicated for all diseases involving Blood. In cases of Blood deficiency, tonification of this point invigorates the vessels and regulates the flow of Qi and Blood.

RESULTS

After three courses of treatment, the patient showed no improvement. The tremors persisted, and the tongue and pulse signs remained about the same. None of the symptoms of Blood deficiency and internal Wind had changed, despite what was believed to be a sound analysis of the clinical manifestations, and the correct selection of points and techniques. Why?

According to the theory of Chinese medicine, Qi, animate though intangible, is easily replenished, while Blood, though tangible, is not readily replenished. In cases of deficiency of Blood, however, Blood may regenerate itself if Qi is first replenished. Applying these principles, CV-6 *(qi hai)* and S-36 *(zu san li)* were therefore added to the point prescription, using tonification at both points. The characters that comprise the name of the point CV-6 *(qi hai)* can be translated as the 'reservoir of Qi'. As its name implies, this is an important point for replenishing Qi. S-36 *(zu san li)* is the lower uniting point of the leg Yang Brightness Stomach channel. This channel is one through which much Qi and Blood circulate, and S-36 *(zu san li)* is the point at which the Qi of this channel gathers. Tonification of this point therefore regulates Qi and Blood.

After two courses of treatment with the modified prescription, marked improvement was noted, with only slight tremors occurring at times of mental tension. The patient's complexion, mental state and appetite were improved, the dizziness was substantially reduced, the pulse grew stronger, and the tongue became a normal red color.

Treatment was continued with the modified prescription every other day for one month in order to consolidate the therapeutic effect. Acupuncture was then discontinued because the condition was considered to have stabilized. One year's follow-up showed no relapse. According to a recent report, the patient, now nineteen years old, was doing well in school. □

Vertigo from Ascendant Liver Yang
(Ménière's Syndrome)

Xuàn Yùn 眩晕

Lan, male, 27 years old. For 4 years, the patient suffered from repeated episodes of vertigo and blurred vision. The symptoms first occurred the day after he had a quarrel with a co-worker. The patient was a moody individual, and said that after the incident he was unable to forget it for a long time. At first, the episodes occurred at 2-3 month intervals, and lasted only about 30-40 minutes, after which the symptoms disappeared. Gradually, however, the episodes increased in severity, and occurred at intervals of only 10 days. Each episode lasted 2-3 days. There were no prodromal symptoms before onset. Vertigo, blurred vision and vomiting, accompanied by tinnitus, pallor and sweating, were the chief complaints. The patient had to lie down with his eyes closed, avoiding the slightest movement of the head, to prevent aggravation of the symptoms. His throat became dry, and his mouth had a bitter taste. Any attempt to drink induced severe vomiting.

Upon examination, the patient's tongue was red, and the coating was yellow. His pulse was wiry and rapid. Audiometer measurement and vestibular function tests established the diagnosis as Ménière's syndrome. Neither sedatives nor block therapy demonstrated any curative effect.

SYNDROME DIFFERENTIATION

In Chinese medicine, vertigo is generally attributed to ascendant Liver Yang due to deficiency of Liver Yin. (For other possible etiologies, see the following case.) There are several causes of ascendant Liver Yang. It can be found in individuals who constitutionally have hyperactive Yang. It may also result from extreme anger or depression. Yet another cause is deficient Kidney Yin. When Kidney Yin (water) is deficient, it is unable to nourish Liver Yin (wood); an imbalance between Liver Yin and Liver Yang ensues, resulting in ascendant Liver Yang.

With this patient, the first sign of vertigo occurred after a fit of anger. Anger harms the Liver by disturbing its function of spreading and regulating Qi; Liver Qi thus becomes stagnant. Prolonged stagnation of Qi transforms into Fire, which consumes Yin. Since the Liver is associated with Wind which is

Yang in nature, deficient Liver Yin results in ascendant Liver Yang which, together with Wind, rises to disturb the head and eyes; hence the symptoms of dizziness and blurred vision. Because the Liver 'opens' through the eyes, ascendant Liver Yang causes blurred vision, and even sensitivity to light in severe cases.

The Liver and Gall Bladder have an interior-exterior relationship; ascendancy of Liver Yang may therefore lead to disharmony of Gall Bladder Qi. Because the Gall Bladder channel passes through the ears, tinnitus then results. Ascendant Liver Yang also generates Liver Fire that flares upward, causing a dry throat, a bitter taste in the mouth, and a red tongue with a yellow coating. Ascendant Liver Yang may likewise cause an upsurge of Stomach Qi, resulting in vomiting and a poor appetite. A wiry and rapid pulse is also a sign of ascendant Liver Yang. The diagnosis was therefore vertigo from ascendant Liver Yang.

TREATMENT

The principles of treatment were to subdue the ascendant Liver Yang, and to clear the Liver Fire.

Points selected:

Liv-3 *(tai chong)*, TB-3 *(zhong zhu)*, G-41 *(zu lin qi)*, G-2 *(ting hui)*, TB-17 *(yi feng)*, P-6 *(nei guan)*, S-36 *(zu san li)*, K-6 *(zhao hai)*, G-20 *(feng chi)*

Four or five of the above points were needled once daily with balanced tonifying-draining manipulation. The needles were retained for fifteen minutes during each session.

Discussion of points:

Four of the points in this prescription, Liv-3 *(tai chong)*, TB-3 *(zhong zhu)*, G-41 *(zu lin qi)* and G-20 *(feng chi)*, have the effect of subduing ascendant Liver Yang and clearing Liver Fire. They are therefore frequently selected for treating the vertigo associated with this disease pattern. G-2 *(ting hui)* on the Gall Bladder channel, and TB-17 *(yi feng)* on the Triple Burner channel, were selected for treating the tinnitus. These are local points on channels that communicate with the ears. P-6 *(nei guan)* and S-36 *(zu san li)* were chosen for treating the vomiting. Because K-6 *(zhao hai)* nourishes Kidney Yin, it was used here for treating the dry throat and bitter taste in the mouth.

RESULTS

After 14 treatments, the severe vertigo was alleviated. However, when the patient was tired, he continued to experience slight blurring of vision, tinnitus and nausea, which subsided after a short rest. To consolidate the therapeutic effect, needling was therefore continued once every 2-4 days.

After 30 treatments, the vertigo and other symptoms were completely relieved. Treatment was therefore terminated. Follow-up 1 year later found the patient to be feeling well, with no recurrence of symptoms. □

Vertigo from Phlegm-Dampness

Xuàn Yùn 眩晕

Gao, male, 60 years old. The patient complained of frequent dizziness, exaggerated by emotional upset, of about 8 years' duration. Each episode, which occurred 3-4 times per day, lasted 1-2 minutes, during which the patient felt as if he were spinning. During the previous 2 months, the dizzy spells lasted the entire day, perhaps because of overwork. His blood pressure soared to 175/105mm Hg, and antihypertensive medication became indispensable.

The four examinations of Chinese medicine found the patient to be well-developed and robust, with a loud voice and strong respiration. He complained of dizziness associated with blurred vision, heaviness of the limbs, an oppressive sensation in the chest, poor appetite, and dryness in the mouth without desire to drink. He often had rattling of mucus in the throat. Bowel movements were normal; there was occasional dribbling at the end of urination. The tongue was red, with a yellowish-white coating in the center. The pulse was slippery and rapid.

SYNDROME DIFFERENTIATION

Vertigo is a disturbance in which the individual has a subjective impression of movement in space, or of objects moving around him. Mild cases may be resolved by merely closing the eyes, while more severe cases may simulate seasickness, and be accompanied by nausea and vomiting. The pathogenesis can be ascribed to any one of three conditions: ascendant Liver Yang; Phlegm-Dampness which interferes with the rising of clear Yang to the head; or deficiency of Blood and Qi which deprives the Brain of nutrients.

This patient suffered from dizziness of several years' duration. However, he did not exhibit the restlessness, bitter taste in the mouth, and wiry pulse that are characteristic of ascendant Liver Yang. Nor did he have such symptoms as lack of energy, pallor, paleness of the nails and tongue, insomnia, excessive dreaming, and frail pulse that are characteristic of deficiency of Blood and Qi. Rather, his symptoms indicated Phlegm-Dampness as the underlying cause.

The presence of Phlegm-Dampness interfered with the rising of clear Yang to the head, resulting in dizziness and blurred vision. The lodging of Phlegm-Dampness in the middle Burner resulted in the oppressive sensation in the chest and epigastrium, and that in the lower Burner resulted in the dribbling after urination. Heaviness of the limbs was evidence of Dampness, and rattling in the throat confirmed the presence of Phlegm. The pulse and tongue signs were also consistent with the pattern of Phlegm-Dampness. Phlegm-Dampness constrains the Qi, which over time will transform into Heat. The yellow tongue coating here reflected this process. In summary, the pattern was one of Phlegm-Dampness, which transformed into Heat.

TREATMENT

The principles of treatment were to eliminate the Phlegm, resolve the Dampness and remove the Heat.

Points selected:

G-20 *(feng chi)*, M-HN-3 *(yin tang)*, P-6 *(nei guan)*, S-36 *(zu san li)*, S-40 *(feng long)*, Sp-9 *(yin ling quan)*, LI-11 *(qu chi)*

Discussion of points:

G-20 *(feng chi)* and M-HN-3 *(yin tang)* are local points in the vicinity of the disorder. G-20 *(feng chi)* acts to clear the head and eyes. M-HN-3 *(yin tang)* is frequently used in the treatment of dizziness and headaches. S-40 *(feng long)* is specifically used to resolve Phlegm, and Sp-9 *(yin ling quan)* to eliminate Dampness. These two points are an effective combination for the treatment of Phlegm-Dampness. P-6 *(nei guan)* is the connecting point of the Pericardium channel, joining this channel with the Triple Burner channel. The Triple Burner is the pathway of Fluids, which, if impaired, causes stasis of Fluids and accumulation of Phlegm. Needling P-6 *(nei guan)* clears the Triple Burner to facilitate the flow of Fluids. S-36 *(zu san*

li) acts to strengthen the Spleen's transporting function so that Phlegm-Dampness is removed. Needling LI-11 *(qu chi)* removes Heat, and in this case was used to eliminate the Heat caused by constrained Qi.

Because this pattern was one of excess, draining manipulation was utilized. The common techniques of raise-thrust and twirling were applied. In twirling the needles, the amplitude was large, and the rate was rapid. In raise-thrusting, the needles were first inserted deeply, and then raised to just below the skin. The needles were thrust gently, and raised with force.

RESULTS

On the first visit, when G-20 *(feng chi)* was needled, the needle sensation was distinctly felt to propagate in the direction of the temples. A strong needle sensation was experienced at the other points as well. The needles were retained for 40 minutes. Upon withdrawal of the needles, the patient felt that his vision was improved, and that the dizziness had diminished. Blood pressure was then 135/90mm Hg. After the second treatment, further improvement was noted; the oral antihypertensive medication was therefore discontinued.

Because of a family row, the patient's blood pressure rose to 170/100mm Hg on the third day, and he became restless. Since this was the result of an upsurge of Liver Qi caused by anger, Liv-3 *(tai chong)*, the source point of the Liver channel, was added to the prescription. After four more treatments, the Liver Qi was soothed, the dizziness improved, and the blood pressure was brought down to 140/90mm Hg. After another week of treatment, the patient was spirited and agile, and his appetite improved. The yellow tongue coating became thin and white.

Up to this point, the patient had received daily treatments for 14 days. The treatment regimen was then reduced to once every other day. After an uneventful course, treatment was discontinued a month later. A follow-up after 6 months showed no recurrence of symptoms.

Note: In order to successfully treat Phlegm, it is important to distinguish the location of the Phlegm, and to determine whether the causal symptoms are those of excess or deficiency. Phlegm is likely to be found either in the Stomach and Intestines, in the chest, or in the limbs. In many cases, Phlegm is not limited solely to one of these locations, but may simultaneously involve different parts of the body, as in the present case.

When Phlegm accumulates in the Stomach and Intestines, there is painful distention in the epigastrium and abdomen. Upon percussion over the epigastrium, there is either a sound indicating that fluid is present, or there are rumbling sounds in the intestines. The pulse is submerged and wiry, and the tongue coating is greasy and white, or greasy and yellow.

Phlegm in the chest and hypochondria results in pain and fullness in this area, which is more pronounced in the hypochondria. There is shortness of breath and heavy breathing. The pulse is submerged and wiry, and the tongue coating is white.

Phlegm in the chest and lungs results in coughing and fullness in the chest, an inability to lie flat, difficulty in breathing, and frothy, copious sputum. The pulse is wiry and tight, and the tongue coating is white and greasy.

Phlegm affecting the limbs causes heaviness of the limbs or aching of the joints, or even slight edema of the limbs. There is an absence of sweating and thirst, and an aversion to cold. Breathing may also be difficult. There is frothy, copious sputum, and the tongue coating is white. The pulse is wiry and tight.

All of the aforementioned patterns are those of excess. There are, in addition, two patterns of deficiency: Yang deficiency of the Spleen and Stomach, and Yang deficiency of the Kidney. The former presents with fullness in the chest and hypochondria, dizziness, no desire to drink (or vomiting after drinking), frequent spitting of clear sputum, or a palm-sized, cold area on the back. The pulse is wiry, thin and slippery, and the tongue coating is white and moist.

Deficiency of Kidney Yang presents with coldness of the limbs, cramps in the lower abdomen, urinary disturbance, palpitations and shortness of breath. The tongue is swollen with a slippery, white coating, and the pulse is thin and weak.

The Organs associated with Phlegm are the Lung, Spleen and Kidney. They control the transportation and distribution of water. When their function is impaired, water may accumulate, giving rise to Phlegm.

With respect to treatment, points are chosen in accordance with the Organ(-s) affected, as well as the location of the Phlegm. For example, to treat Phlegm in the chest, the principle is to clear the Lung and transform the Phlegm. Among the points that may be used are B-13 *(fei shu)*, LI-4 *(he gu)*, CV-12 *(zhong wan)* and S-40 *(feng long)*. For Phlegm in the Spleen and Stomach, the principle is to strengthen the Spleen to transform the Phlegm. Points such as CV-12 *(zhong wan)*, P-6 *(nei guan)*, S-36 *(zu san li)*, S-40 *(feng long)*, Sp-1 *(yin bai)*, Sp-6 *(san yin jiao)*, B-20 *(pi shu)* and B-21 *(wei shu)* are utilized.

It should also be noted that Phlegm affects the flow of Qi, and that in protracted cases, Phlegm may transform into Heat. The treatment strategy should take these factors into account as well. □

Wind-Stroke
(Sequelae of Cerebrovascular Accident)

Zhòng Fēng 中风

Zhou, male, 57 years old. The patient's history was recounted by his son. The patient was found to have hypertension 3 years ago. Since that time, his blood pressure fluctuated between 180/100 and 210/120mm Hg. For 2 weeks before coming to the hospital, he suffered from dizziness, blurred vision, light-headedness, numbness of the fingertips and a feeling of heaviness in the limbs. One day during the second week, the patient suddenly fell and became comatose. He was then taken to the hospital.

Upon examination at the hospital, the patient's blood pressure was found to be 200/120mm Hg. The diagnosis was cerebral vascular accident secondary to hypertension. Sodium nitroprusside was administered by intravenous drip, and his blood pressure was reduced slightly to 200/110mm Hg. However, seven days later he was still disoriented. His speech was extremely slurred, with a loud, rattling sound in his throat, as if a foreign substance were lodged in it. He had complete dysphagia to the point that even a mouthful of fluid would bring about spasmodic coughing and vomiting. His blood pressure was still high at this time, measuring 190/110mm Hg.

Further inquiry revealed that the patient's urine was scanty and deep yellow in color, and that his stools were dry and infrequent. His pulse was wiry and slippery, and he had a stiff tongue with a yellow, greasy coating.

SYNDROME DIFFERENTIATION

In Chinese medicine, strokes are sometimes named according to their causal factor; thus, there is Wind-stroke, Summer Heat-stroke, etc. This patient's condition, beginning with dizziness, light-headedness, blurred vision, numbness of the fingertips and heaviness of the limbs, and followed by sudden loss of consciousness, falls in the category of Wind-stroke. It is the result of extreme disharmony between the Yin and Yang of the Liver, whereby Liver Yang surges upward, and together with Phlegm, obstructs the channels and the senses. In this case, Phlegm arose because Heat (Liver Yang) congealed the Fluids into Phlegm. Because the Spleen's transporting function was disturbed by the ascending Liver Yang, Phlegm accumulated.

Wind-stroke is further subdivided into channel-stroke and Organ-stroke. The former is an early (and therefore milder) stage of the disorder, and the symptoms are mostly limited to the trunk and extremities; consciousness remains intact. In the latter type, the condition is grave, with loss of consciousness; even with appropriate treatment, mental deterioration is apparent.

This case was one of Organ-stroke. The acute types of Organ-stroke are differentiated as 'closed' (hyperspastic) and 'abandoned' (atonic). Besides unconsciousness, in Wind-stroke of the closed type the patient has clenched hands and teeth, a red face and feverish body, snoring, rattling in the throat, scanty, yellow urine, and constipation. In abandoned-type Wind-stroke, the symptoms include closed eyes, open mouth and hands, a pale face, weak breathing, and incontinence of urine and stool.

This patient presented with unconsciousness associated with slurred speech, rattling in the throat, difficulty in swallowing, deep yellow urine, and constipation. These were all signs of excess. The syndrome was therefore Wind-stroke of the closed type due to ascendance of Liver Yang and accumulation of Phlegm, which obstructed the senses.

TREATMENT

The principles of treatment were to pacify the Liver, extinguish the Wind, resolve the Phlegm, clear the senses, open the 'closed' symptoms and restore speech.

Points selected:

GV-20 *(bai hui)*, Liv-3 *(tai chong)*, K-1 *(yong quan)*, CV-22 *(tian tu)*, S-40 *(feng long)*, P-6 *(nei guan)*, L-11 *(shao shang)*, H-5 *(tong li)*, CV-23 *(lian quan)*

A pyramid needle was used to prick GV-20 *(bai hui)*, K-1 *(yong quan)*, L-11 *(shao shang)* and Liv-3 *(tai chong)*. These points were superficially punctured to let out a few drops of blood. Filiform needles were used at all other points, which were drained.

Discussion of points:

Needling GV-20 *(bai hui)* pacifies the Liver, extinguishes Wind and clears the senses. Liv-3 *(tai chong)*, the transporting point of the Liver channel, also pacifies the Liver and extinguishes Wind. CV-22 *(tian tu)* and CV-23 *(lian quan)* are effective in resolving Phlegm and opening the closed symptoms in order to clear the throat and restore speech. S-40 *(feng long)*, the connecting point of the Stomach channel, is also effective in resolving Phlegm. P-6 *(nei guan)* calms the Spirit, regulates Qi, resolves Phlegm, clears the senses, and is used symptomatically for difficulty in swallowing. H-5 *(tong li)* calms the Spirit and regulates Heart Qi. It is particularly effective in treating stiffness of the tongue, and is frequently used for slurred speech due to Wind-stroke.

K-1 *(yong quan)*, the well point of the Kidney channel, has the functions of reviving from fainting, clearing Heat and pacifying the Liver. L-11 *(shao shang)*, the well point of the Lung channel, also revives from fainting and clears the throat. These two points are quite painful when needled. The pain, however, clears the senses and raises the Spirit. They are therefore frequently used in treating the comatose, and patients with impaired mental function.

RESULTS

Two hours after needling, some improvement was noted in the rattling in the throat and the movement of the tongue, as well as in the mental state of the patient. He could also swallow liquids. The next morning, the patient was able to utter simple sentences, and reported that the sensation of obstruction in his throat had diminished. His blood pressure was then found to be 180/100mm Hg.

Because consciousness was fully restored, GV-20 *(bai hui)*, K-1 *(yong quan)* and L-11 *(shao shang)* were discontinued. A filiform needle was substituted for the pyramid needle at Liv-3 *(tai chong)* to drain the excess Yang.

Two new points, H-7 *(shen men)* and K-6 *(zhao hai)*, were then added to the prescription. H-7 *(shen men)* clears the Heart channel and is used in treating diseases of the Spirit and mind. K-6 *(zhao hai)* clears the Kidney channel and nourishes Yin. Because the Heart 'opens' through the tongue, and the Kidney channel courses along the throat and terminates at the root of the tongue, stimulation of these two points also relieves stiffness of the tongue. H-7 *(shen men)* and K-6 *(zhao hai)* were tonified, because even though ascendant Liver Yang and the abundance of Phlegm are manifestations of excess, deficiency of Heart and Kidney Yin was the root of this condition. In cases of this type, Chinese medicine emphasizes that the acute symptoms should be treated first, and then the root cause. After the patient had regained consciousness, it was therefore appropriate to add H-7 *(shen men)* and K-6 *(zhao hai)* to nourish the Heart and Kidney Yin.

After five daily treatments with this modified prescription, the stiffness of the tongue was resolved, his speech became clearer, and he could swallow without difficulty. His mental acuity was by then fully restored.

Seven more treatments were administered to consolidate the therapeutic effect, and treatment was then discontinued. During a three-month follow-up, the condition remained stable.

Note: The causal factor in both this and the following case was Yin deficiency, which led to ascendant Liver Yang, and thus Wind-stroke. In the present case, the patient had lost consciousness. Treatment was therefore initially aimed at restoring consciousness (opening the senses). Once consciousness was restored, treatment was then focused upon resolving the root, or causal factor.

Unlike the present case, in which the patient was first seen one week following the onset of Wind-stroke, the patient in the following case was first seen six months post-stroke. The patient in the present case underwent fourteen treatments, after which the symptoms were alleviated. The patient in the following case, on the other hand, required forty-four treatments before limb function was essentially restored. This underscores the rule that the sooner therapy is begun following onset of Wind-stroke, the faster and better the recovery.

In China at the present time, acupuncture is recognized as an accepted therapy in stroke rehabilitation, and there are no stroke-related conditions for which it is contraindicated. □

Wind-Stroke
(Sequelae of Cerebrovascular Accident)

Zhòng Fēng 中风

Cao, male, 61 years old. The patient had suffered from hypertension with dizziness and headache for over 10 years. Six months ago, following a moment of over-excitement, he was suddenly afflicted with motor disturbance of the right arm and leg, accompanied by slurred speech, pulling of the corner of the mouth to the left, and drooling. He was admitted to a hospital and diagnosed as having suffered cerebral thrombosis. After treatment with a combination of traditional Chinese and western medicine for 2 months, the condition was stabilized. The patient was discharged from the hospital and referred to our acupuncture clinic for further treatment. He did not come to the clinic, however, until 4 months later, when he realized that his condition was not getting any better by itself.

On his first visit, the patient complained of light-headedness, palpitations and insomnia. His speech was impaired, and the corner of his mouth was drawn to the left. There was paresis of the extremities on the right, with myodynamia (muscular strength) of grade 2 (out of 5) in the arm, and grade 3 in the leg. He could not move the fingers of his right hand, nor could he stand or walk. The leg muscles showed increased tonus. The tongue was red, and the pulse was wiry, thin and slippery.

SYNDROME DIFFERENTIATION

In Chinese medicine, diseases manifested primarily by sudden onset of drawing at the corner of the mouth to one side, inability to move the arm and leg on one side, and difficulty in articulating speech are attributed to movement of internal Wind of the Liver. In this case, the accompanying symptoms of dizziness and headache indicated deficiency of Kidney Yin, which led to deficiency of Liver Yin, and in turn caused the ascending of Liver Yang. The ascending Liver Yang transformed into internally-generated Wind. The emotional excitement triggered an upward surge of this internal Wind, and led to a rebellious flow of Qi and Blood upward, which obstructed the channels in the head, and caused light-headedness. Heat in the form of Liver Yang caused the Fluids to congeal into Phlegm, and because the Spleen's

147

transporting function was disturbed by the hyperactive Liver Yang, the Phlegm stagnated. Stagnation of Wind-Phlegm in the channels impeded the circulation of Qi and Blood in the extremities, thus depriving them of vigor and nourishment, and causing their immobility. Stagnation of Wind-Phlegm in the channels of the head also caused the mouth to slant awry. The ascendant Liver Yang induced Fire of the Heart to flare upward, resulting in palpitations and insomnia. The red tongue, and the wiry, thin and slippery pulse were further signs that this case was one of ascendant Liver Yang, and obstruction of the channels by Wind-Phlegm.

TREATMENT

Treatment was directed at nourishing the Yin to check the ascendant Liver Yang, and resolving the Phlegm in order to remove the obstruction from the channels.

Points selected:

G-20 *(feng chi)* bilaterally, CV-23 *(lian quan)*, S-4 *(di cang)*, S-6 *(jia che)*, LI-15 *(jian yu)*, LI-11 *(qu chi)*, LI-4 *(he gu)*, M-UE-22 *(ba xie)*, S-31 *(bi guan)*, S-32 *(fu tu)*, S-36 *(zu san li)*, S-40 *(feng long)*, S-41 *(jie xi)*, Sp-6 *(san yin jiao)*, Liv-3 *(tai chong)*

All but the first point were needled on the right side only in accordance with the principle of local point selection. Balanced tonifying-draining manipulation was used. Treatment was administered once daily.

Discussion of points:

The key to treatment in this case was in subduing the ascendant Liver Yang, and the resulting internal Wind. G-20 *(feng chi)* is an important point for dispelling Wind. Because this function was so important in this case, this point was needled bilaterally. CV-23 *(lian quan)* is primarily used for conditions of the throat, and for slurred speech.

Sp-6 *(san yin jiao)* is the point of intersection of the three leg Yin channels. Liv-3 *(tai chong)* is the transporting point of the Liver channel. Using these two points together has the effect of nourishing the Yin to check the ascendant Liver Yang.

LI-15 *(jian yu)*, LI-11 *(qu chi)* and LI-4 *(he gu)* are important points on the arm Yang Brightness (Large Intestine) channel, and S-4 *(di cang)*, S-6 *(jia che)*, S-31 *(bi guan)*, S-32 *(fu tu)*, S-36 *(zu san li)*, S-40 *(feng long)* and S-41 *(jie xi)* are all major points on the leg Yang Brightness (Stomach) channel. The Yang Brightness channels are abundant in Qi and Blood. The extremities must be supplied with Qi and Blood from the Yang Brightness channels in order to properly function. In patients afflicted with hemiplegia, needling points on the Yang Brightness channels helps regulate the flow of Qi and Blood, nourishes the limbs, and resolves stagnation in the channels. S-4 *(di cang)* and S-6 *(jia che)* are used primarily for clearing the channels of the face, and are important points for treating the pulling at the corner of the mouth and of the eyes, which are symptoms associated with hemiplegia. M-UE-22 *(ba xie)* is a set of points specifically used for immobility of the finger joints.

Points on the head and face were needled first, followed by those on the arm, and then the leg. Points on the arm were treated sequentially from LI-15 *(jian yu)*, progressing downward along the channel. Points on the leg were needled in the same manner. The sequential treatment of points on a limb was performed by the relay method to clear the channel. Thus, LI-15 *(jian yu)* was needled so that the needle sensation was transmitted to LI-11 *(qu chi)*, and then LI-11 *(qu chi)* was needled so that the needle sensation reached LI-4 *(he gu)*. The same method was used on the leg, i.e., in the order of S-31 *(bi guan)*, S-32 *(fu tu)*, S-36 *(zu san li)* and S-41 *(jie xi)*. The relay method is very effective in resolving obstruction of the channels, and is thus useful in treating hemiplegia.

RESULTS

After 20 daily treatments, the pulling at the corner of the mouth was improved. Myodynamia in the affected limbs was also improved, from grade 2 to grade 3 in the arm, and from grade 3 to grade 4 in the leg. The patient could walk slowly with the aid of a cane. Treatment was suspended for 1 week because of a cold. A cold is an external excess, and in this case was a new, compounding condition which might have influenced the efficacy of treatment if the needling were continued with the same set of points. In such cases, acupuncture may be suspended to allow the cold to run its course, or to allow treatment with medication. Alternatively, a new set of points may be selected to treat the cold.

Two weeks after treatment was resumed, the nasolabial grooves became symmetrical, and the actions of the muscles at the corners of the mouth were restored. Myodynamia in the arm reached grade 4, and that in the leg returned to normal. However, the patient was still unable to freely move the distal joints in the affected arm.

Since the condition had already improved significantly, the points on the head, face and leg, as well as LI-15 *(jian yu)* and LI-11 *(qu chi)* on the arm, were dropped. In their place, a new set of points was selected to open the channels at the distal end of the affected arm: TB-5 *(wai guan)*, LI-5 *(yang xi)*, LI-4 *(he gu)*, SI-3 *(hou xi)*, TB-4 *(yang chi)* and M-UE-22 *(ba xie)*. These points were needled once daily for ten days, after which normal movement of the right arm and fingers was essentially restored. Treatment was then terminated, and the patient was advised to continue physical therapy exercises at home. Follow-up six months later found the patient's condition to be stable. □

Wind-Stroke
(Wallenberg's Syndrome)

Zhòng Fēng 中风

Li, male, 65 years old. Symptoms of dizziness, vomiting with hiccough, hoarseness and difficulty in swallowing appeared abruptly 1 year ago. At the time of onset, there was no loss of
consciousness, and the patient remained ambulant. He was diagnosed as having suffered a cerebral infarction resulting in Wallenberg's syndrome. After 1 month's treatment, the vomiting,
dizziness and hiccough subsided, but there was no improvement in the hoarseness and difficulty in swallowing. He was treated for several months with herbs for invigorating the Blood,
but with no apparent improvement. The patient decided to try acupuncture.

The four examinations of Chinese medicine found the patient to be emaciated, with
a blank expression, and a low, hoarse voice.
He was ambulant, and could move his arms
freely. The patient was on a liquid diet because of the difficulty in swallowing, which
was accompanied by frequent coughing and
choking. At times, intravenous feeding was
required to maintain nutrition. The tongue
was slightly purple with a greasy, white coating. The pulse was wiry and slippery.

SYNDROME DIFFERENTIATION

This disease pertains to the channel-stroke
type of Wind-stroke. According to the classics, "By age 40, Yin is naturally reduced by
half" (*Simple Questions*, chapter 5). This
process of aging can result in ascendant
Liver Yang, which transforms into Wind that
disturbs the senses (also known as the upper
orifices) and the Brain. Another cause of
Wind-stroke is when, from excessive eating
or over-indulgence of alcohol, food and
water accumulate, and fail to transform into
nutrient Essence. Instead, they transform
into Phlegm, which obstructs the channels.
Circulation of Qi and Blood are thus hindered, giving rise to this condition.

This patient admitted to overindulgence
of alcohol. The dizziness, vomiting, hoarseness, difficulty in swallowing and wiry pulse
were signs of upward disturbance by Liver
Wind. The slippery pulse and the greasy
tongue coating indicated the presence of
Phlegm. The slightly purple tongue signified
long-term Qi deficiency from a protracted
disease, and Blood stasis.

As this was a case of channel-stroke, the following channels were affected: the Governing vessel, which travels up the spinal cord to GV-16 *(feng fu)*, and there enters the Brain; the Bladder channel, which enters the Brain at the vertex of the head; the Conception vessel, which passes through the throat region; and the branch of the Stomach channel which starts at S-5 *(da ying)* and ends at S-9 *(ren ying)*, passing through the throat region.

TREATMENT

The principles of treatment were to subdue the Wind and resolve the Phlegm, and to clear the channels to facilitate the circulation of Qi and Blood.

Points selected:

GV-20 *(bai hui)*, B-7 *(tong tian)*, GV-19 *(hou ding)*, GV-15 *(ya men)*, GV-16 *(feng fu)*, G-20 *(feng chi)*, CV-23 *(lian quan)*, S-9 *(ren ying)*, CV-22 *(tian tu)*, Liv-3 *(tai chong)*

Balanced tonifying-draining manipulation through raise-thrust and twirling techniques was applied at all points, except where otherwise indicated below. Treatment was administered daily, and the needles were retained for 20 minutes during each session.

Discussion of points:

GV-20 *(bai hui)* is used in the treatment of Wind-stroke because of its location at the vertex, below which is the Brain; needling this point thus clears the Brain. The combination of this point with B-7 *(tong tian)* and GV-19 *(hou ding)* regulates the Qi and Blood of the head, and opens the senses. The combination of GV-16 *(feng fu)*, the 'residence of Wind', with G-20 *(feng chi)*, the 'pool of Wind', subdues the Wind. Liv-3 *(tai chong)* was also chosen to subdue the Liver Wind. GV-15 *(ya men)* and CV-23 *(lian quan)* are important points for treating hoarseness. S-9 *(ren ying)* is effective for treating difficulty in swallowing.

Needle insertion at GV-20 *(bai hui)*, B-7 *(tong tian)* and GV-19 *(hou ding)* was oblique to a depth of about 0.5 unit. Slight twirling was applied, which produced a local sensation of distention. GV-16 *(feng fu)* and GV-15 *(ya men)* were needled to a depth of 1 unit. The needles were raise-thrust and twirled slightly, which produced a sensation of local distention and soreness. Needle insertion at G-20 *(feng chi)* was directed toward the opposite eye to a depth of 1.2 units. The needle sensation was transmitted to the same side of the head, and to the orbit.

At CV-23 *(lian quan)* the needle was directed toward the base of the tongue to a depth of 1.3 units. This produced a sensation of soreness and distention at the root of the tongue. At S-9 *(ren ying)* the needle was inserted perpendicularly 1.2 units deep; care was taken to avoid piercing the carotid artery. The needle sensation at this point traveled up and down the channel. Needle manipulation was avoided. At CV-22 *(tian tu)* the needle was introduced along the posterior surface of the sternum to a depth of 1.5 units. Manipulation was also avoided at this point. Insertion of the needle produced a feeling of painful distention below the Adam's apple, and behind the sternum.

RESULTS

After ten treatments, the family reported improvement in the patient's coughing and choking, and the patient was able to eat soft food; however, the hoarseness remained. The patient received further treatment once every two days, for a total of thirty-two treatments. By this time, the patient himself reported that the coughing and choking were very infrequent, and that soft food was tolerable. The intravenous feeding was therefore dispensed with. There was also improvement in the hoarseness. Because the patient wished to return home, herbs were prescribed for use at home to further resolve the Phlegm and clear the channels. He did not return to the clinic thereafter.

Note: Compared with the two previous cases, this patient's condition was protracted (one year's duration). Even after thirty-two treatments, although most of his symptoms had resolved, he still experienced some hoarseness. In treating stroke victims, therapy should therefore begin as early as possible to achieve the best results. □

CHAPTER THREE
Pain

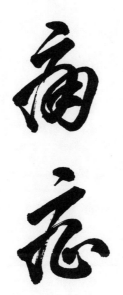

Crane's Knee Wind
(Rheumatoid Arthritis)

Hè Xī Fēng 鹤膝风

Li, male, 42 years old. The patient first noticed swelling and pain in both knees 3 years ago. The condition worsened over the course of time, to the extent that movement of the knees was restricted, and the patient was unable to stand erect. The condition was diagnosed at another hospital as rheumatoid arthritis. Various methods to treat the condition were tried, including Chinese herbs, anti-inflammatory agents and acupuncture, but without success. The patient was then referred to this clinic as a last resort.

Examination revealed swelling and pain in both knees, but the overlying skin was not edematous, nor was it particularly tight or tender to the touch. Movement was restricted, with flexion limited to 90°, and there was an inability to fully extend the knees. There was frank atrophy of the quadriceps, such that the knees resembled those of a crane. The patient's complexion was pasty. Urine and stools were normal. The patient was sensitive to cold, and the legs below the knees were cold to the touch. The tongue was pale and swollen, and the coating was thin and white. The pulse was thin and deficient.

X-ray showed periarticular osteoporosis of both knees, but no erosion of the bony substance. Laboratory tests showed Hgb 7.8g, ESR 26mm/hr, and antistreptolysin 'O' titer within normal range. A chest X-ray was negative.

SYNDROME DIFFERENTIATION

In Chinese medicine, painful obstruction results when external pathogenic influences take advantage of a condition of deficiency and invade the body. In this case, the invasion was one of Damp-Cold. Dampness caused the swelling and pain, and the limitation in movement. Cold caused contraction, and interfered with the Blood supply in the affected areas. The obstruction to the flow of Qi and Blood gave rise to pain and muscular atrophy. Because the swelling and atrophy caused the knees to resemble those of cranes, the ancient Chinese referred to this type of condition as 'crane's knee Wind.'

The other symptoms, including the pasty complexion, sensitivity to cold, coldness in the legs, the pale tongue with a thin, white coating, and the thin, deficient pulse, were all manifestations of Kidney Yang deficiency. This condition renders an individual more susceptible to invasion by Damp-Cold. Externally-contracted conditions in those with Kidney Yang deficiency tend to localize in the lower back or lower extremities. The patient's condition was therefore one of Kidney Yang deficiency, resulting in Damp-Cold lodging in the knees.

TREATMENT

Treatment was aimed at warming the Kidney and supplementing the Kidney Yang, resolving the Cold and dispelling the Dampness.

Points selected:

B-11 *(da zhu)*, B-17 *(ge shu)*, B-23 *(shen shu)*, GV-4 *(ming men)*, CV-6 *(qi hai)*, Sp-10 *(xue hai)*, M-LE-27 *(he ding)*, S-35 *(du bi)*, M-LE-16 *(xi yan)*, S-34 *(liang qiu)*, G-34 *(yang ling quan)*, Sp-9 *(yin ling quan)*

Treatment was administered on alternating days, and the needles were retained for 20 minutes during each session. There was an intermission of 5 days after every 2 weeks of treatment. Tonifying manipulation was utilized at all points, and warm needle moxibustion was applied at B-23 *(shen shu)*, GV-4 *(ming men)*, M-LE-27 *(he ding)*, S-35 *(du bi)* and M-LE-16 *(xi yan)*.

Discussion of points:

B-11 *(da zhu)* is the meeting point of the bones, and is indicated for diseases of the joints. B-17 *(ge shu)* is the meeting point of Blood; needling this point tonifies and in-vigorates the Blood, thereby improving the circulation in the affected areas, and promoting the dispersion of Damp-Cold.

B-23 *(shen shu)*, GV-4 *(ming men)* and CV-6 *(qi hai)* were chosen to regulate the Kidney, supplement the Kidney Yang and facilitate the dispersion of Damp-Cold. The Kidney controls the bones. When the Kidney is strong, diseases of the bones and joints heal rapidly.

The local points were chosen to promote the local circulation of Qi and Blood in order to reduce the swelling and pain.

RESULTS

Marked improvement was observed after three months of treatment. The swelling subsided, the range of motion increased, the coldness of the lower extremities diminished, and the pulse became stronger. Because the condition was responding well, treatment was continued with the same set of points, and the same combination of needling and moxibustion. After three more months of treatment, the swelling of the knees was alleviated, and full flexion and extension were almost completely restored, although there was still occasional stiffness. The leg muscles had increased in size, and both the sensitivity to cold as well as the coldness in the lower extremities had disappeared. The complexion and the tongue appeared normal, and the pulse was moderately strong. Laboratory tests showed Hgb 9.8g. X-rays of the knees were normal. The patient was followed up for six months, with no recurrence of symptoms. □

Facial Pain
(Trigeminal Neuralgia)

Tóu Tòng 头痛

Qiu, male, 47 years old. The patient had suffered from pain on the right side of his face for 7 years. He consulted many doctors for help, but to no avail. On one occasion, the pain was mistaken for a dental condition, and a lower molar was extracted; the pain, however, was not relieved at all. After the condition was correctly diagnosed as trigeminal neuralgia, block therapy was administered several times, but provided only temporary relief. About 2 weeks before he came to the acupuncture clinic, recurrence of the condition was induced by exposure to a draft. The patient began experiencing paroxysmal attacks of pain on the right side of his face. Several dozen episodes occurred each day, and the pain was unbearable. Even intramuscular injections of meperidine provided only temporary relief.

At the clinic, the patient held his head and face in agony with his hands, and rushed time and again toward a wall to bump his head against it. He was disheveled, and the right side of his face was streaked with tears. Saliva flowed continuously from his mouth. A trigger point was found on the right temple at M-HN-9 *(tai yang)*, and there was a burning sensation over the painful area. Other symptoms included yellow urine, a red tongue with a thin, yellow coating, and a wiry and rapid pulse.

SYNDROME DIFFERENTIATION

In traditional Chinese medicine, trigeminal neuralgia is regarded as a type of facial pain manifested primarily by spasmodic pain in the cheek. It is most frequently seen in the 40-60 year-old age group. This condition is attributed to one of the following patterns:

- Wind-Cold attacking the Yang Brightness channels (Large Intestine and Stomach), and the muscles along these channels. Cold has a constricting nature; when it strikes the channels and muscles, it causes them to constrict. The flow of Qi and Blood is thus obstructed, leading to pain. A patient presenting with this pattern usually suffers from severe pain when exposed to cold, which is generally relieved by warmth. Accompanying symptoms include thin nasal discharge, a white tongue coating, and a floating pulse.

- Wind-Heat attacking the channels and muscles of the face. This impedes the flow of Qi and Blood, resulting in pain. Other symptoms include a burning sensation at the site of pain, salivation, tearing, aggravation of symptoms when exposed to heat, a thin, yellow tongue coating, and a wiry, rapid pulse.

- Emotional disturbance such as excessive worry or anger which impairs the Liver and causes stagnation of Liver Qi. Over a period of time, the stagnant Liver Qi transforms into Fire which blazes upward, causing pain in the face. Distinguishing symptoms include irritability, restlessness, dizziness, flushed face, a bitter taste in the mouth, hypochondrial pain, a red tongue with a yellow coating, and a thin, wiry pulse.

This patient suffered from facial pain of several years' duration which had been induced by exposure to a draft. The pain was unbearable and was accompanied by such Heat symptoms as a burning sensation in the affected area, a red tongue with a thin, yellow coating, and a wiry, rapid pulse. The diagnosis was accordingly facial pain caused by invasion of the face by Wind-Heat.

TREATMENT

A passage in *Simple Questions* (chapter 54) instructs: "When the flow of Qi and Blood is impeded and the channels are obstructed, bleeding should be effected by needling." Because the present case was one in which the flow of Qi and Blood was obstructed, bloodletting was indicated. This was accomplished through rapid prickings which were performed with a pyramid needle.

Points selected for bloodletting:

TB-18 *(qi mai)*, the 12 well points, M-HN-9 *(tai yang)*

Discussion of points:

TB-18 *(qi mai)* lies in the center of the mastoid process in back of the ear. It belongs to the Triple Burner channel, which has an internal branch that traverses the ear and cheek. It was pricked to a depth of 0.2-0.3 unit, and 0.5cc of purple-black blood was expelled. The expulsion of the dark, stagnant blood opened and regulated the flow of Qi in the channels of the ear and face.

The 12 well points are located at the ends of the fingers and toes, and are commonly used for bloodletting. Stimulating these points regulates the Qi of the 12 primary channels, and conforms to the treatment principle of selecting points which are remote from the site of the disease. In this case, the well points were pricked to a depth of 0.1 unit, and squeezed until the dark blood turned bright red. The trigger point, M-HN-9 *(tai yang)*, was the site at which the obstructed Qi and Blood had concentrated. It was pricked to a depth of 0.2 unit, and 1cc of purple-black blood was expelled.

Only by combining local points with those which were remote from the site of the disease could the flow of Qi and Blood be freed of obstruction, thus eliminating the pain. Although bloodletting at these points helped promote the flow of Qi and Blood, it could not eliminate the pathogenic Wind-Heat. Other points were therefore added for this purpose.

Points selected for needling:

GV-16 *(feng fu)*, G-20 *(feng chi)*, LI-4 *(he gu)* and L-7 *(lie que)* were needled bilaterally, and TB-17 *(yi feng)* was needled on the right side alone.

Discussion of points:

G-20 *(feng chi)* and GV-16 *(feng fu)* are both important points for dispelling Wind. TB-17 *(yi feng)* was used to disperse the Wind-Heat which had accumulated in the head and face. LI-4 *(he gu)* and L-7 *(lie que)* are two of the 'four dominant points' which were found by the ancients to have a wide variety of applications (see Introduction). A rhyme in the book, *Gatherings From Outstanding Acupuncturists,* reads: "The face and the mouth are governed by *he gu.* / For the head and the neck, there is *lie que* to resort to." As the rhyme suggests, these two points are effective in treating diseases of the face, mouth, head and neck. The use of these points in this case removed the stagnation of Qi and Blood in the channels of the head and face. The needles were pointed obliquely upward (proximally), which induced an upward-radiating needle sensation.

Because the condition here was one of excess, draining manipulation was applied, using raise-thrust and twirling techniques. And because the pain was quite severe, the needles were retained for one hour during each treatment to enhance the therapeutic effect.

RESULTS

During the first treatment of bloodletting and acupuncture, the pain gradually subsided. In fact, it had already become tolerable before the needles were removed. Over the next five days, bloodletting and acupuncture were administered once daily, and the condition continued to improve. The period between attacks increased to as long as one day, but the pain recurred, especially when the trigger point was irritated. It was suggested that the bloodletting may have been too frequent at the outset. Because the condition of the patient had already improved, the frequency of bloodletting was reduced to every other day, while needling was continued on a daily basis.

After six more days of treatment, the pain basically disappeared; nor did tapping the trigger point precipitate a recurrence. To consolidate the therapeutic effect, needling was continued once every other day for two weeks, by which time the pain was eliminated. The patient was followed up for two years, with no recurrence of symptoms. □

Headache from Phlegm-Dampness

Tóu Tòng 头痛

Liu, male, 57 years old. The patient suffered from episodes of head and neck pain, and a heavy feeling in the head, for more than 3 years. Two months ago, he was admitted to a hospital because the condition had worsened. The accompanying symptoms included constant fatigue, general weakness, tinnitus in the left ear, and fullness in the chest and epigastrium. He had sputum in the throat that was difficult to expectorate, halitosis, and recurring oral ulcers. His appetite was normal. Stools were loose and unformed. He had dribbling of urine, which was slightly yellow in color, and had a foul odor. The tongue was red, with a thin coating in the front, but a yellow, greasy coating in the middle. The pulse was soggy. The patient was diagnosed as having cerebral arteriosclerosis, deficient blood supply from the vertebrobasilar artery, cervical spine disease and hyperlipemia. No improvement was observed after 2 months in the hospital. The patient thereupon turned to acupuncture therapy.

SYNDROME DIFFERENTIATION

The head is regarded as the confluence of all the Yang channels. The Qi and Blood of all the Organs also meet in the head. Therefore, invasion by external Wind-Cold, Wind-Heat or Wind-Dampness, or damage to the Organs caused by internal factors, may all induce headache.

A headache of external origin is characterized by sudden onset, and is accompanied by signs of an exterior condition. A headache of internal origin is characterized by slow onset and long duration, with manifestations of disturbance of the internal Organs.

This patient's headache was one of internal origin, as evidenced by the lack of exterior symptoms, and by the presence of tinnitus, and fullness in the chest and epigastrium.

Headaches of internal origin are of three types: ascendant Liver Yang, Phlegm-Dampness, and Blood stasis. This patient's headache was accompanied by a feeling of heaviness in the head, which is characteristic of Dampness. Long-standing, stagnant Phlegm-Dampness transforms into Heat, which attacks the head and keeps the clear Yang away. This leads to headache and a feeling of heaviness in the head, tinnitus, fatigue, and a dry mouth with foul breath. Stagnant Phlegm-Dampness also causes fullness in the chest and epigastrium, unformed stools, and dribbling, foul-smelling urine. A red tongue with a greasy, yellow coating, and a soggy pulse are also indicative of Phlegm-Dampness. The diagnosis was therefore headache due to long-standing Phlegm-Dampness, which had transformed into Heat.

TREATMENT

The Spleen is the source of Phlegm. The function of the Spleen is to transform and transport food and water. When the Spleen fails to function properly, food and water will aggregate to form Phlegm. The principle of treatment in this case was therefore to strengthen the function of the Spleen in order to resolve the Phlegm and clear the Heat.

Points selected:

GV-20 *(bai hui)*, M-HN-9 *(tai yang)*, G-20 *(feng chi)*, P-6 *(nei guan)*, Sp-4 *(gong sun)*, Sp-9 *(yin ling quan)*, S-40 *(feng long)*, LI-11 *(qu chi)*, S-44 *(nei ting)*, S-36 *(zu san li)*

Treatment was administered once daily.

Discussion of points:

GV-20 *(bai hui)* and M-HN-9 *(tai yang)* are local points for treating headache. G-20 *(feng chi)* is located near the base of the skull, and is especially useful for head and neck pain. P-6 *(nei guan)* and Sp-4 *(gong sun)* may be used for treating diseases of the chest, Heart and Stomach, and are often chosen to regulate the functions of the Spleen and Stomach. Sp-9 *(yin ling quan)* is an important point for dispelling Dampness. S-40 *(feng long)* is used primarily for resolving Phlegm. LI-11 *(qu chi)* is effective for clearing Heat. S-44 *(nei ting)* is the gushing point of the Stomach channel; gushing points are used to regulate Heat in the body. The combination of S-44 *(nei ting)*, Sp-9 *(yin ling quan)*, S-40 *(feng long)* and LI-11 *(qu chi)* has the ef-

fect of dispelling Dampness, resolving Phlegm and clearing Heat.

S-36 *(zu san li)* is the lower uniting point of the Stomach, and is often used to strengthen the Spleen.

The signs and symptoms of the patient were those of excess due to internal obstruction by Phlegm-Dampness, hence draining manipulation was used at G-20 *(feng chi)*, Sp-9 *(yin ling quan)*, S-40 *(feng long)*, LI-11 *(qu chi)* and S-44 *(nei ting)*. The needles were inserted quickly, retained for 20 minutes, and then slowly withdrawn. The other points in the prescription were needled with balanced tonifying-draining manipulation. M-HN-9 *(tai yang)* was needled perpendicularly with a 1-unit needle, which produced a sensation of local soreness and distention.

RESULTS

The pain in the neck disappeared after three treatments. The headache also diminished, but the other symptoms persisted. G-20 *(feng chi)* was then dropped. Needling of the other points was continued for ten more days until the oral ulcers and halitosis were alleviated. However, the tinnitus, heavy feeling in the head, and sputum in the throat were still not relieved. Therefore, three more points were added: M-HN-1 *(si shen cong)* for heaviness in the head, SI-19 *(ting gong)* for tinnitus, and CV-22 *(tian tu)* for sputum in the throat.

Daily treatment was continued with the modified point prescription for another two weeks, with marked improvement in the symptoms. During this time, the yellow tongue coating disappeared. The frequency of treatment was then reduced to once every other day. After ten more treatments, all of the symptoms disappeared, and the treatment was terminated. The patient returned three months later for a check-up, and reported that he had experienced no further headaches. ☐

Headache from Stagnation of Qi and Blood

Tóu Tòng 头痛

Li, female, 30 years old. Five years ago after catching a cold post partum, the patient suffered a severe headache which lasted several hours. Medication temporarily relieved the symptoms, but the headache occurred frequently thereafter, particularly on windy or rainy days, or after physical exertion. Analgesic tablets were usually sufficient to relieve the symptoms. During the past year, however, the headaches increased in frequency, and occurred on almost a daily basis for several hours in the forehead and on both sides of the head. The pain was stabbing in nature, and the patient would often press her head against the wall until a double dose of analgesic tablets eased the pain. Vitamins and herbs were prescribed, but with no apparent effect. A particularly severe headache occurred 3 days ago after physical exertion, accompanied by intense nausea. A double dose of analgesic tablets did not help, and meperidine was effective for only a few hours. The patient then came to the acupuncture clinic.

The patient's demeanor was gloomy. Her head was wrapped with a piece of cloth to shield her from drafts and light. She was tired, restless and irritable. Her tongue was light red with a thin, white coating, and her pulse was wiry.

SYNDROME DIFFERENTIATION

The onset of this patient's condition occurred post partum, after an attack by Wind. Deficiency of Qi and Blood is very common in post partum women if proper care is not taken. At this time, external pathogenic influences can easily invade the body and obstruct the channels, which causes pain. Because the nature of Wind is to float upward, the upper part of the body is often the target of invasion by pathogenic Wind. The top of the forehead is traversed by a branch of the leg Yang Brightness (Stomach) channel, and the sides of the head by the Lesser Yang (Triple Burner and Gall Bladder) channels. When Wind resides in the Yang Brightness and Lesser Yang channels, pain will occur in the forehead and the sides of the head.

In this patient, the condition was first induced by Wind, thus the headaches often recurred when she was exposed to wind. On rainy days, Qi and Blood have a tendency to flow less freely in the channels. Physical exhaustion depletes the Qi, which reduces its capacity to impel the flow of Blood. This in turn results in stagnation and pain. It is for these reasons that the patient's headaches often occurred on rainy days, or after physical exertion.

When Qi in the leg Yang Brightness (Stomach) channel is obstructed, the Stomach does not function properly, and nausea ensues. When Qi is obstructed in the Lesser Yang (Triple Burner and Gall Bladder) channels, the regulatory functions of the Gall Bladder and Triple Burner are compromised, and restlessness and irritability result.

A gloomy demeanor indicates stasis of Blood. A wiry pulse reflects Wind and pain. The tongue coating in this case was not markedly abnormal, suggesting that the disease was still in the channels, and had not penetrated to the internal Organs.

TREATMENT

Points on the affected channels formed the basis for the prescription.

Points selected:

M-HN-3 *(yin tang)*, G-8 *(shuai gu)*, G-20 *(feng chi)*, LI-4 *(he gu)*, TB-8 *(san yang luo)*, S-37 *(zu san li)*, M-HN-9 *(tai yang)*

Balanced tonifying-draining manipulation was applied at all points except M-HN-9 *(tai yang)*, which was pricked to bleed. Treatment was administered once daily. The needles were retained for 30 minutes at each session, during which time they were manipulated once.

Discussion of points:

G-8 *(shuai gu)*, G-20 *(feng chi)* and TB-8 *(san yang luo)* are points on the Lesser Yang channels of the arm and leg. LI-4 *(he gu)* and S-36 *(zu san li)* are points on the Yang Brightness channels of the arm and leg. Needling these points clears their respective channels to facilitate the flow of Qi. The combination of G-20 *(feng chi)* and LI-4 *(he gu)* dispels Wind. S-36 *(zu san li)* regulates the Stomach and suppresses nausea. M-HN-3 *(yin tang)* was chosen as a local point at the site of the headache. M-HN-9 *(tai yang)* is an important point for treating headaches. To remove the local stasis of Blood, this point was quickly pricked with a pyramid needle to bleed a few drops of blood.

RESULTS

After the first treatment, the headaches substantially diminished, and the patient slept much better. The nausea also disappeared. Bloodletting at M-HN-9 *(tai yang)* was then discontinued, and the use of a filiform needle at this point was substituted, using balanced tonifying-draining manipulation. After the second treatment, the headaches disappeared, and the remaining symptoms improved. Seven more treatments were administered to consolidate the therapeutic effect.

On follow-up seven years later, the patient reported that she no longer suffered from headaches, even on windy or rainy days, or after physical exertion. Mild headaches did occasionally occur after colds, but responded well to analgesic tablets. □

Lower Back Pain from
Invasion of Damp-Cold

Yāo Tòng 腰痛

Chen, female, 37 years old. The patient complained of lower back pain of 4 years' duration, which she first experienced after living in a damp house for about 6 months. Since then, the pain had been intermittent, and was aggravated during rainy weather, when she was tired, or when she lay in bed for long periods of time. Light exercise and hot compresses relieved the pain. During the past year, she noticed pain in the middle of her back below the level of the 7th thoracic vertebra as well, which often awakened her at night. She was hospitalized, but X-ray examination of the spine revealed no abnormality. Blood count was within normal limits. She was diagnosed as having lumbar strain. Block therapy, massage, physical therapy and herbal medication were ineffective. She finally turned to acupuncture.

Examination disclosed that her tongue had dark red eruptions and a scanty coating, and that her pulse was thin and choppy.

SYNDROME DIFFERENTIATION

Lower back pain may be acute or chronic. The long duration (four years) of the condition in this case reflected its chronic nature. Chronic lower back pain may be caused by Damp-Cold, or by deficiency of the Kidney, or may result from prolonged strain of the muscles of the lower back.

The patient had lived in a damp house for half a year before she first experienced lower back pain. Clearly, Damp-Cold had invaded her back during this time, and had caused the lower back pain. Because of the stagnant nature of Damp-Cold, when it invades the channels the normal flow of Qi and Blood is impeded. This explains why the pain was aggravated at night, or when the patient lay in bed for long periods of time, since the flow of Qi and Blood was then slowed down. It also explains why the pain diminished when the flow of Qi and Blood was invigorated by light exercise, or by the application of hot compresses. The eruptions on the tongue, and the thin, choppy pulse were further evidence of Blood stasis.

In summary, this case of lower back pain was due to invasion of the channels by Damp-Cold, which resulted in stasis of Blood.

TREATMENT

The principle of treatment was to warm the channels in order to dispel the Damp-Cold and normalize the flow of Qi and Blood.

Points selected:

B-23 *(shen shu)*, B-25 *(da chang shu)*, B-40 *(wei zhong)*, M-BW-35 *(jia ji)* at the 7th, 9th and 11th thoracic vertebrae

Treatment was administered once daily. Balanced tonifying-draining manipulation through raise-thrust and twirling techniques was applied at all points. The needles were retained for 20 minutes during each session.

Discussion of points:

Both B-23 *(shen shu)* and B-25 *(da chang shu)* are located on the lower back; needling these two points helps eliminate Damp-Cold and normalize the flow of Qi and Blood. B-40 *(wei zhong)* is a point on the Bladder channel, which courses along the two sides of the spine and through the lumbar region. Its efficacy in the treatment of diseases involving the back has long been recognized. The M-BW-35 *(jia ji)* vertebral points were selected because the patient complained of pain in the middle back; these points were used to promote the flow of Qi and Blood in that region.

With the patient lying prone, B-23 *(shen shu)* and B-25 *(da chang shu)* were first needled, and then a moxibustion box containing a 1-inch moxa stick was applied over these 2 points. The needle sensation at B-40 *(wei zhong)* extended down to the heel. At the M-BW-35 *(jia ji)* vertebral points, a distinct sensation of soreness and distention was felt locally.

RESULTS

There was no apparent improvement after five treatments. Although the patient felt relaxed after each morning's treatment, the pain returned in the afternoon, and disturbed her sleep at night.

Upon review, two reasons were considered for the apparent failure of the treatment thus far: (1) because this case involved Damp-Cold, the duration of moxibustion was not long enough; and (2) the prone position was inappropriate, as experience had shown that lumbar strain responds better when the patient is treated in a sitting position, since the needling sensation is stronger.

During the ensuing treatments, the patient was therefore asked to straddle a chair, with her back bent naturally, while the points on the back were needled for ten minutes. Warm needle moxibustion with 1-inch moxa stubs was then applied at each point. The patient felt a penetrating warmth, and the skin became flushed. After the moxa stubs were consumed, circular moxibustion was applied for another five minutes at each point. Because the patient was treated in a sitting position, the use of B-40 *(wei zhong)* was discontinued.

After two treatments with this modified regimen, the patient reported marked improvement in the pain, and said that she slept well through the night. After three more treatments, the pain beside the lower thoracic vertebrae disappeared, and she felt only occasional pain in the lower back. Although her work prevented her from returning to the clinic for three days, her condition had remained reasonably stable when she returned. Because the pain in the middle back was eliminated, the use of the M-BW-35 *(jia ji)* vertebral points was discontinued. For the final five treatments, only B-23 *(shen shu)* and B-25 *(da chang shu)* were treated with warm needle moxibustion. By then the back pain had essentially resolved, and she could move her body freely. Follow-up for six months showed no relapse. □

Lower Back Pain from Trauma
(Acute Lumbar Sprain)

Yāo Tòng 腰痛

Wu, male, 42 years old. Two days ago, the patient sprained his back while moving a heavy object. A dragging pain was felt at the time. The next day it became so severe that he was unable to straighten up, and the pain intensified with the slightest movement. Tenderness was present in the middle of the superior edge of the iliac crest, and at the lateral border of the sacrospinal muscles on both sides. Lumbar pain was elicited by raising either leg when extended, but Laseque's sign was negative on both sides. X-ray examination revealed no abnormality in the lumbar vertebrae.

The four examinations of Chinese medicine found the patient to have a pained expression. He was unable to straighten his back, and remained bent forward. The back muscles were stiff, and movement was limited in all directions. Severe tenderness was elicited near the points B-23 *(shen shu)*, B-25 *(da chang shu)* and B-26 *(guan yuan shu)*. The tongue had a thin, white coating, and the pulse was wiry.

spinal column through the lumbar region, and then down into the popliteal fossa. The lumbar sprain in this case obstructed the flow of Qi in the Bladder channel, thus the tenderness at B-23 *(shen shu)*, B-25 *(da chang shu)* and B-26 *(guan yuan shu)*. Because the disorder involved only the sinews and channels, and not the internal Organs, the tongue coating was normal. The wiry pulse indicated pain, which was related to the sprain in the lumbar region.

SYNDROME DIFFERENTIATION

The etiology of the disorder was trauma. The pain was fixed in one place and was aggravated by pressure, indicating stagnation of Qi and Blood, and an excess syndrome.

The Bladder channel runs parallel to the

TREATMENT

Points were chosen primarily along the Bladder channel. Draining manipulation was used to relieve the stagnation in order to invigorate the Blood and promote the flow of Qi.

Points selected:

B-23 *(shen shu)*, B-25 *(da chang shu)*, B-26 *(guan yuan shu)*, M-BW-23 *(yao yi)*, B-40 *(wei zhong)*

Draining manipulation was applied once daily through raise-thrust and twirling techniques. The needles were retained for 20 minutes during each session.

Discussion of points:

Points along the Bladder channel were chosen in accordance with the principle of selecting points on the channel affected by the disorder. Local points in the vicinity of the disorder were used in combination with remote ones.

B-23 *(shen shu)*, B-25 *(da chang shu)* and B-26 *(guan yuan shu)* can be used to regulate the flow of Qi in the Bladder channel, and thus relieve pain. M-BW-23 *(yao yi)*, a miscellaneous point, is effective in treating both acute lumbar sprain and chronic muscle strain in that area. B-40 *(wei zhong)* is one of the 'four dominant points', and is effective in treating back pain (see Introduction).

At B-23 *(shen shu)* the needle was inserted perpendicularly to a depth of about 1 unit. The needle sensation was one of local soreness and distention, which was transmitted up and down the back along the course of the Bladder channel. Needle insertion at B-25 *(da chang shu)* was perpendicular to a depth of about 1.3 units, producing a sensation of soreness and distention which shot down to the sacrococcygeal region. At B-26 *(guan yuan shu)* the needle was inserted perpendicularly to a depth of about 1.3 units, producing soreness and distention which radiated to the buttock. Needle insertion at M-BW-23 *(yao yi)* was perpendicular to a depth of about 1.3 units, producing soreness and distention which was transmitted in the direction of the iliac crest. B-40 *(wei zhong)* was needled perpendicularly to a depth of about 0.5 unit, producing an electric shock-like sensation which shot toward the calf and the arch of the foot.

RESULTS

After the first treatment, the pain in the back was substantially alleviated. The patient could straighten his back, and could move it slightly. Treatment was continued on successive days for a total of five treatments, by which time the pain in the back had disappeared completely, and free movement of the back was restored. The patient was instructed not to move heavy objects, nor to tire himself. He was followed up for one month, during which time he remained free of back pain. □

Lower Back Pain from Trauma
(Acute Lumbar Sprain)

Yāo Tòng 腰痛

Zhao, male, 40 years old. Two days ago while working, the patient sprained his lower back. The next day the pain intensified, especially on the right side, and was aggravated by coughing. He took some Chinese pills intended for injuries from falls and contusions, and applied a local pain-relieving plaster. These proved to be ineffective, however, and on the second day he was carried by a family member to the acupuncture clinic for treatment.

On examination, the patient had a pained expression. There was no scoliosis of the back. Tenderness and guarding were present over both sides of the lumbar region, and were more marked on the right. Both sides of the lumbar region were stiff because of spasm, which limited his motion in bending forward, backward, and to both sides, as well as twisting at the waist. The tongue was purple and dull, and the pulse was choppy. X-ray showed no abnormality in the lumbar vertebrae.

SYNDROME DIFFERENTIATION

Lower back pain is a common clinical condition. It can be caused by external Damp-Cold, deficiency of the Kidney, or trauma. In lower back pain from Damp-Cold, the pain is accompanied by sensations of heaviness, soreness and numbness which may involve the legs, and the symptoms are aggravated by rainy or cold weather. In lower back pain due to deficiency of the Kidney, the pain is indistinct and continuous, and the patient will complain of soreness and weakness in the lower back and legs. Lower back pain due to Blood stasis is brought on by poor posture, overexertion, strenuous exercise or trauma. Stabbing pain is the rule, and the affected area is tender to the touch. The onset is usually acute.

The present case resulted from a back sprain, which led to stagnant Qi and stasis of Blood, causing severe pain in the lower back. The spastic stiffness and limited motion were attributed to a poor supply of Qi and Blood in the muscles and channels. The dull, purple tongue and choppy pulse also reflected stagnant Qi and stasis of Blood. All of these signs and symptoms indicated a condition of excess.

TREATMENT

The principle of treatment was to eliminate the stagnation in the channels and disperse the stasis of Blood to relieve the pain.

Points selected:

B-40 *(wei zhong)*, B-59 *(fu yang)*, B-23 *(shen shu)*, B-25 *(da chang shu)*, B-65 *(shu gu)*

All points were needled bilaterally. Since this was a condition of excess, draining manipulation was applied.

Discussion of points:

B-40 *(wei zhong)*, B-59 *(fu yang)* and B-65 *(shu gu)* are points on the Bladder channel, which runs along both sides of the spinal column and passes through the lumbar region. In treating lower back pain, the use of these three points facilitates the flow of Qi and Blood, and eliminates stagnation in the channel. B-40 *(wei zhong)* is particularly effective in treating conditions of the lower back. B-65 *(shu gu)*, the 'son' point of the Bladder channel, and B-59 *(fu yang)*, the accumulating point of the Yang Heel channel, is an effective combination for draining excess and eliminating stagnation from the lower back. These points were chosen in accordance with the principles of selecting points along the channel(s) affected by the condition, and selecting points below to treat diseases above.

B-23 *(shen shu)* and B-25 *(da chang shu)* were chosen as local points to eliminate stagnation in the channel, thus relieving the muscle spasms.

The respiration tonifying and draining method was used here. In this technique, needle insertion, manipulation and withdrawal are all synchronized with the patient's breathing. For draining, the needle is inserted during inhalation, and after the needle sensation is obtained, the needle is raised-thrust or twirled each time the patient inhales. The raising, thrusting and twirling are of wide amplitude and high frequency.

The needle is not manipulated during exhalation. After the needle has been retained for an appropriate time, it is withdrawn during exhalation. For tonification (not indicated here), the needle is inserted during exhalation, and after the needle sensation is obtained, the needle is raised-thrust or twirled each time the patient exhales. Needle manipulation is of small amplitude and low frequency, and is not performed during inhalation. After needle retention, it is withdrawn during inhalation.

In this case, B-65 *(shu gu)* was needled first. With the patient in a sitting position, a 1-unit needle was inserted quickly. After the needle sensation was obtained, draining manipulation was applied for five minutes. During manipulation, the patient was asked to stand and slowly limber his waist by bending and twisting, with gradually increasing speed. The needle was then retained for ten minutes, after which the procedure was repeated. The other points were then needled. This type of treatment is sometimes known as 'acupuncture with exercise', and is believed to enhance the action of eliminating stagnation in the channels.

At B-40 *(wei zhong)* a 1-unit needle was inserted perpendicularly, with the needle sensation extending distally. At B-59 *(fu yang)* a 1.5-unit needle was inserted perpendicularly, producing a local needle sensation. At B-23 *(shen shu)* and B-25 *(da chang shu)*, 2-unit needles were used, with the needle tips directed slightly toward the spinal vertebrae at an angle of 80^0. The needles were inserted 1.8 units deep, and the needle sensation was transmitted to the buttocks and the back of the thighs. At all of these points, the needles were retained for 30 minutes.

RESULTS

Immediately after the first treatment, the patient was sweating slightly, and reported that he felt relaxed, and that the pain was "half gone." He could already stoop a bit. When he came to the clinic the next day, he could walk with the aid of a cane. He was treated again in the same manner, and afterward said that the pain was greatly relieved.

On the third day, the use of B-65 *(shu gu)* was discontinued, as this point is used primarily for acute pain. Therapy continued for three more days, by the end of which the pain had completely disappeared, and the patient was able to move about freely. □

Painful Obstruction
(Ankylosing Spondylitis)

Bì Zhèng 痹症

Lu, male, 34 years old. Five years ago, the patient began to experience aching in the spine associated with general weakness and lassitude. Over a period of 3 years, the pain gradually increased. The patient noticed that his spine protruded backward, and that there was difficulty in expanding the chest, and in bending forward. The condition worsened until he was unable to lie on his back. He was X-rayed at another hospital and the condition was diagnosed as ankylosing spondylitis. Various therapies were administered over the course of about 6 months, including periarticular block with steroids, oral administration of both Chinese herbs and western anti-inflammatory drugs, physical therapy and acupuncture. However, there was no improvement, and the patient was referred to this clinic.

Examination found that the patient lacked spirit, and had a lusterless face. He complained of pain in the back that radiated to the sides of the ribcage. There was marked tenderness over the spinous processes of the 5th through 12th thoracic vertebrae. The patient was bent forward, and full extension of the spine was impossible. He was unable to sleep when the pain was severe.

Accompanying symptoms included dizziness, decreased appetite, fatigue, thirst without desire to drink, and clear, copious urine. The tongue was pale, with tooth marks along the edges, and the coating was thin and white. The pulse was thin and wiry.

Laboratory tests showed Hgb 8.6g, ESR 46mm/hr, and antistreptolysin 'O' titer less than 500 units. Otherwise, the blood tests were normal. Urinalysis and body temperature were also normal. X-ray findings of the heart and lungs were negative. X-ray of the thoracic spine showed blurring of the apophysial joints from the 6th through the 11th thoracic vertebrae, with generalized demineralization of their bodies, but no erosion.

SYNDROME DIFFERENTIATION

The Kidney controls the bones. When the Kidney is deficient, the bones are susceptible to invasion by external pathogenic influences. The Spleen and Stomach are the source of Qi and Blood. When the Spleen is deficient, the normal Qi will likewise be deficient, since it depends upon the nourishment of Qi and Blood. This also renders the body susceptible to invasion by external pathogenic influences. In this patient, the lusterless face, dizziness, reduced appetite, pain in the back, clear and copious urine, fatigue, pale tongue and thin pulse were all evidence of deficiencies of both the Kidney and the Spleen.

Deficiency of normal Qi led to invasion by Wind, Cold and Dampness. These pathogenic influences invaded the Governing vessel and Bladder channel, since this was the area in which the symptoms appeared. Because of deficiency of the Kidney, the vertebrae were specifically affected. With the flow of Qi and Blood obstructed in these two channels, pain and limited back motion resulted.

TREATMENT

Points selected:

GV-14 *(da zhui)*, B-17 *(ge shu)*, B-20 *(pi shu)*, B-23 *(shen shu)*, CV-6 *(qi hai)*, S-36 *(zu san li)*, Sp-6 *(san yin jiao)*

The points were needled once daily, and the needles retained for 20 minutes. Ten treatments comprised 1 course of therapy, with 2-3 days' rest between courses. Tonifying manipulation was applied at all points except GV-14 *(da zhui)*, where balanced tonifying-draining manipulation was used.

Discussion of points:

GV-14 *(da zhui)* intersects with all the Yang channels of the leg and arm. Since the Bladder channel and Governing vessel are Yang channels, and because the condition appeared along the course of the Governing vessel, GV-14 *(da zhui)* was chosen in order to clear the channels and restore the flow of Qi. B-17 *(ge shu)* is the meeting point of Blood; needling this point promotes the circulation of Blood, and thus relieves pain.

B-20 *(pi shu)* and B-23 *(shen shu)* are the associated points on the back for the Spleen and Kidney respectively. When stimulated, both Organs are strengthened, which in turn strengthens the bones and sinews.

CV-6 *(qi hai)* is the 'sea' in which Qi is produced. In this case, it was needled to strengthen the deficient Kidney. (CV-4 *[guan yuan]* could also have been used.) S-36 *(zu san li)* is a point which is commonly used for tonifying deficient conditions. Sp-6 *(san yin jiao)* is noted for its effect in strengthening the Spleen, tonifying the Kidney and resolving Dampness. The combined use of these three points was intended to tonify both the Blood and Qi.

RESULTS

After 30 treatments, some improvement was noticed, particularly in the patient's general condition. He appeared to be more spirited, slept better, and had a better appetite. The back pain was also somewhat alleviated; ESR was 32mm/hr. The tongue and pulse remained about the same as before.

In order to hasten the restoration of channel flow and stop the pain, the following points were added: B-11 *(da zhu)*, M-BW-35 *(jia ji)* from the 5th to the 12th thoracic vertebrae. B-11 *(da zhu)* was chosen because it is the meeting point of the bones. The vertebral points M-BW-35 *(jia ji)* are local points adjacent to the affected area, and were used to promote the flow of Qi. Balanced tonifying-draining manipulation was applied at these points; manipulation remained the same at the other points in the prescription. Treatment was administered once every other day.

After another two months of treatment, marked improvement was observed. The complexion became ruddy, and the dizziness disappeared. The pain in the spine was substantially reduced, and the difficulty in bending forward and expanding the chest was no longer noticeable. Laboratory tests then showed that Hgb had increased to 10.2g, and ESR was reduced to 24mm/hr. The tongue was redder, and the pulse was moderate. It was evident that the normal Qi was being restored, and that the pathogenic influences were declining.

Efforts were then concentrated on relieving the stiffness and pain in the spine. The following prescription was used: B-11 *(da zhu)*, GV-14 *(da zhui)*, GV-10 *(ling tai)*, GV-9 *(zhi yang)*, GV-11 *(shen dao)*, GV-8 *(jin suo)*, GV-7 *(zhong shu)*, GV-6 *(ji zhong)*, M-BW-35 *(jia ji)* from the 5th to the 12th thoracic vertebrae. These points were chosen in order to continue to promote the flow of Qi and Blood in the Governing vessel. Treatment was administered once every other day, and balanced tonifying-draining manipulation was applied at all points.

After another two months of treatment with this modified prescription, the pain subsided, and free motion of the back was restored. ESR was reduced to 10mm/hr. The patient was followed up for one year, with no recurrence of symptoms. □

Painful Obstruction
(Cervical Disc Degeneration)

Bì Zhèng 痹症

He, male, 58 years old. The patient had suffered from stiffness and pain in the nape of the neck and shoulders for 6 months. The pain, which radiated to both upper extremities, had worsened during the past month. Movement of the neck was limited, and the pain was particularly excruciating on rotation when tipping the head backward. Numbness and weakness were noted in the thumb and index finger of both hands. There was marked tenderness on both sides of the spinous processes of the 5th and 6th cervical vertebrae. Tenderness was also apparent along the medial borders, and above and below the spine, of both scapulae. Applying pressure to these areas relieved the tenderness. Biceps reflex of both arms was diminished. X-ray showed disappearance of the anterior curvature of the cervical spine, narrowing of the interspace between the 5th and 6th cervical vertebrae, and osteophytic formations at the vertebral margins. The diagnosis was degeneration of the intervertebral disc between the 5th and 6th cervical vertebrae, and osteosis.

The patient was obese. His tongue was swollen, with tooth marks along the edges. The tongue coating was thin and white, and the pulse was submerged and frail.

SYNDROME DIFFERENTIATION

This disease occurs more frequently after forty years of age because of general deterioration of the Liver and Kidney. The Liver governs the muscles and sinews, while the Kidney governs the bones. When Liver and Kidney Qi are deficient, the muscles, sinews and bones will lack nourishment, and the functioning of the extremities will thus be diminished. If this condition persists, circulation of Qi in the channels will be impeded, which will further disrupt the functioning of the extremities.

In this case, the pain which was partially relieved upon pressure, the swollen, tooth-marked tongue, and the submerged, frail pulse all indicated Qi and Blood deficiency. Because of this deficiency, the thumbs and index fingers were numb and weak. Since the areas affected are traversed by several channels (Governing, Small Intestine, Large Intestine, Triple Burner, Bladder and Gall

Bladder), the pattern was one of impairment of the flow of channel Qi, and deficiency of the Liver and Kidney.

TREATMENT

Treatment was directed first at relieving the symptoms of pain and stiffness along the channels, and then at resolving the underlying cause.

Points selected:

GV-14 *(da zhui)*, M-BW-35 *(jia ji)* between the 5th and 6th cervical vertebrae, B-10 *(tian zhu)*, SI-14 *(jian wai shu)*, B-14 *(jue yin shu)*, G-21 *(jian jing)*, SI-11 *(tian zong)*, LI-15 *(jian yu)*, LI-4 *(he gu)*, LI-11 *(qu chi)*

All of the points were needled once daily with tonifying manipulation through raise-thrust and twirling techniques.

Discussion of points:

The first seven points are local points in the vicinity of the pain and stiffness. They were used to promote the flow of Qi in the affected channels, and thereby relieve the pain. The last three points, LI-15 *(jian yu)*, LI-11 *(qu chi)* and LI-4 *(he gu)*, were used to relieve the pain in the upper arm, and to resolve the numbness and weakness in the thumbs and index fingers. These symptoms all occurred along the arm Yang Brightness (Large Intestine) channel.

At GV-14 *(da zhui)* the needle was slanted slightly upward, and the sensation produced was one of distention extending up and down the spine, and to both shoulders. M-BW-35 *(jia ji)* between the 5th and 6th cervical vertebrae was needled perpendicularly 1.3 units deep, and the sensation was one of local distention and soreness. At B-10 *(tian zhu)*, needling produced a sensation of local distention and soreness, extending downward. Needling SI-14 *(jian wai shu)*, B-14 *(jue

yin shu)* and G-21 *(jian jing)* produced a sensation of local distention and soreness. SI-11 *(tian zong)* was needled obliquely, with the tip pointed laterally; distention and soreness in the scapular region radiated to the lateral aspect of the arm. LI-15 *(jian yu)* was needled obliquely downward, with the sensation extending toward the elbow. At LI-4 *(he gu)* the needle sensation reached the thumb and index finger. When LI-11 *(qu chi)* was needled, the sensation of local distention and soreness traveled along the forearm, and was occasionally felt in the shoulder or fingers.

RESULTS

After five treatments, some improvement was noted in the pain and stiffness of the neck and shoulder, as well as the pain in the arm, and the numbness and weakness in the thumbs and index fingers. After twenty treatments with the same set of points, all of the symptoms were "half gone," as described by the patient.

B-18 *(gan shu)* and B-23 *(shen shu)* were then added to the original point prescription. The former was used to nourish Liver Blood, thereby strengthening the Kidney, and thus the bones. The frequency of treatment was reduced to once every other day, since the symptoms had diminished in intensity.

After another 15 treatments (for a total of 35), the pain and stiffness in the neck, shoulders and arms had resolved, and the neck had become supple and moved freely. The numbness and weakness in the thumbs and index fingers had virtually disappeared. Biceps reflex was normal, and X-ray showed that the anterior curvature of the cervical spine had been partially restored. The patient was followed up for 6 months, with no recurrence of pain. □

Painful Obstruction
(Cervical Disc Degeneration)

Bì Zhèng 痹症

Wei, male, 51 years old. The patient suffered from a painful, stiff neck for 3 months. The pain extended to the occipital region, and the left arm felt heavy, numb and sore. When the neck was extended backward, an electric shock-like sensation was felt in the left arm and fingers. Chinese herbs and western drugs failed to relieve the pain.

Examination revealed limited movement of the neck. The patient was unable to look up at the ceiling, and his chin could not touch his chest. There were clicking sounds when the neck was forced to move, and the lateral aspects of both the 5th and 6th cervical vertebrae were tender. Both the compression and brachial plexus traction tests were positive. The tongue was dark red, and the pulse was moderate and submerged.

Blood pressure, blood lipid levels and ECG were normal. X-ray revealed a reduction in the curvature of the cervical spine, hyperplasia of the posterior lower margin of the 4th through 7th cervical vertebrae, and a narrowing of the 5th and 6th cervical intervertebral spaces.

SYNDROME DIFFERENTIATION

The Governing vessel courses through the posterior aspect of the neck and along the midline of the spinal column from the coccyx to the skull. It governs the Yang Qi of the entire body, and is the confluence of all the Yang channels. According to the *Yellow Emperor's Inner Classic: Simple Questions* (chapter 1), "Yang declines in women at age 42, and in men at age 48." This patient was over 48 years of age at the time his symptoms first appeared. The Yang Qi had begun to wane, leading to deficiency of Qi in the Governing vessel. This caused stiffness and limited movement of the neck.

The deficiency of Qi also rendered the Governing vessel susceptible to invasion by pathogenic Wind, Cold and Dampness, all of which accumulated in the neck and hindered the circulation of Qi. This process often affects the Bladder and Large Intestine channels, which was the case here. Obstruction always leads to pain, hence the patient suffered from pain in the neck, which extended to the left arm.

TREATMENT

The principles of treatment were to facilitate the flow of Qi in the Governing vessel, and to dispel the Wind, Cold and Dampness. Points were chosen along the affected channels.

Points selected:

GV-14 *(da zhui)*, B-11 *(da zhu)*, LI-15 *(jian yu)*, LI-11 *(qu chi)* and LI-4 *(he gu)* on the left side only

Treatment was administered once daily, with ten sessions comprising one course of therapy.

Discussion of points:

GV-14 *(da zhui)* is the point of intersection of the Governing vessel and the Yang channels of the arm and leg. This point was needled to clear the Governing vessel, and to eliminate the Wind, Cold and Dampness. The needle was inserted quickly, and then advanced slowly to a depth of about 1.5 units, or until the needling sensation was obtained. In this case, the needle point was first directed slightly upward, and then downward after the needling sensation was obtained. Rapid raise-thrust manipulations of small amplitude were performed until the patient felt a sore, numb sensation extending downward along the Governing vessel. This was followed by rhythmic twirling of the needle for about one-half minute. The needle was then raised to just below the surface of the skin, and pointed to the left. It was again raised-thrust and twirled for about one minute to produce a sore, numb sensation, which this time extended to the left shoulder and arm. The needle was then removed.

B-11 *(da zhu)* is the point of intersection of the Small Intestine channel on the Bladder channel. It is also the meeting point for the bones. Needling this point promotes the circulation of Qi in all the Yang channels,

relaxes the sinews, invigorates the collateral vessels and strengthens the bones. It is especially useful for treating pain and stiffness in the neck and back. The needle at this point was inserted obliquely downward to a depth of 0.3-0.5 unit. The 'burning the mountain' tonification technique was applied until a sensation of heat was transmitted to the upper arm.

LI-15 *(jian yu)*, LI-11 *(qu chi)* and LI-4 *(he gu)* are effective in the treatment of neck pain. After needling GV-14 *(da zhui)* and B-11 *(da zhu)*, these three points were needled in the order listed to enhance the needling sensation, which was transmitted from the neck to the hand via the shoulder and arm. Draining manipulation was used to eliminate the Wind, Cold and Dampness.

RESULTS

The patient felt a very strong needling sensation during the first session, and afterward felt much relieved. After ten sessions, the stiffness in the neck was completely alleviated, although a slight numbness in the left arm remained. The radiating, electric shock-like sensation along the left arm was still present when the neck was extended backward. After twenty treatments with the same set of points, there was further improvement in all of the symptoms, and the neck was more flexible. After a total of thirty sessions, the patient was able to move his neck freely, and all other symptoms had disappeared. There was no recurrence of pain during a six month follow-up, although X-ray continued to show no change in the bony hyperplasia of the cervical vertebrae.

Physical exercises were recommended to consolidate the therapeutic effect. At the outset, the patient was advised that the exercises should be limited, and then gradually increased in motion and duration, to prevent overstraining. □

Painful Obstruction
(Lateral Humeral Epicondylitis)

Bì Zhèng 痹症

Wang, female, 50 years old. For about 6 months, the patient, a street sweeper, had suffered from pain in her left elbow, especially when trying to grip with her left hand. Because of the pain and associated weakened grip, she was unable to work or do her daily household chores. A surgeon diagnosed the condition as lateral humeral epicondylitis ('tennis elbow'). Various therapies were tried over a period of 2 months, including nerve block, massage and physical therapy, but without success. She therefore sought acupuncture therapy as a last resort.

Examination showed the presence of local tenderness over the left lateral humeral epicondyle. Pain was also elicited by resisting dorsiflexion of the patient's hand. The pulse was weak, and the tongue was pale with a thin, white coating.

SYNDROME DIFFERENTIATION

At 50 years old, the patient's Qi and Blood were declining, as reflected in her tongue and pulse. In addition, the prolonged occupational strain of street-sweeping had injured her Qi and Blood, resulting in disruption of flow, particularly in those parts of her body strained by work, such as the elbow. This gave rise to pain. The condition was protracted due to the deficiency and stagnation of Qi and Blood.

TREATMENT

The principle of treatment was to warm the channel and invigorate the Blood.

Points selected:
LI-11 *(qu chi)*, LI-4 *(he gu)*, points of tenderness

At the points of tenderness, after the needles were inserted, 1-unit moxa stubs were burned on the handle of each needle until the surrounding skin became flushed. Treatment was administered once daily. All points were tonified through raise-thrust and twirling manipulation. The needles were retained for 20 minutes during each session.

Discussion of points:
The points of tenderness were localized sites of stagnant Qi and Blood. Needling these points eliminated the stagnation. LI-11

(qu chi) was chosen as a local point because of its proximity to the affected area. LI-4 *(he gu)* was needled for its effect in arresting pain.

RESULTS

After ten treatments, some improvement was noticed. However, it was still painful for the patient to make a fist or twist a towel. Ginger-mediated moxibustion was therefore utilized. Ginger has a warming effect which facilitates the flow of Qi and Blood. Slices of ginger, each measuring approximately 2cm in diameter and 1cm in thickness, were perforated with many tiny holes, and one slice was placed over each point of tenderness. Moxa cones, measuring about 1.5cm in diameter at the base, were then burned atop the ginger for as long as the patient could tolerate. When the pain became intolerable, the cones were temporarily removed with a pair of forceps, and then replaced after a short respite. When the cones were consumed, the ginger slices were removed. The other two points in the prescription, LI-11 *(qu chi)* and LI-4 *(he gu)*, were then needled.

This modified regimen was also administered once daily. Marked improvement was attained after seven treatments. The patient was then able to perform ordinary household chores. Treatment was continued for another week, and she was then discharged and advised not to overstrain her arm. □

Painful Obstruction
(Perifocal Inflammation of the Shoulder)

Bì Zhèng 痹症

Huang, male, 52 years old. Two months before coming to the clinic, the patient had worked in the draft of an electric fan, which had been placed to the right of his desk. At first he felt a slight discomfort in his right shoulder, which gradually became quite painful. Two weeks later, the pain became so severe that it interfered with his sleep. Movement of the shoulder joint was also limited. The pain was alleviated with aspirin and butazolidin, as well as block therapy with procaine and cortisone, but movement of the joint remained restricted, and the pain returned when the treatment was discontinued. The patient then turned to acupuncture therapy.

Examination showed an absence of redness or swelling in the right shoulder. Abduction was limited to 70⁰. He could raise his right arm to his ear, but was unable to stretch it backward. He needed help in getting dressed. His right shoulder and upper arm were sensitive to wind and cold, and he experienced numbness and distention in the fingers of his right hand. The tongue was dark red with a thin, white coating, and the pulse was wiry and tight.

SYNDROME DIFFERENTIATION

The patient suffered primarily from pain and limited motion of the shoulder joint. This condition falls in the category of painful obstruction, a group of disorders characterized by pain due to obstruction of the channels by external pathogenic influences. In this case, the condition was caused by invasion of the shoulder region by Wind, Cold and Dampness. Because this condition is frequently found in patients who are middle-aged, it is also known as the '50-year-old shoulder'.

There are three types of painful obstruction, based upon which of three pathogenic influences predominates. When Wind predominates, the joints and muscles are painful, and the pain is not fixed in one place. The pain radiates to the neck, back or fingers, and is accompanied by numbness and distention. When Cold predominates, the pain is severe, and the patient becomes intolerant of cold. When Dampness predominates, the site of the pain is fixed, and there is local swelling and a feeling of heaviness.

Since the patient in this case had a history of continuous exposure to a cool draft, the pain was severe, there was numbness and distention in the fingers, and no swelling in the shoulder, the condition was diagnosed as painful obstruction due to Wind and Cold. When the skin and pores were relaxed during hot weather, these pathogenic influences entered the skin while it was exposed to the continuous draft from the fan. The Wind and Cold then obstructed the flow of Qi and Blood in the local channels, thus resulting in pain and restricted movement of the shoulder.

TREATMENT

To relieve the pain, draining manipulation and moxibustion were used to clear the channels, promote the flow of Qi, invigorate the circulation of Blood and dispel the Wind and Cold.

Points selected:

S-38 *(tiao kou)*, B-57 *(cheng shan)*, M-UE-48 *(jian nei ling)*, LI-10 *(shou san li)*, TB-5 *(wai guan)*, LI-15 *(jian yu)*, TB-14 *(jian liao)*

Treatment was administered once daily.

Discussion of points:

Joining S-38 *(tiao kou)* to B-57 *(cheng shan)* has been effective in our experience for treating pain and restricted movement of the shoulder. With the patient in a sitting position, the needle is first inserted at S-38 *(tiao kou)*. When the needle sensation is obtained, the needle is inserted further in the direction of B-57 *(cheng shan)* until the needle sensation is obtained at that point. Draining manipulation is then applied by twirling the needle. Insertion is to a depth of 2.0-2.5 units. After manipulating the needle for 1-2 minutes, and with the needle still in place, the patient is asked to slowly flex, abduct and then extend his arm. (This is called 'acupuncture with exercise'.) The

movements should be slow at first, and then gradually become faster. Overexertion should be avoided. As the shoulder is exercised, needle manipulation is continued. Some improvement in the symptoms can generally be felt within 3-5 minutes. This method, however, is primarily suited for cases with a relatively short history, and not for patients with chronic conditions, or for those who are aged and infirm.

Stimulation of the local points LI-15 *(jian yu)*, TB-14 *(jian liao)* and M-UE-48 *(jian nei ling)* facilitates the flow of Qi in the local channels, and invigorates the circulation of Blood. Applying moxibustion at these points has the effect of warming and dispersing the Cold. Needling LI-10 *(shou san li)*, a point somewhat distant from the site of the pain, alleviates pain in the shoulder and arm. TB-5 *(wai guan)*, another distant point, was used to disperse the Wind.

RESULTS

During the first session, when S-38 *(tiao kou)* was joined to B-57 *(cheng shan)*, the patient was asked to exercise his right shoulder while the acupuncturist continued to twirl the needle. The patient immediately felt the pain diminish, and two minutes later, the range of motion in the shoulder increased. He was able to abduct the arm to 120°, could lift the arm to reach the top of his head, and could stretch it backward to touch the sacral region with the back of the hand. After six minutes, the needle was removed.

The other points were then needled with raise-thrust and twirling manipulation for one minute after needle sensation was obtained. At LI-15 *(jian yu)* and TB-14 *(jian liao)*, after the needles were inserted, warm needle moxibustion was applied, and the needles were retained for thirty minutes.

After three sessions, the pain was markedly reduced, and the range of motion in the right shoulder was further improved. Because the joining of S-38 *(tiao kou)* to B-57 *(cheng shan)* is used only for acute, severe pain (and is itself quite painful), its use was discontinued at this time. After three more treatments with the remaining points, the pain disappeared, the numbness and distention in the fingers decreased, and the ability of the right arm to lift, abduct and extend backward was basically restored. However, some discomfort was still felt when the shoulder was moved over a wider range. After ten treatments, all symptoms were alleviated, and there was no further restriction in motion. Treatment was therefore discontinued. The patient was followed up for three months, and there was no recurrence of symptoms. □

Painful Obstruction
(Sciatica)

Bì Zhèng 痹症

Li, male, 52 years old. The patient had previously sprained his back. He had always been fond of sports, and a month ago, while playing golf, he sprained his back again. Continuous pain developed in his lower back on the left side and left buttock, and spread downward along the posterior and lateral aspects of the leg to the ankle. The range of motion at the waist was limited, and bending backward or to the left caused great pain. Because he could not lie flat on his back, he had to lie on one side when sleeping, and it was difficult to turn over. Walking, stooping, squatting and even sitting were painful. Palpation revealed slight tenderness just to the left of the spinous processes of the 4th and 5th lumbar vertebrae, and there was a point of extreme tenderness on the left buttock, about 2cm above G-30 (huan tiao). Lasèque's test was positive on the left (less than 30°). X-ray showed slight narrowing of the intervertebral space between the 4th and 5th lumbar vertebrae. The condition was diagnosed as intervertebral disk protrusion and sciatica of the left side. Block therapy and massage were ineffective, and the patient asked to be treated with acupuncture.

The four examinations of traditional Chinese medicine found the patient to be robust, but with a pained expression on his face. He was bent forward, with his left hip and leg flexed, and he limped when he walked, favoring his left leg. There was a tender point on the left buttock which, when pressed, caused a severe, sharp pain to radiate down the posterior and lateral aspects of the left leg. Walking was extremely painful, and the patient could only move a few steps at a time. His tongue had a white coating, which was thick and slippery, and the pulse was wiry.

SYNDROME DIFFERENTIATION

This patient was suffering from a condition that falls in the category of painful obstruction. The sprain had caused localized stagnation of Qi and stasis of Blood, and the obstruction to the flow of Qi and Blood caused the pain. The wiry pulse reflected the presence of pain, and the severe tenderness in the lower back and buttock indicated a pattern of excess. (If the pattern had been one of deficiency, the pain would have diminished upon pressure.)

In this case, the pathways of two channels were important in determining the location of the obstruction. The Bladder channel travels parallel with and lateral to the spine to the lumbar region. A branch then traverses the buttock, descends along the back of the thigh to the popliteal fossa, and then continues downward over the back of the leg and around the lateral malleolus to the lateral aspect of the little toe. The primary areas of pain in this case were on or near the course of the Bladder channel. The Gall Bladder channel travels over the lateral side of the thigh and leg, and then continues downward in front of the lateral malleolus to the lateral aspect of the tip of the fourth toe. The pain along the lateral aspect of the leg in this case conformed to the course of the Gall Bladder channel.

The diagnosis was therefore stagnation of Qi and stasis of Blood due to back sprain, with resulting painful obstruction to the flow of Qi in the Bladder and Gall Bladder channels.

TREATMENT

Points were chosen primarily along the Bladder and Gall Bladder channels, together with the M-BW-35 *(jia ji)* vertebral points. Draining manipulation was utilized to promote the flow of Qi and to invigorate the circulation of Blood in order to relieve the pain.

Points selected:

M-BW-35 *(jia ji)* at the 4th and 5th lumbar vertebrae, the point of tenderness on the buttock, G-30 *(huan tiao)*, B-57 *(cheng shan)*, B-37 *(yin men)*, B-40 *(wei zhong)*, G-34 *(yang ling quan)*, G-40 *(qiu xu)*, B-64 *(jing gu)*

All points were needled on the left side only. Treatment was administered once daily. The needles were retained for 20 minutes, during which time they were manipulated once or twice.

Discussion of points:

The principle used in point selection was to combine local points with remote ones. The M-BW-35 *(jia ji)* vertebral points, the point of tenderness on the buttock, G-30 *(huan tiao)*, B-37 *(yin men)*, B-40 *(wei zhong)*, B-57 *(cheng shan)* and G-34 *(yang ling quan)* were local points, chosen because of their proximity to the locations of pain. The other two points, B-64 *(jing gu)* and G-40 *(qiu xu)*, were remote points, and were of secondary importance in this prescription. B-64 *(jing gu)* is the source point of the Bladder channel, and G-40 *(qiu xu)* is the source point of the Gall Bladder channel. Source points are those places where channel Qi concentrates; needling these points thus facilitated the flow of Qi in the channels. Draining with strong stimulation eliminated the stasis of Blood and invigorated the flow of Qi to alleviate the pain. Deep puncture at the M-BW-35 *(jia ji)* vertebral points was used for the same effect locally. In addition, these points were used to balance the pull on both sides of the lumbar vertebrae, so that the mildly protruded disk could be reduced spontaneously.

All points were needled with 30-gauge filiform needles. At the M-BW-35 *(jia ji)* vertebral points, 2-unit needles were inserted perpendicularly, 0.5 unit lateral to the spinous processes of the 4th and 5th lumbar vertebrae, to a depth of about 1.5 units. The needle sensation extended to the buttock, and to the back of the thigh.

The point of greatest tenderness on the buttock is usually located superomedially to G-30 *(huan tiao)*. A cord-like structure can often be felt in this area, and upon pressure, pain is elicited which extends to the leg. A 2.5-unit needle was inserted perpendicularly at this point to a depth of about 2 units. The needle sensation extended to the posterior aspect of the leg, sometimes reaching as far as the ankle. G-30 *(huan tiao)* was needled perpendicularly with a 3-unit needle to a depth of about 2.5 units. The needle sensation at this point also extended to the back of the leg, and occasionally reached as far as the arch of the foot.

At B-37 *(yin men)*, B-40 *(wei zhong)* and B-57 *(cheng shan)*, the needle sensation extended in the same direction as that at G-30 *(huan tiao)*. G-34 *(yang ling quan)* was needled to a depth of about 1 unit, eliciting a sensation that extended along the lateral aspect of the leg toward the front of the lateral malleolus. G-40 *(qiu xu)* was needled to a depth of about 1 unit, producing a sensation of local soreness and distention. At B-64 *(jing gu)*, an oblique insertion was made to a depth of about 0.5 unit, producing a sensation of local soreness and distention.

RESULTS

After five treatments, the pain in the lower back, buttock and leg was improved. The back and leg could be stretched to a greater extent, and the patient's limp was also less pronounced. When lying supine, the left leg could be raised to 45⁰. The patient was able to lie on his back at night when sleeping. Treatment was continued using the same points.

After 20 treatments, the patient could straighten his back, and fully stretch his leg. When lying supine, the left leg could be raised to 70⁰. The areas affected by pain were reduced in number. The lower back was pain-free, but there was still some pain in the buttock, the posterior and lateral aspects of the thigh, and at G-39 *(xuan zhong)*. Even at these sites, however, the pain was only half as severe as it had originally been.

In view of the reduction in pain, the original prescription was modified by dropping B-57 *(cheng shan)* and G-34 *(yang ling quan)*, and adding G-31 *(feng shi)* and G-39 *(xuan zhong)*. After 20 more treatments with the modified prescription, the pain was basically eliminated, and the patient was able to move his back and leg freely. He was advised to avoid strenuous exercise involving the back and the legs, and not to tire himself.

One month later when he came for a follow-up examination, slight pain was still present on the outer thigh, and around G-39 *(xuan zhong)* on the lower leg. Treatment was therefore resumed at G-30 *(huan tiao)*, B-37 *(yin men)*, G-31 *(feng shi)*, G-34 *(yang linq quan)* and G-39 *(xuan zhong)*. These points were all drained, and the needles retained for 20 minutes. Treatment was administered once every other day for 1 week, by which time the residual pain had disappeared completely. The patient was reexamined 2 months later, and no recurrence of pain was reported. □

Painful Obstruction
(Senile Panarthralgia)

Bì Zhèng 痹症

Guo, female, 60 years old. Arthralgia of the elbows, wrists, knees and ankles first appeared 2 years ago, without apparent cause. Phenylbutazone, meclofenamate and medicinal herbs brought some relief, but the condition was exacerbated by physical exertion or changes in the weather. During the past 6 months, the pain increased in severity, and had extended to the neck, shoulders and upper spine. In the past 2 months, the patient was unable to do housework owing to limited movement of the shoulder, elbow and knee joints. Laboratory tests of ESR, rheumatoid factor and anti-streptolysis 'O' showed normal values. Because drug therapy had proved to be ineffective, she decided to try acupuncture.

The four examinations of Chinese medicine found the patient to be slightly overweight, with a dull complexion. The multiple painful joints were normal in appearance, and there was no swelling noted. Pain prevented her from being able to raise either of her arms above chest level. The elbows could not be flexed more than 60⁰, and were unable to bear any weight. Knee joint motion varied between 0-60⁰ of flexion. Even with assistance, the patient could walk no more than ten meters before the pain became intolerable.

The pain was worse in cold weather, and at night. The patient felt weak and sweated spontaneously. She was sensitive to cold and wind. The tongue was a dull, pale color, with a white coating. The pulse was deep, thin and wiry.

SYNDROME DIFFERENTIATION

The chief complaint of the patient was multiple joint pain that worsened upon exposure to cold. In the elderly, the protective Qi is deficient, which renders the channels vulnerable to invasion by Wind, Cold and Dampness. These pathogenic influences obstruct the flow of Qi, and the obstruction of the channels leads to pain. Deficiency of Qi combined with obstruction of the channels by pathogenic influences causes insufficient nourishment of the sinews, leading to limited movement of the joints.

In this case, the weakness, sensitivity to cold and wind, and spontaneous sweating indicated deficiency of Qi. Deficiency of Qi led to poor circulation of Blood, hence the dull complexion and the dull, pale tongue. The deep, thin pulse was a sign of deficiency, and the wiry pulse was a sign of pain.

TREATMENT

The points selected were primarily local points on the Yang channels, and were chosen to clear the obstruction from the channels, and to replenish the Qi.

Points selected:

G-20 *(feng chi)*, B-10 *(tian zhu)*, LI-11 *(qu chi)*, TB-5 *(wai guan)*, LI-4 *(he gu)*, SI-3 *(hou xi)*, G-34 *(yang ling quan)*, S-35 *(xi yan)*, M-LE-16 *(du bi)*, B-62 *(shen mai)*, S-36 *(zu san li)*

All points were needled with balanced tonifying-draining manipulation except S-36 *(zu san li)*, which was tonified with warm needle moxibustion. Treatment was administered once daily, and the needles were retained for 20 minutes. Ten sessions comprised 1 course of therapy, with 3 days' rest between courses.

Discussion of points:

Balanced tonifying-draining manipulation was utilized because the patient had symptoms of both deficiency (Qi) and of excess (stagnation of pathogenic influences in the channels). S-36 *(zu san li)* is one of the 'four dominant points' of the body (see Introduction). In this case, it was first needled with tonifying manipulation, after which warm needle moxibustion was applied to replenish the Qi. G-34 *(yang ling quan)* is the meeting point of the sinews and is often used for motor disorders of the muscles and sinews. SI-3 *(hou xi)* and B-62 *(shen mai)* are the confluent points of the Governing vessel and Yang Heel channel respectively. They are effective in the treatment of pain. G-20 *(feng chi)* and TB-5 *(wai guan)* were chosen to dispel the pathogenic influences, and thus to clear the obstruction from the channels.

RESULTS

After ten treatments, there was some alleviation of pain, but it was still severe at night. No improvement of joint motility was evident. After the second course of therapy, the weather turned cold and the symptoms worsened, with involvement of the fingers and toes. The patient became extremely sensitive to the cold.

The treatment principle was then reconsidered, and it was concluded that the patient's deficient constitution was of primary importance. Because the channels were 'empty' (deficient of Qi), the pathogenic influences easily invaded the body and obstructed the channels. More emphasis should therefore have been placed upon dispelling the pathogenic influences, accompanied by efforts to tonify the Qi.

To this end, G-20 *(feng chi)* and TB-5 *(wai guan)* were replaced with GV-14 *(da zhui)*, B-23 *(shen shu)* and K-7 *(fu liu)*, while the other points in the prescription remained as before. The three new points were tonified, and warm needle moxibustion was applied at B-23 *(shen shu)*. Needling GV-14 *(da zhui)* has the effect of invigorating the circulation of Qi. Since B-23 *(shen shu)* is the associated point on the back for the Kidney, and K-7 *(fu liu)* is the 'mother' point of the Kidney channel, the combined use of these two points replenishes Kidney Qi and warms Kidney Yang, which is the foundation of Yang for the entire body. After ten daily sessions of treatment with this modified prescription, the pain was markedly reduced, although limited motility of the joints still remained.

At that time, due to ingestion of cold, raw food, the patient began to experience painful diarrhea. The treatment was therefore shifted to deal with the new ailment. Needling of the previous points was temporarily discontinued, since acute symptoms take priority in treatment. The points selected for the new ailment were S-25 *(tian shu)*, CV-6 *(qi hai)*, S-36 *(zu san li)* and Sp-4 *(gong sun)*.

These points were tonified, and moxibustion was applied at CV-6 *(qi hai)*. The diarrhea was relieved after three sessions.

Treatment of the painful obstruction (arthralgia) was then resumed as before. After two more courses of therapy, the pain abated during the day, and the shoulders, elbows and knees could move slightly. The patient was able to walk 30 meters with assistance, and the weakness and spontaneous sweating were much improved. After a total of 50 sessions of treatment, the pain in all joints disappeared. The arms could be raised overhead, and the elbow and knee joints could be flexed to 100°. The patient was able to walk 100 meters with the help of a cane, and could move about in the house. Only the knee joints had slight pain upon extreme variations in the weather. Thirty more sessions of needling with the same set of points were conducted to consolidate the therapeutic effect. Follow-up for six months found the condition to be stable. □

Painful Obstruction of Blood
(Acromelalgia)

Xuè Bì 血痹

Zhu, female, 34 years old. The patient complained of paroxysmal burning pain, redness and swelling in both arms below the elbows for over 3 months. The pain abated in the presence of cold, and was aggravated by warmth. It was more severe at night, and at times was so unbearable that her sleep was disturbed. Her condition was diagnosed at a hospital as acromelalgia. She had no history of underlying disorders. She was given vitamin B$_1$ and physical therapy, after which the symptoms were somewhat alleviated. Recently, however, the pain became worse and failed to respond to oral analgesics. She therefore asked to be treated with acupuncture.

Examination revealed that the patient was of normal development, and was moderately nourished. Physical examination of the heart, lungs, liver and spleen found nothing unusual. The abdomen was soft. Redness of the skin was present on both arms below the elbows, and slightly warm to the touch. The joints of the upper extremities could be moved freely. Gripping things with either hand aggravated the pain, and produced numbness. The pulse was wiry and thin, and the tongue was red with a thin, white coating.

SYNDROME DIFFERENTIATION

Acromelalgia, also called erythromelalgia, is rare as a primary disorder, especially when occurring in the upper extremities. Modern medicine attributes its cause to a disturbance in the sympathetic nervous system, but its etiology is still unknown. Traditional Chinese medicine classifies this condition as painful obstruction of Blood, which is usually induced by invasion of Cold. When the channels are attacked by Cold, the flow of Qi and Blood becomes stagnant. If unresolved, Cold stagnates in the channels and is then transformed into Heat, which in this case was believed to be the cause of the redness and raised temperature of the skin below the elbows. This also explains why the pain abated in the presence of cold, and was aggravated by warmth. The severe pain in the forearms at night was a sign of Blood stasis, which also accounted for the slight numbness in those areas. The red tongue signified stagnant Heat, and the wiry pulse indicated pain. In summary, this case was one of accumulation of Heat in the channels with Blood stasis due to stagnation of Qi. The original invasion of Cold was obscured by its transformation into Heat.

TREATMENT

Draining manipulation was applied with the aim of eliminating the Heat, opening the channels, invigorating the Blood and resolving the stasis.

Points selected:

GV-14 (da zhui), LI-11 (qu chi), TB-5 (wai guan), LI-4 (he gu). These points were needled once daily. Bloodletting by pricking the fingertip points M-UE-1 (shi xuan) was performed every other day.

Discussion of points:

GV-14 (da zhui) is the point of intersection of the Governing vessel with the Yang channels of the arm and leg. This point has the effect of eliminating Heat. Needling LI-11 (qu chi) and LI-4 (he gu) clears Heat and opens the channels, thereby alleviating pain. Needling TB-5 (wai guan) likewise dispels Heat and opens the channels. Bloodletting by pricking the fingertip points M-UE-1 (shi xuan) with a pyramid needle helps to invigorate the Blood, resolve stagnation, dispel Heat and open the channels.

At GV-14 (da zhui) the needle was inserted perpendicularly to a depth of about 1.2 units, producing a sensation of local soreness and distention. LI-11 (qu chi) was needled perpendicularly to about 1.3 units, producing a sensation of soreness and numbness which ex-

tended along the Large Intestine channel to the tip of the index finger. TB-5 (wai guan) was needled perpendicularly to a depth of about 0.8 unit, producing a sensation of soreness and numbness which extended in the direction of the middle finger. At LI-4 (he gu) the needle was inserted to a depth of about 1 unit, producing a needle sensation of soreness and numbness which extended toward the thumb and index finger.

Draining manipulation through raise-thrust and twirling techniques was applied. The fingertip points M-UE-1 (shi xuan) were pricked to let 1-2 drops of blood from each point.

RESULTS

After seven treatments, most of the pain in the forearms had disappeared. The redness of the skin was improved, although numbness in the hands persisted. The pulse was still wiry and thin, and the tongue retained its thin, white coating; but the tongue itself was no longer red. Judging from the pulse and the remaining symptoms, it was concluded that the Heat in the channels and the stasis of Blood had largely dissipated. Accordingly, GV-14 (da zhui) and M-UE-1 (shi xuan) were withdrawn from the point prescription, leaving LI-11 (qu chi), TB-5 (wai guan) and LI-4 (he gu). These points continued to be needled daily, using the same draining methods as before. After another seven treatments, the pain in the forearms, redness of the skin and numbness in the hands had all disappeared. The patient was followed up for one year, during which there was no recurrence of symptoms. □

Painful Obstruction of the Bone
(Calcaneal Spur)

Gŭ Bì 骨痹

Liang, female, 54 years old. During the 3 months prior to her visit to the clinic, the patient felt increasing pain in her right heel. Upon walking, a severe pain was felt where her right heel touched the ground; the pain was less pronounced when her right leg was lifted. Walking or standing on both feet was difficult. X-ray examination revealed a conical osseous proliferation of the calcaneus at the insertion of the plantar fascia. The diagnosis was calcaneal spur.

The four examinations of Chinese medicine revealed that the patient was obese and quiet. She walked with a slow gait, and could not endure walking or standing for long. Digital pressure at the center of the right heel produced severe pain, and upon deep pressure, a hard mass was palpable. She also had soreness in the lower back, and weakness in the legs. She tired easily and felt dizzy. Her tongue was pale with a thin, white coating, and her pulse was submerged, thin and without strength.

SYNDROME DIFFERENTIATION

Bone spurs fall under the category of painful obstruction in traditional Chinese medicine. In *Simple Questions* (chapter 43), painful obstruction of the bone is described as pain or swelling of a joint or an area of a bone. The patient here was diagnosed with this condition owing to the deep, hard, localized mass, which was palpable on deep pressure.

The patient was obese, and most obese people suffer some degree of deficiency. More specifically, the patient's symptoms of soreness in the lower back and weakness in the legs, dizziness and fatigue, the pale tongue with a thin, white coating and the submerged, thin and weak pulse all pointed to deficient Yin of both the Liver and the Kidney.

The Liver governs the sinews, and the Kidney governs the bones and stores Essence. Because of the Yin deficiency in both of these Organs, the sinews, channels and marrow were deprived of nourishment, thus leading to pain in the heel. The course of the Kidney channel starts under the small toe, runs obliquely across the arch, and enters the heel from behind the medial malleolus before ascending along the medial surface of the leg. Because the Kidney channel passes through the heel, Kidney deficiency resulted in an inadequate flow of Qi to this area, which became intolerant of strain. Finally, because of the patient's obesity, great stress was placed on the heels, causing Blood stasis and stagnant Qi, which led to severe tenderness upon pressure.

In summary, the condition manifested in symptoms of excess from Blood stasis and stagnant Qi, with deficiency of Liver and Kidney Yin as the root cause.

TREATMENT

In treating this case, consideration was given both to the manifestations and the root cause. The point of pain, and points associated with the Kidney, formed the basis of the prescription. Both acupuncture and moxibustion were used to open the channels, remove the Blood stasis and stagnant Qi, and replenish the Kidney in order to consolidate the foundation.

Points selected:

The point of pain in the center at the bottom of the heel, K-3 *(tai xi)*, B-60 *(kun lun)*, B-57 *(cheng shan)* and B-23 *(shen shu)*, all on the right side. Treatment was administered once daily, and the needles were retained for 20 minutes.

Discussion of points:

The point of pain over the heel was selected as a local point. Deep puncture at this point relieves pain by removing local stagnant Qi and Blood stasis. Warm needle moxibustion was then applied at this point to warm and open the channel, thus promoting the flow of Qi and Blood to help remove the stagnation and stasis.

K-3 *(tai xi)* is the source point of the Kidney channel, and B-23 *(shen shu)* is the associated point on the back for the Kidney;

tonifying these two points replenishes Kidney Qi. It should be noted that one approach to treating deficiency of an Organ is to tonify its 'mother' Organ. Since the Kidney is the 'mother' of the Liver, tonifying the former strengthens the latter. In addition, because the Kidney is interior-exteriorly related to the Bladder, needling B-60 *(kun lun)* and B-57 *(cheng shan)* on the Bladder channel helps facilitate the flow of Qi and Blood in the heel region.

Thirty-gauge filiform needles were used at all of the points. The point of pain on the heel was needled perpendicularly with a 1.5-unit needle to a depth of about 1 unit, reaching the periosteum. No raise-thrust or twirling of the needle was utilized, as this would have been too painful.

The point of pain remained stationary. After the needles were inserted at the other points, warm needle moxibustion was applied at this point. Two 1-unit stubs were used during each session.

K-3 *(tai xi)* was needled perpendicularly with a 1-unit needle to a depth of about 0.4 unit; tonifying manipulation was then applied. The needle sensation resembled an electric shock, which was transmitted to the medial aspect of the heel and arch. B-60 *(kun lun)* was needled obliquely toward the heel with a 1.5-unit needle to a depth of about 1 unit; moderate tonifying-draining manipulation was applied. The needle sensation was one of soreness and distention, which was transmitted to the lateral aspect of the heel. B-57 *(cheng shan)* was needled perpendicularly to a depth of about 1.2 units; moderate tonifying-draining manipulation was applied. The needle sensation of soreness and distention was transmitted to the region above the Achilles' tendon. B-23 *(shen shu)* was needled perpendicularly with a 1.5-unit needle to a depth of about 1.2 units; tonifying manipulation was applied, and the needle sensation of soreness and distention was transmitted both up and down the channel.

RESULTS

After three treatments, the pain was substantially alleviated. When she walked, the patient could touch the ground with her right heel without much pain. The soreness in the lower back, weakness in the legs, and dizziness were also improved. After eleven treatments using the same set of points, the pain in the right heel disappeared altogether, and the patient could walk freely. The other symptoms had also improved significantly. However, X-ray showed that the calcaneal spur remained the same as before.

Treatment was then discontinued. When the patient returned to the clinic one month later, she reported that the pain in her heel had not recurred, and that she was quite pleased with the result.

Note: Although the pain was alleviated during the course of treatment, the spur was not resolved. It is probable that the pain will return, at which time acupuncture should be used again. □

Painful Obstruction of the Bone
(Costal Chondritis)

Gǔ Bì 骨痹

Qian, male, 36 years old. One year ago, during house-moving, the patient was inadvertently exposed to a draft while perspiring. Three days later, persistent pain was felt over the right chest. During the next few days, a swelling appeared in that area, with distinct tenderness. The diagnosis was costal chondritis. Local injections of procaine and prednisone were tried, together with oral administration of analgesics. However, the condition persisted for more than 10 months, and was aggravated by fatigue, and by changes in the weather.

Examination revealed a tender swelling, about the size of an almond, over the right 4th and 5th costochondral junctions. The pain increased upon coughing, lying on the right side, deep breathing, or abduction of the right arm. The skin over the mass was normal, and no fluctuation was felt on palpation. Laboratory findings were within normal limits. The patient's face was pale yellow. The tongue was dark red with a thin, white coating, and the pulse was submerged and choppy.

SYNDROME DIFFERENTIATION

The patient reported that he was constitutionally weak. His complexion and pulse revealed deficiency of Qi and Blood. When this deficiency was aggravated by fatigue, the undernourished bone and adjacent tissue became susceptible to invasion by Wind-Cold. Once in the channels, the Wind-Cold interfered with the flow of Qi and Blood. Pain and local tenderness were signs of excess, while the dark red tongue and choppy pulse were manifestations of Blood stasis. The root of the condition was therefore deficiency of Qi and Blood, and the manifestations reflected Qi stagnation and Blood stasis. It was therefore a syndrome of both excess and deficiency. The condition was called painful obstruction of the bone because of the swelling over an area of bone.

TREATMENT

To relieve the pain, treatment was directed at invigorating the Blood to resolve the stasis, and expelling the Cold to restore free-flowing in the channel. This was achieved by the combined use of draining manipulation and ginger-mediated moxibustion.

Points selected:

CV-17 *(tan zhong)*, K-22 *(bu lang)*, K-23 *(shen feng)*, two points of pain over the 4th and 5th costochondral junctions, L-1 *(zhong fu)*, P-6 *(nei guan)*

Treatment was administered once daily.

Discussion of points:

CV-17 *(tan zhong)* is the meeting point of Qi. Stimulating this point promotes the flow of Qi, which helps in expelling the pathogenic Wind-Cold. K-22 *(bu lang)* and K-23 *(shen feng)* are local points in the vicinity of the swelling. As points on the Kidney channel, their use strengthens the normal Qi in order to expel the pathogenic influences, and thereby resolve the stagnation and relieve the pain. Points of pain are those places at which the pathogenic influences lodge. Stimulating these points invigorates the Blood and disperses the stasis. L-1 *(zhong fu)* is the alarm point of the Lung; when needled with balanced manipulation, it promotes the flow of Qi, thereby invigorating the Blood. P-6 *(nei guan)* is effectively used to relieve pain involving the Heart, Stomach or chest.

After arrival of Qi, draining manipulation through twirling was applied at points in the vicinity of the lesion — K-22 *(bu lang)*, K-23 *(shen feng)* and the two points of pain. At the other three points, balanced tonifying-draining manipulation was used. The needles were retained for twenty minutes.

Ginger-mediated moxibustion was administered for 5-10 minutes at all points except P-6 *(nei guan)* and L-1 *(zhong fu)*. These 2 points were used primarily to promote the flow of Qi in the Lung and Pericardium channels, both of which traverse the affected area. In this case, it was felt that needling alone at these points was sufficient to promote the flow.

RESULTS

After three treatments, the pain and swelling were substantially alleviated. To enhance the tonification aspect of the treatment, S-36 *(zu san li)* was added to strengthen the Qi and Blood, and to help the normal Qi dispel the pathogenic influences. After five more treatments, the swelling subsided, and the patient's complexion resumed a normal appearance, as did his tongue. The pulse was wiry, and moderate in rate. To consolidate the effect, the same treatment was continued for three more days. After a total of eleven treatments, the condition had completely resolved. Follow-up for one year showed no relapse. □

Painful Obstruction of the Sinews

Jīn Bì 筋痹

Su, male, 52 years old. The patient, a packing laborer, suffered from pain and swelling over the back of his right wrist for 2 weeks. There was no history of trauma, only of overwork and fatigue. The pain was aggravated by movement of the fingers, and by abduction of the wrist. The pain radiated toward the back of the hand and the lateral aspect of the forearm. Movement of the thumb, index and middle fingers was impaired. Application of a traditional preparation, Anti-Dampness Analgesic Plaster (shāng shī zhǐ tòng gāo), was ineffective. The patient therefore sought acupuncture therapy.

The four examinations of Chinese medicine found a well-developed patient, with healthy facial color. There was swelling and redness over the extensor pollicis longus, extensor indicis proprius and extensor digitorum communis tendons. Pain increased upon movement of the fingers and dorsiflexion of the wrist; with the latter movement, a fine, grating sound of the tendons was heard. The tongue was pink with a thin, white coating. The pulse was moderate in rate, but wiry. The diagnosis was painful obstruction of the sinews.

SYNDROME DIFFERENTIATION

This case developed without a history of severe trauma, but from overuse of the hand, which was required in the patient's work. It is noted in *Simple Questions* (chapter 23) that prolonged walking damages the sinews. The word 'walking' may refer to movement involving any joint. In this case, there were no symptoms of invasion by external pathogenic influences, nor were there signs of disease in the internal Organs. The syndrome was therefore one of stagnation of Qi and stasis of Blood in the channels due to damaged sinews (tendons).

The pain and swelling resulted from the stagnation of Qi and stasis of Blood. The prolonged stasis generated Heat, which caused redness in the affected area. The fine grating sounds occurred because the swelling caused the tendons to rub against each other during movement. Because the pain and swelling occurred in the paths of the Large Intestine and Triple Burner channels, the pathology was localized in these two channels. Thus, the final diagnosis was painful obstruction of the sinews, with stagnation of Qi and stasis of Blood in the Large Intestine and Triple Burner channels.

TREATMENT

The principle of treatment was to promote the flow of Qi and dissipate the stasis of Blood.

Points selected:

LI-4 *(he gu)*, LI-5 *(yang xi)*, TB-5 *(wai guan)* and three points of pain in the area of swelling

Draining manipulation was applied at all points, and the needles were retained for 20 minutes during each session.

Discussion of points:

The three points of pain were chosen based on the traditional principle, 'wherever the pain, there is the point'. LI-4 *(he gu)*, LI-5 *(yang xi)* and TB-5 *(wai guan)* are local points on the channels in which the flow of Qi was impeded. Needling these points was aimed at promoting the flow of Qi. Draining manipulation was used because the pattern was one of excess.

At the points of pain, the needles were inserted at an angle of 15^0 to a depth of 0.8 unit, with the tips directed toward the wrist. The first needle was inserted lateral to the extensor pollicis longus tendon, the second needle medial to the extensor indicis proprius tendon, and the third needle in the swelling over the extensor digitorum communis tendon. Draining manipulation was applied by twirling the needles. The sensation produced was one of local distention. At LI-4 *(he gu)* the needle sensation radiated toward the thumb, index finger and wrist. When LI-5 *(yang xi)* was needled, the sensation was one of local soreness. At TB-5 *(wai guan)* the sensation radiated toward the back of the hand and forearm along the path of the Triple Burner channel.

RESULTS

The pain and swelling were substantially reduced after the first treatment. The grating sounds also diminished. After five daily treatments, all symptoms disappeared, and free movement of the fingers and wrist was restored. Acupuncture was then discontinued. The patient was advised to avoid overwork in the future. Follow-up one month later found no abnormalities. □

CHAPTER FOUR
Disorders of the Eyes, Ears, Nose and Throat

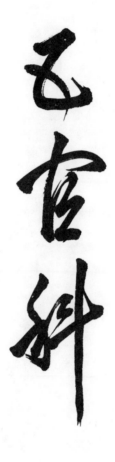

Absence of Facial Sweating
(Hemifacial Anhidrosis)

Bàn Miàn Wú Hàn Zhèng 半面无汗症

Shen, male, 42 years old. For 18 years the patient suffered from left-sided migraine headaches, with a frequency of 1-2 attacks per month. Absence of sweating (hemifacial anhidrosis) of the same side set in about 1 year ago. Various doctors were consulted, but the cause of the ailment could not be ascertained.

Upon examination, the left side of the face was dry, with no trace of sweat. However, the right side was moist and slightly flushed. The demarcation was very clear along the midline of the face, from the midpoint between the eyebrows to the middle of the chin. The tongue and pulse were normal, and no other abnormalities were found.

SYNDROME DIFFERENTIATION

This was a rare disease. In traditional Chinese medicine, the head and face is the area of confluence of all the Yang channels. When Qi in the Yang channels is obstructed, disturbing the circulation of Qi and Blood, headache results. This is because obstruction leads to pain. Prolonged headache aggravates the obstruction, which in turn affects the secretion of sweat.

The secretion of sweat is also related to the opening and closing of the sweat pores. Since the skin, including the sweat pores, is controlled by the Lung, stagnation of Qi in the Lung will affect the normal function of the sweat pores. The absence of sweating can thus result from failure of the pores to open. Furthermore, sweat is one of the five Fluids (sweat, saliva, spittle, tears and nasal discharge*), and is controlled by Kidney Qi. The Kidney is responsible for sending clear Fluids to the Lung, which then distributes them in various forms, including sweat. When stagnation occurs in the Kidney channel, the distribution of sweat is hindered, leading to the absence of sweating.

---

*In Chinese medicine, saliva is controlled by the Spleen, and spittle by the Kidney.

The diagnosis was accordingly obstructed Qi and Blood in the Yang channels of the head and face, together with stagnation of Qi in the Lung and Kidney channels.

TREATMENT

Treatment was directed at clearing the channels and opening the sweat pores. Both local and distant points were chosen.

Points selected:

LI-4 *(he gu)*, L-7 *(lie que)*, K-7 *(fu liu)*, M-HN-9 *(tai yang)*

Treatment was administered once every other day.

Discussion of points:

LI-4 *(he gu)* is a point on the Yang Brightness (Large Intestine) channel of the arm, a channel rich in Qi and Blood which travels up to the face. Needling this point stimulates the circulation of Qi and Blood in the Yang channels of the head and face. It is therefore frequently used for diseases affecting this part of the body. Needling LI-4 *(he gu)* also effects the opening of the sweat pores and promotes sweating, and is therefore used for treating patterns of Cold accompanied by the absence of sweating.

L-7 *(lie que)* is the connecting point of the Lung channel. Needling this point promotes the flow of Lung Qi and opens the sweat pores. K-7 *(fu liu)*, a Kidney channel point, is useful for treating all forms of abnormal sweating (absence of sweating, diminished sweating, spontaneous sweating, night sweats). M-HN-9 *(tai yang)* is commonly used for treating diseases of the head, face and eyes (e.g., painful red eyes, headache, facial paralysis, trigeminal neuralgia) since it acts to clear the head and eyes, and to open the Yang channels of the head and face. In this case, M-HN-9 *(tai yang)* was chosen as a local point to open the Yang channels.

In his book, *Great Compendium of Acupuncture and Moxibustion,* the renowned Ming dynasty acupuncturist, Yang Jizhou, noted: "For diminished sweating, first tonify LI-4 *(he gu)*, and then drain K-7 *(fu liu)*." We followed Yang's method for needling LI-4 *(he gu)* and K-7 *(fu liu)* in this case, and then needled L-7 *(lie que)* with balanced tonifying-draining manipulation. Each of these points was needled bilaterally, and the needles retained for 5-10 minutes. At M-HN-9 *(tai yang)* only the left side was needled. The needle was inserted transversely under the skin, then joined to S-7 *(xia guan)* and S-6 *(jia che)*, a distance of about 3 units. Twirling (large amplitude) and raise-thrust manipulation was applied until the skin began to sweat.

RESULTS

The treatment did not begin to take effect until the fourth session, when sweat appeared on the left side of the face. During the seventh session, there was sweating over the entire forehead, and on both eyelids and cheeks. Treatment was then discontinued. On follow-up three months later, the sweating was still normal, and the patient had experienced no headaches in the meantime. □

Difficulty in Swallowing

Yē Gé 噎嗝

> Chen, female, 43 years old. Five days ago, in a hurry to get to work, the patient swallowed some boiling hot milk. She immediately felt a continuous burning pain behind the sternum. The pain was subsequently aggravated whenever she swallowed food or drink. She was treated with Qi-regulating herbs, but to no avail. She then sought acupuncture treatment.

The patient's chief complaints were difficulty in swallowing, and an unbearable burning pain behind the sternum. The tongue had a thin, white coating, and the pulse was slightly rapid.

SYNDROME DIFFERENTIATION

The symptoms in this case resembled those known in traditional Chinese medicine as 'difficulty in swallowing', characterized by a feeling of obstruction in the throat, or in severe cases by vomiting, when attempting to swallow. Although the symptoms in the present case were relatively mild in that the patient could still swallow (albeit with difficulty), the same principles can be applied in analyzing this condition.

The most prominent symptom here was pain. Neither the tongue coating nor the nature of the pulse showed any specific patho-logical changes. The condition was therefore best understood by applying the principle in Chinese medicine that obstruction leads to pain.

At the level of the channels, it is the obstruction to the flow of Qi and Blood that gives rise to pain. It can therefore be inferred that the obstruction of the channels in this case resulted from stagnation of Qi and stasis of Blood due to the searing effect of the boiling milk.

TREATMENT

Treatment was aimed at promoting the flow of Qi and invigorating the Blood to remove obstruction from the channels. Since the location of the burning pain was behind the sternum, the topographical characteristics of this part of the body were taken into consideration when planning the prescription.

Points selected:

B-13 *(fei shu)*

Balanced tonifying-draining manipulation was applied. The needles were retained for 20 minutes, and were manipulated once every 5 minutes.

Discussion of points:

The Lung is situated in the thoracic cavity, and the Lung channel traverses the throat. Chest pain and difficulty in swallowing can be treated via the Lung. B-13 *(fei shu)*, whose domain corresponds to the thoracic region, was selected for this purpose. B-13 *(fei shu)* is the associated point of the Lung on the back. The associated points are effective in treating diseases not only of the specific Organ with which each is associated, but also of the region of the trunk topographically related to that Organ.

The use of B-13 *(fei shu)* also satisfied another principle of acupuncture: in treating diseases which are Yin in nature, points on the Yang aspects of the body may be selected, and vice versa. Since the chest pertains to Yin, and the back to Yang, pain in the chest may be regarded as a Yin disorder, which can therefore be treated by needling points such as B-13 *(fei shu)* on a Yang channel of the back.

Because the lung is situated directly below B-13 *(fei shu)*, the needle was inserted gently, and slanted slightly toward the spine, to a depth of only 0.5 unit, in order to avoid penetrating the lung. An acupuncture maxim is worth mentioning here: "Points on the chest and back are like ice, while those on the abdomen are like wells." This means that because the muscles in the chest wall and the back are thin like ice, and are close to the heart and lung, care must be taken not to pierce too deeply; whereas because the muscles in the abdominal wall are thick, needle insertion there is like dipping into a deep well.

RESULTS

When the needles were removed after the first treatment, the patient was asked to drink some lukewarm water to find out how the treatment had worked. The patient reported that when she swallowed, the pain behind the sternum was much better. Two more treatments were administered on the following two days, after which the symptoms disappeared completely. Treatment was therefore terminated. □

Discharge of Pus from the Ear

Tīng Ěr 聤耳

Wei, male, 21 years old. The patient had suffered sporadic discharge of pus from the left ear for 2 years. Recently, there was a relapse in the condition, and the patient therefore sought acupuncture treatment.

Upon examination, it was noted that a thin, white, purulent discharge exuded from the patient's left ear canal. The pars tensa of the tympanic membrane was perforated, and the external auditory canal and periphery of the tympanic membrane were also congested.

The patient complained of dizziness, tinnitus, impaired hearing, irritability, dryness of the mouth, and soreness and weakness in the lower back and knees. The tongue was red with a thin, yellow coating, and the pulse was wiry, thin and rapid.

SYNDROME DIFFERENTIATION

The chief complaint of the patient was discharge of pus from the ear canal. When diagnosing any condition in traditional Chinese medicine, one must first decide whether the nature of the disease is one of excess or deficiency.

If the condition is one of excess, the symptoms manifest more abruptly, and run a comparatively short course. When there is pus, it is thick and yellow. In addition, the patient will often experience a sharp, burning pain in the ear, as well as headache and fever. All of these symptoms are due to the invasion of the ear by Wind and intense Heat and Dampness from the Liver and Gall Bladder.

In the case of deficiency on the other hand, the pattern is one of gradual onset and a protracted course, with exacerbations and remissions. The pus is usually thin and white, and the patient often experiences dizziness, tinnitus, irritability, dryness of the mouth, and soreness and weakness in the lower back and knees. These symptoms are due to deficiency of Kidney Yin, leading to upward-flaring of Fire into the ear. Because the patient here presented with these symptoms, the condition was attributed to Kidney Yin deficiency causing upward-flaring of Fire into the ear.

TREATMENT

The principles of treatment were to tonify the Kidney and clear the Fire in order to restore function to the ear.

Points selected:

G-2 *(ting hui)*, TB-17 *(yi feng)*, TB-2 *(ye men)*, G-40 *(qiu xu)*, K-3 *(tai xi)*, all on the left side

Tonification through twirling manipulation was applied at all points. The needles were retained for 20 minutes during each session. Treatment was administered once daily, with 10 treatments comprising 1 course of therapy.

Discussion of points:

G-2 *(ting hui)* and TB-17 *(yi feng)* are both situated in depressions in the vicinity of the ear. They are commonly used as local points in treating various ear disorders. During needling, the patient was asked to open his mouth in order to make the depressions more distinct, thus facilitating location of the points, as well as insertion and manipulation of the needles.

G-40 *(qiu xu)* and TB-2 *(ye men)* are both Lesser Yang channel points. These channels run from behind the ear into the ear, and then exit in front of the ear. Stimulation of these two points helps clear the Fire induced by deficient Kidney Yin, and clear the stagnant Qi from the Lesser Yang channels, thus acting to rid the ear of obstruction. (It should be noted that regardless of whether the pattern is one of excess or deficiency, the flow of Qi in the Lesser Yang channels will be affected, leading to hearing impairment and purulent discharge from the ear. Needling points on the Lesser Yang channels is therefore fundamental to the treatment of this disorder.)

K-3 *(tai xi)* is the source point of the Kidney channel. Since the Kidney 'opens' through the ears, needling this point tonifies the Kidney, nourishes the Yin and clears the deficiency-induced Fire from the ear. While this point could have been needled bilaterally, in this case only the left side was needled.

The combination of points used in this case demonstrates the principles of combining anterior with posterior points (G-2 *[ting hui]* in front of the ear with TB-17 *[yi feng]* behind), and superior with inferior points (TB-2 *[ye men]* on the arm with G-40 *[qiu xu]* and K-3 *[tai xi]* on the leg). Utilization of these two methods enhances the therapeutic effect.

RESULTS

After two treatments, the discharge of pus from the ear was reduced considerably. After seven treatments, no more pus was observed, and the ear became dry and clean. Congestion in the external auditory canal and the eardrum disappeared. Hearing was also improved. Because the symptoms were resolved, acupuncture therapy was therefore discontinued after one course of therapy. On follow-up six months later, the patient reported no recurrences. □

Glaucoma-Like Condition

Qīng Guāng Yǎn 青光眼

Zheng, male, 63 years old. The patient suffered from high intraocular pressure of both eyes for 1 year, accompanied by headache, blurred vision and painful distention, particularly in the left eye. Over the past 3 months, the pain in the head and eyes worsened, sometimes accompanied by nausea and vomiting. Hospital tests found visual acuity of 20/16 in the right eye and 20/25 in the left, and intraocular pressure of 32mm Hg in the right eye and 40mm Hg in the left. There was marked nasal contraction in the visual field of the left eye. Blood pressure was 130/90mm Hg.

The four examinations of Chinese medicine found painful distention in the head and the eyes, particularly on the left side, with blurred vision in both eyes, dizziness, nausea and occasional vomiting. The patient was ill-tempered, and the symptoms worsened when he became irritated. He was thirsty and preferred cold beverages. The tongue was red with a thin, yellow coating, and the pulse was slippery, wiry and rapid.

SYNDROME DIFFERENTIATION

Glaucoma-like condition is due to Wind, Fire or Phlegm. It may be caused by anger, which leads to upward-flaring of Liver Fire (or Wind), or by overwork or eyestrain, which consumes Liver and Kidney Yin, followed by the rising of Fire from deficiency.

This patient had an irritable temperament, and was advanced in age. According to *Simple Questions* (chapter 5): "By age 40, Yin diminishes by half, and life is weakened." When Yin is deficient, Yang Fire will flare upward. In addition, anger injures the Liver and causes Liver Fire to ascend. Because the eyes are the external 'openings' of the Liver, the upward-flaring of Liver Fire leads to painful distention in the head and eyes, and to blurred vision.

The Gall Bladder channel traverses the sides of the head. Because the Liver and Gall Bladder are interior-exteriorly related, Fire in the Liver channel may thus surge upward through the Gall Bladder channel, causing headache on both sides. The function of the Liver is to smoothen and regulate the flow of Qi and Blood. Emotional disturbance leads to the obstruction of Liver Qi, which may then transform into Fire that flares upward to attack the head and eyes. This explains why the patient's symptoms were aggravated by emotional upset or anger.

The Liver pertains to wood, and the Stomach to earth. In the mutual control cycle of the five phases, exuberance of Liver Fire results in the over-control of earth by wood. Thus, when the Stomach is attacked by Liver Fire, food is not digested well. It transforms into Phlegm-Dampness, which induces nausea and vomiting. This is further evidenced by a slippery quality in the pulse. A wiry pulse indicates a Liver disorder; a rapid pulse is a symptom of Fire. Thus, a rapid and wiry pulse is associated with Liver Fire. A red tongue with a yellow coating is also a sign of Liver Fire. In sum, this patient's condition was one of Liver Fire attacking the Stomach, and stagnation of Phlegm-Dampness.

TREATMENT

Points were chosen primarily from the Liver, Gall Bladder and Stomach channels, supplemented by points near the eyes. Draining manipulation was applied in order to clear the Liver of Fire, pacify the Stomach and suppress the rebellious Qi.

Points selected:

B-2 *(zan zhu)*, M-HN-9 *(tai yang)*, G-20 *(feng chi)*, CV-12 *(zhong wan)*, P-6 *(nei guan)*, S-36 *(zu san li)*, Liv-2 *(xing jian)*, K-3 *(tai xi)*

All points were needled bilaterally. Treatment was administered every other day, and the needles were retained for 20 minutes during each session. Ten treatments comprised 1 course of therapy, with 2-3 days' rest between courses.

Discussion of points:

B-2 *(zan zhu)* and M-HN-9 *(tai yang)* are located in the vicinity of the eyes. Draining these points clears the Fire from the head and eyes, and relieves painful distention. Because glaucoma-like condition involves the anterior part of the eye, shallow points such as these were chosen instead of such deep points as B-1 *(jing ming)* or M-HN-8 *(qiu hou)*, which are generally used for conditions involving the posterior part of the eye.

G-20 *(feng chi)* is an important point for treating pain in the head and eyes. Liv-2 *(xing jian)* is the gushing point of the Liver channel; needling this point has the function of clearing Heat from the channel. It has been shown that needling Liv-2 *(xing jian)* rapidly reduces the intraocular pressure of the eyes.* K-3 *(tai xi)* is both the source point and the transporting point of the Kidney channel; tonifying this point replenishes Kidney Yin. Strong Kidney Yin strengthens Liver Yin, and strong Liver Yin will in turn check Liver Yang, or Liver Fire. P-6 *(nei guan)*, CV-12 *(zhong wan)* and S-36 *(zu san li)*, needled with balanced tonifying-draining manipulation, pacifies the Stomach to promote its digestive function. This resolves the Phlegm, and thereby arrests the nausea and vomiting.

B-2 *(zan zhu)* was needled to a depth of 0.3-0.4 unit, and M-HN-9 *(tai yang)* to a depth of 1 unit. At G-20 *(feng chi)* the needle was inserted toward the opposite eye to a depth of about 1.2 units, and the needle sensation was transmitted to the orbital region on the same side of the head. Draining manipulation was applied at these three points through raise-thrust and twirling techniques.

Liv-2 *(xing jian)* was needled to a depth of about 0.7 unit. Rapid raise-thrust draining manipulation was applied for about 30 seconds, but twirling of the needle was avoided because of the pain it causes at this point.

---

*Journal of Traditional Chinese Medicine, 1963; 8:299.

CV-12 *(zhong wan)* and S-36 *(zu san li)* were needled to a depth of 1.2 units, and P-6 *(nei guan)* to a depth of 0.7 unit. Balanced tonifying-draining manipulation was applied at these three points after the needle sensation was obtained. The needle sensation at S-36 *(zu san li)* was transmitted to the front of the ankles, while that at P-6 *(nei guan)* was transmitted up and down the arm. At CV-12 *(zhong wan)* the sensation was one of local pain and distention. K-3 *(tai xi)* was needled to a depth of 0.4 unit. This point was tonified, and the needle sensation was transmitted to the mid-sole.

RESULTS

By the end of the first course, there was marked amelioration of the pain in the head and eyes. The vomiting was arrested, and the patient no longer complained of thirst and irritability. The intraocular pressure dropped to 25mm Hg in both eyes. After 42 treatments with the same set of points, all of the symptoms disappeared. Intraocular pressure was 18mm Hg in the right eye and 20mm Hg in the left, visual acuity was 20/16 in the right and 20/13 in the left, and the visual field was restored to normal. Needling was continued once a week for another month to consolidate the effect. Treatment was then terminated, and the patient was advised to avoid fatigue and emotional upset. He was followed up for 3 months, during which time the intraocular pressure remained stable. □

Loss of Voice

Shī Yīn 失音

Shen, female, 27 years old. Hoarseness began after a cold that involved a sore throat, and was accompanied by a thick voice, coughing and thirst. After taking western drugs (erythromycin and expectorants), the cough and sore throat resolved, but the hoarseness developed into loss of voice. Spraying of tincture of benzoin provided no relief; nor did ingestion of either warm, acrid Chinese herbs, or cool, bitter ones that ventilate the Lung and clear internal Heat. The disease became chronic for over 6 months.

The patient complained of restlessness, disturbed sleep, tinnitus, a dry throat, and weakness and soreness in the lower back and in the knees. She was emaciated, her cheeks were flushed, and the palms and soles of the feet were hot. Severe hoarseness caused her to speak with difficulty. The tongue was red with no coating, and the pulse was thin and rapid.

SYNDROME DIFFERENTIATION

The chief complaint of the patient was hoarseness that developed into loss of voice. In Chinese medicine, loss of voice from hoarseness is classified either as excessive in nature, caused by external factors, or as deficient in nature, caused by internal factors.

Hoarseness caused by external pathogenic influences is associated with symptoms of excess, and is characterized by an abrupt onset and a short course. It is generally caused by Wind, Cold or Heat that invades the Lung system (upper respiratory tract). Recovery is comparatively swift after proper treatment. Hoarseness caused by internal factors is associated with symptoms of deficiency. It often runs a chronic course of long duration due to injury of the body Fluids from Heat in the Lung, or Yin deficiency of the Lung and Kidney. Treatment is relatively difficult.

Depending on the signs and symptoms, hoarseness may therefore be categorized as one of four types:

- Wind-Cold. Hoarseness begins abruptly with a non-productive cough, fullness in the chest, stuffy nose, headache, chills

210

and fever. The tongue coating is thin and white, and the pulse is floating.

- Wind-Heat. The onset of hoarseness is abrupt, making talking difficult. Other symptoms include cough with yellow sputum, sore throat and thirst. The pulse is floating and rapid, and the tongue coating is thin and yellow.

- Lung Heat with injured Fluids. Hoarseness is accompanied by a dry throat, thirst, non-productive cough and dry lips. The tongue is red, and the pulse is rapid.

- Yin deficiency of the Lung and Kidney. Hoarseness may cause aphonia, and is accompanied by a dry throat. The emaciated patient feels restless and cannot sleep well. The cheeks are flushed, and the palms and soles are hot. There is dizziness, tinnitus, and soreness and weakness in the lower back and knees. The tongue is red and without coating. The pulse is thin and rapid.

In this particular case, hoarseness occurred after a cold, and was accompanied by a thick voice, sore throat, coughing and thirst. These symptoms are of the Wind-Heat type, caused by invasion of the Lung by external Wind-Heat, and by the failure of Lung Qi to properly descend. If herbs of a pungent and cooling nature had been used at the outset to dispel the Wind-Heat from the exterior of the body, the symptoms would have improved. Instead, pungent and warming, and bitter and cooling herbs were erroneously prescribed. Not only did these fail to dispel the Wind-Heat, they also prolonged the stagnation of Heat, which wasted and damaged the body Fluids or Yin.

It should be pointed out that the chief manifestations of the disease were in the throat and vocal cords. According to Chinese medicine, hoarseness is related to dysfunction of the Lung and Kidney, for the voice is produced by the Lung system, and is rooted in the Kidney. The Lung channel leads to the epiglottis, and the Kidney channel controls the base of the tongue and the pharynx. The Lung controls the Qi which produces the voice; the Kidney stores Essence, the abundance of which is transformed into Qi. When there is sufficient Essence in the Kidney, and sufficient Qi in the Lung, Essence and Qi will ascend to support the epiglottis, agitating the vocal cords to produce the voice. Insufficiency of Qi in the Lung and Essence in the Kidney will cause hoarseness or aphonia.

The duration of the disease in this patient exceeded six months, and deficiency always follows a disease of long duration. Her initial symptoms of Wind-Heat had transformed into Yin deficiency of the Lung and Kidney. The emaciation, flushed cheeks, hot palms and soles, restlessness and insomnia were all typical manifestations of internal Heat from deficient Yin. The Kidney resides in the lower back and 'opens' externally through the ears. Thus, deficient Kidney Yin caused weakness and soreness in the lower back and knees, and tinnitus. Long-term stagnation of Heat in the Lung led to dysfunction of the Lung, whose Qi then failed to agitate the vocal cords for emission of sound. The deficient Kidney Yin could no longer support the pharynx and base of the tongue, and also led to the dry throat. The red tongue, and the thin, rapid pulse were further evidence of internal Heat from deficient Yin.

The diagnosis was therefore Yin deficiency of the Lung and Kidney, and deficient Qi of the Lung, accompanied by Heat.

TREATMENT

For deficiency of Lung and Kidney Yin (the underlying cause of the disease), treatment was directed at nourishing the Kidney Yin, tonifying the Lung and replenishing its Qi.

At the same time, the accompanying Heat in the Lung was drained.

Points selected:

L-9 *(tai yuan)*, L-7 *(lie que)*, L-10 *(yu ji)*, K-6 *(zhao hai)*, K-7 *(fu liu)*, K-3 *(tai xi)*, CV-22 *(tian tu)*, B-13 *(fei shu)*

All points were needled with slight raise-thrust and twirling manipulation, and the needles were retained for 15-20 minutes during each session. Treatment was administered once every other day, with 7 sessions comprising 1 course of therapy. Rest intervals of 2-3 three days were allowed between courses. For the duration of treatment, the patient was advised to eat regularly, but to abstain from pungent stimulants, such as spicy foods and alcohol.

Discussion of points:

L-9 *(tai yuan)* is the source point of the Lung channel. This point tonifies the Lung and replenishes its Qi. L-7 *(lie que)* ventilates the Lung and arrests coughing. L-10 *(yu ji)* is the gushing point of the Lung channel, and is effective in clearing Heat from the Lung, and in relieving hoarseness. K-6 *(zhao hai)*, K-2 *(fu liu)* and K-3 *(tai xi)* are Kidney channel points. These three points tonify the Kidney and replenish Yin. It is also noteworthy that L-7 *(lie que)* is connected with the Conception vessel, and K-6 *(zhao hai)* with

the Yin Heel channel, as the points of confluence of these miscellaneous channels. The Conception vessel and Yin Heel channel traverse the Lung system, pharynx and diaphragm, and are especially useful in treating disorders in those areas.

CV-22 *(tian tu)* belongs to the Conception vessel. B-13 *(fei shu)* belongs to the Bladder channel, and is the associated point on the back for the Lung. When these two points are combined, one on the front and the other on the back, they have a regulatory effect on diseases of the Lung system and pharynx. The depth of needle insertion at both points in this case was about 0.5 unit.

RESULTS

After five treatments, the patient reported that the dryness in the throat, tinnitus, restlessness and insomnia were improved, but that the hoarseness remained. After two courses of therapy, the hoarseness began to diminish, and the patient could talk in a low voice. After four courses, her voice was fully restored. Other symptoms, such as the hot palms and soles, flushed cheeks, and soreness in the lower back, all gradually resolved. On follow-up one year later, the patient was doing well. □

Nasal Discharge from Deficient Lung Qi
(Allergic Rhinitis)

Bí Yuān 鼻淵

Gu, female, 37 years old. For 5 years, the patient suffered from a sensation of slight coldness in her back, and was prone to catch cold, whatever the season. More recently, when exposed to cold air or an irritating smell, she would experience severe itching in the nose, followed by repeated sneezing. Between attacks, her nose was often obstructed, and would discharge a profuse, thin, white fluid. She also suffered from general lassitude and spontaneous sweating. Her tongue was pale with a thin, white coating. Her pulse was frail and thin. An otorhinolaryngologist diagnosed the condition as chronic allergic rhinitis. Conventional treatment was unsuccessful, and the patient was referred for acupuncture therapy.

SYNDROME DIFFERENTIATION

The principal symptoms were those of the nose. In traditional Chinese medicine, the nose is regarded as the 'opening' of the Lung. When the Lung functions normally, respiration is smooth, the nose is unobstructed and the sense of smell is intact. When the Lung is invaded by external pathogenic influences, or when there is deficiency of Lung Qi, then the flow of Lung Qi will be impaired, and symptoms will develop. Generally, diseases caused by external pathogenic influences are those of excess, and diseases caused by deficient Qi are those of deficiency.

Lung diseases caused by external pathogenic influences are of four types: Wind-Cold, Wind-Heat, Dry-Heat and Damp-Heat.

Symptoms of Wind-Cold include nasal obstruction with a thin, white discharge, sneezing, fever, chills, headache, cough and the absence of sweating. The pulse is floating and tight.

Symptoms of Wind-Heat include nasal obstruction with a thick, yellow discharge, fever, cough, sweating and thirst. The pulse is floating and rapid.

Symptoms of Dry-Heat include dryness in the nose, nasal obstruction with a scanty, yellow discharge (sometimes blood-tinged), a bitter taste in the mouth, dry throat, dry stools, deep yellow urine and thirst. The tongue is red, and the pulse is thin and rapid.

Symptoms of Damp-Heat include nasal obstruction with a profuse, thick and foul discharge, an impaired sense of smell, heaviness of the head, headache, a bitter taste in the mouth, reduced appetite and deep yellow urine. The tongue is red with a yellow, greasy coating, and the pulse is slippery and rapid.

Differentiation among these patterns of excess depends primarily upon differences in their associated systemic symptoms, and in the color, density and quantity of the nasal discharge.

Deficient Lung Qi is also manifested by local and systemic symptoms. Local symptoms include nasal obstruction, itching in the nose, nasal discharge and sneezing. Systemic symptoms include general lassitude and fatigue, lack of spirit and apathy, spontaneous sweating and a propensity for catching cold. The latter symptom is attributed to the Lung's function of controlling the skin: deficicnct Lung Qi results in weakening of the skin's function of warding off externally-contracted diseases, which allows invasion by external pathogenic influences.

In this case, the patient's symptoms were those of deficient Lung Qi. Although the local symptoms of nasal obstruction, sneezing and the thin, white discharge were the same as those associated with invasion by Wind-Cold, the absence of characteristic exterior symptoms, such as fever, chills, headache, the absence of sweating and a floating pulse, ruled out that diagnosis. Moreover, the course of the disease in this case was longer than that of an invasion by Wind-Cold, which usually has a sudden onset and a shorter course. In addition, the chill experienced in cases of deficient Lung Qi is usually felt as a localized sensation of coldness in the back, whereas the chill associated with Wind-Cold is often more severe, and involves the entire body.

TREATMENT

Treatment was directed at strengthening the Lung Qi and clearing the nasal passages using both acupuncture and moxibustion.

Points selected:

B-13 *(fei shu)*, L-9 *(tai yuan)*, LI-20 *(ying xiang)*, LI-4 *(he gu)*

Treatment was administered once daily. Mild moxibustion was administered at B-13 *(fei shu)*, and the other points were needled with balanced tonifying-draining manipulation. Twelve treatments comprised one course of therapy.

Discussion of points:

B-13 *(fei shu)* is the associated point on the back for the Lung. Mild moxibustion at this point strengthens the Qi of the Lung channel, and increases the body's resistance to disease. L-9 *(tai yuan)* is the source point of the Lung channel. Needling this point tonifies the Lung. LI-20 *(ying xiang)* is located beside the nostrils. Both this point and LI-4 *(he gu)* are on the Large Intestine channel, which winds around the nose. Both points are therefore frequently used in treating disorders of the nose.

The rationale was to treat the root or underlying cause—in this case deficient Lung Qi—by tonification of B-13 *(fei shu)* and L-9 *(tai yuan)*, and to treat the manifestations or symptoms—in this case nasal obstruction—by needling LI-20 *(ying xiang)* and LI-4 *(he gu)*. This combination of points is consistent with the principles of acupuncture therapeutics: selection of points in accordance with the pattern of the disease, the channel involved, and the presenting symptoms.

Mild moxibustion differs from circular moxibustion. The latter is administered by rotating the moxa stick around and above the point, and is used for problems involving an extensive area, such as rheumatic or muscular pain, and skin conditions. Mild moxibustion is administered by gradually moving the moxa stick away from the skin surface until the patient feels that the level of heat is comfortable. The stick is then held steadily above the point until there is local erythema, and a subjective feeling of warmth.

RESULTS

After seven treatments, the itching and sneezing were substantially reduced, and after five more treatments there was gradual relief of nasal obstruction and discharge. After an intermission of five days, a second course of twelve treatments was administered with the same set of points. Complete relief was obtained, including alleviation of the coldness in the back.

Follow-up after two years revealed that although there had been several relapses, the symptoms were considerably reduced in severity. The patient had not returned to the clinic because she felt that her problem did not warrant further treatment. □

Nasal Discharge from Heat in the Lung
(Chronic Maxillary Sinusitis)

Bí Yuān 鼻淵

Kang, female, 20 years old. For 2 years, the patient suffered from a stuffy nose with malodorous, purulent discharge, which necessitated changing her handkerchief several times a day. The discharge formed crusts in the nasal cavity, sometimes streaked with blood. Her voice had a nasal sound as though she were suffering from a bad cold. She was often light-headed. She preferred coolness, and had an aversion to heat. Her mouth was dry, and she was fond of cold beverages. She was constipated and her urine was scanty. The tip of her tongue was red, and the coating was thin and yellow. The pulse was rapid. She was diagnosed in a hospital as having chronic maxillary sinusitis, and was treated by puncture and irrigation more than 10 times, without effecting a cure. She then decided to try acupuncture.

SYNDROME DIFFERENTIATION

In Chinese medicine, conditions with a turbid (purulent) nasal discharge are referred to as *bí yuān*, denoting a pool in the nose. Such conditions are often due to prolonged accumulation of Wind-Heat in the Lung and the nose. When Wind-Heat becomes stagnant after the nasal passages have been blocked, the result is formation of mucus and continuous discharge. Another cause is Damp-Heat injuring the Spleen and Stomach, which disrupts the metabolism of water and nutrients, and results in the accumulation of these pathogenic influences in the nose, and the formation of discharge.

In cases of Wind-Heat, the nasal discharge is yellow, thick and profuse; when severe, there may be redness and painful swelling around the nostrils, and a stuffy nose. Accompanying symptoms include headache, fever, aversion to wind, cough, a red tongue with a white coating, and a floating, rapid pulse. In cases of Damp-Heat, the yellow, turbid and profuse nasal discharge has a foul odor. The nose is stuffy, accompanied by headache and a sensation of heaviness in the head, fullness of the stomach with poor appetite, a bitter taste and a sensation of stickiness in the mouth, lack of desire to drink, yellow urine, a red tongue with a yellow, greasy and slippery coating, and a slippery and rapid, or soft and rapid pulse.

This case presented with neither the exterior symptoms of Wind-Heat, nor with the symptoms associated with Damp-Heat injuring the Spleen and Stomach, which causes the accumulation of these pathogenic influences in the nose. Due to the protracted course of the disease, the exterior symptoms of Wind-Heat had already penetrated to the interior of the body, and the upward movement of Lung Heat had injured the nasal passages, blocking them, and leading to the formation of the purulent discharge. The upward movement of Heat had also caused the discomfort in the head.

The presence of interior Heat accounted for all of the symptoms, including the preference for coolness and aversion to heat, the feeling of dryness in the mouth and desire for cold beverages, and the constipation and scanty urine. The thin, yellow tongue coating and the rapid pulse also pointed to an interior Heat syndrome. The tip of the tongue reflects the condition of the Heart and Lung; the redness at the tip of this tongue thus signified the presence of interior Heat.

In summary, the long-standing, purulent discharge from the nose in this case was the result of accumulation of Heat in the Lung and the nasal passages.

TREATMENT

Treatment was aimed at dispelling the Heat from the Lung, and opening the nasal passages.

Points selected:

LI-11 *(qu chi)*, L-7 *(lie que)*, LI-4 *(he gu)*, L-10 *(yu ji)*, LI-20 *(ying xiang)*, M-HN-3 *(yin tang)*, S-44 *(nei ting)*

Since the patient was suffering from a condition of excess (invasion of Heat), draining through raise-thrust and twirling manipulation was administered. This was in accordance with the principle that excess should be treated by draining. Treatment was performed once daily.

Discussion of points:

LI-11 *(qu chi)* and LI-4 *(he gu)* are Large Intestine channel points. The Large Intestine and Lung channels are exterior-interiorly related. LI-11 *(qu chi)* relieves Heat, and LI-4 *(he gu)* relieves Heat and clears the Lung. These two points were thus chosen to dispel the Heat from the Lung. L-7 *(lie que)* is the connecting point of the Lung channel, connecting it with the Large Intestine channel. L-7 *(lie que)* was selected in this case for treating the discomfort in the head, since this point is used primarily in treating disorders of the head and neck.

L-10 *(yu ji)* is the gushing point of the Lung channel, and was chosen to dispel the Heat from the Lung. The gushing points are traditionally used for dispelling Heat *(Classic of Difficulties,* chapter 68).

LI-20 *(ying xiang)* is used primarily for treating disorders of the nose, and has the action of opening the nasal passages. In this case, it was chosen as a local point. M-HN-3 *(yin tang)* was chosen for treating both the discomfort in the head, and the stuffy nose. S-44 *(nei ting)* is the gushing point of the Stomach channel, and is therefore useful in dispelling Heat. Since the Stomach channel begins beside the nose, using this Stomach channel point on the foot helped to dispel the Heat from the nasal passages.

At L-7 *(lie que)* a 1-unit needle was inserted obliquely upward, which transmitted the needle sensation in that direction. At L-10 *(yu ji)* a 1-unit needle was inserted perpendicularly until the needle sensation was obtained locally. At LI-20 *(ying xiang)* a 1.5-unit needle was inserted obliquely toward the root of the nose to a depth of 1 unit, where a fairly strong local needle sensation was obtained. As soon as this point was needled, the patient felt her nose clear. At M-HN-3 *(yin tang)* a 1-unit needle was inserted obliquely downward toward the tip of the nose. At S-44 *(nei ting)* a 1-unit needle was inserted perpendicularly, producing a strong local needle sensation.

RESULTS

After ten daily treatments, the stuffiness of the nose improved, and the purulent discharge diminished. After fifteen treatments, the discomfort in the head subsided, but there was still a small amount of purulent discharge from the nose. The patient then left on a business trip, and treatment was therefore suspended for eight days, during which time there was no exacerbation of the condition. Therapy resumed when she returned. After another twenty treatments with the same set of points, all of the symptoms were alleviated. During a follow-up period of one and one-half years, there was no recurrence. □

Sparks Before the Eyes
(Photopsia)

Shén Guāng Zì Xiàn 神光自现

Wei, male, 42 years old. The patient, an office worker, had a history of migraine since youth. At age 30, he began to suffer from occasional diplopia, and upon undue eye strain would see golden sparks, followed by a bursting pain in the head and severe pain in the eyes, as if they were falling out. This was accompanied by nausea, vomiting and loss of appetite. The episodes occurred at 20-30 day intervals, each lasting 3-5 days. He was examined at an EENT clinic, and the condition was diagnosed as photopsia. Because the patient often overstrained his eyes during work, the condition worsened. He therefore sought acupuncture therapy.

Examination revealed that the patient's tongue was red. His pulse was wiry, thin and rapid at the front and middle positions, and frail at the rear position.

SYNDROME DIFFERENTIATION

The primary symptoms of this disorder were headache and sparks before the eyes. Chinese medicine regards the eyes as the 'openings' for the Liver. When Liver Yin is deficient, the eyes are deprived of nourishment, causing sensations of dancing sparks and flashes of light. Deficient Liver Yin leads to ascendant Liver Yang, resulting in severe pain in the head and eyes. Ascendant Liver Yang in turn affects the Spleen, causing nausea, vomiting and loss of appetite.

A long-standing deficiency of Liver Yin can also affect the Kidney, thereby producing deficient Kidney Yin. This was reflected in the present case by the nature of the pulse. Although it was wiry, thin and rapid at the front and middle positions, signifying deficient Liver Yin and resultant ascendant Liver Yang, it was frail at both rear positions, which indicated that the Kidney was deficient.

In summary, this condition was due to Yin deficiency of the Liver and Kidney, which caused ascendant Liver Yang.

TREATMENT

The principles of treatment were to replenish the Liver and Kidney Yin, and to check the ascendant Liver Yang.

Points selected:

Liv-3 *(tai chong)*, K-3 *(tai xi)*, Sp-6 *(san yin jiao)*, S-36 *(zu san li)*, B-1 *(jing ming)*, M-HN-8 *(qiu hou)*, M-HN-9 *(tai yang)*, G-37 *(guang ming)*, G-20 *(feng chi)*, GV-20 *(bai hui)*, LI-4 *(he gu)*

Treatment was administered once daily, with ten treatments comprising one course of therapy.

Discussion of points:

Liv-3 *(tai chong)* is the source point of the Liver channel, and K-3 *(tai xi)* is the source point of the Kidney channel. Tonification of these points strengthens the Liver and Kidney. Sp-6 *(san yin jiao)* is the point of intersection of the three Yin channels of the leg (Liver, Kidney and Spleen), and acts to replenish these Organs. S-36 *(zu san li)* has a general strengthening action. Needling these four points therefore not only strengthens the Liver and Kidney, but also improves the function of the Spleen and Stomach, thus alleviating the nausea and vomiting, and improving the appetite.

B-1 *(jing ming)*, M-HN-8 *(qiu hou)* and M-HN-9 *(tai yang)* are local points in the vicinity of the eye, and are often used in treating eye diseases. At B-1 *(jing ming)* the needle was inserted perpendicularly to a depth of 0.1-0.3 unit; raise-thrust and twirling techniques were avoided. M-HN-8 *(qiu hou)* was needled with the patient in a supine position, and with his eyes held open. The eyeball was pushed upward with the thumb, and the needle inserted along the lower surface of the eyeball, directed obliquely toward the back of the orbit to a depth of 1.0-1.5 unit. At M-HN-9 *(tai yang)* the needle was inserted transversely 1.0-1.5

units under the skin, joining to G-8 *(shuai gu)*. The combined use of these three points is effective in treating conditions of the head and eyes, such as pain and photopsia.

G-37 *(guang ming)* and G-20 *(feng chi)* were used to treat the root of the condition, ascendant Liver Yang. Both points are on the Gall Bladder channel, which has an exterior-interior relationship with the Liver channel. GV-20 *(bai hui)* and LI-4 *(he gu)* were chosen for their functions of clearing the senses and relieving headache.

RESULTS

On the morning after the fifth treatment, the patient felt dizzy, and sensed that an attack of photopsia was imminent. However, following treatment that day, he said that he felt fine, and that his sense that an attack was imminent had disappeared. After the first course of treatment, an intermission of three days was allowed before the second course began. During the second course of treatment, an attack occurred suddenly, which lasted half a day. It was accompanied by headache and a sensation of distention in the eyes. However, both symptoms were less pronounced than before acupuncture therapy began. Nevertheless, flashes of light and dancing sparks were still experienced during the attack. Treatment was continued with the same set of points for a total of thirty sessions. By that time, all symptoms had disappeared, and therapy was therefore discontinued.

The patient was followed up for one year, and no further recurrences were reported. □

Squint
(Strabismus)

Xié Shì 斜视

Chen, male, 22 years old. The patient often lay on his side during infancy, and was found to have a fixed cross right eye at age 1½. His parents thought he was too small to go to the hospital, and hoped that the eye would become normal when he grew older. However, at age 10 the squint remained, and he was referred to an eye clinic. Physical examination revealed esotropia of 45° in the right eye, with limited abduction. Vision in the right eye was 20/200. The diagnosis was congenital paralytic esotropia of the right eye. Because of misgivings about surgery on the part of the patient and his family, corrective glasses were prescribed. After wearing the glasses for 12 years, the squint had still not resolved. Instead, the right eyeball appeared sunken into the socket, and diplopia had set in. The family became quite concerned, and turned to acupuncture on the recommendation of friends.

The patient was thin and small in stature. His facial expression was neutral, and his mind was clear in conversation. His appetite was good, and bowel function was normal. The right eye was dull and fixed in the medial corner of the eye. The tongue was light red, with a thin, white coating.

SYNDROME DIFFERENTIATION

The primary mechanism leading to squint in Chinese medicine is the failure of Qi and Blood to nourish the sinews and Blood vessels near the eye. Dysfunction of the sinews and Blood vessels causes limitation of movement of the eyeball. The etiology of this condition is attributed to one of the following factors: invasion of the channels by external Wind-Heat, causing spasm of the sinews and vessels, which impairs the circulation of Qi and Blood; obstruction of the channels by Phlegm-Dampness; or innate constitutional weakness, such that the Qi and Blood are unable to warm and nourish the sinews and vessels.

The history of this patient revealed no signs of Wind-Heat, such as fever, headache, a red tongue with a yellow coating, and a rapid pulse. Nor did he experience an oppressive sensation in the chest, nausea or vomiting, fatigue, a greasy tongue coating or a slippery pulse, all of which would have indicated the presence of Phlegm-Dampness. Rather, his small stature and weak pulse suggested that the condition was caused by an innate constitutional weakness. Lying on his side for long periods of time during infancy may have caused stagnation of Qi and Blood, and resulted in a lack of nourishment to the sinews and Blood vessels near the eye.

TREATMENT

Treatment was directed at clearing the channels, and regulating the Qi and Blood.

Points selected:
G-1 *(tong zi liao)*, S-2 *(si bai)*, M-HN-9 *(tai yang)*, TB-23 *(si zhu kong)* and M-HN-8 *(qiu hou)* were needled on the right side only. S-36 *(zu san li)* and Liv-3 *(tai chong)* were needled bilaterally.

The patient's innate constitutional weakness indicated a deficiency of true Qi. Deficiency should be replenished. The points were therefore tonified by twirling the needles slowly, and with small amplitude.

Discussion of points:
The local points in the vicinity of the eye were chosen to clear the channels. The remote point S-36 *(zu san li)* belongs to the Stomach channel, which is abundant in Qi and Blood; needling this point regulates the Qi and Blood. Liv-3 *(tai chong)* is the source point of the Liver channel. Since the Liver 'opens' to the exterior through the eyes, this point is useful in treating eye diseases.

Needling was administered once daily for 20 days, but with no apparent effect. The situation was then reevaluated. Although acupuncture was regarded as a useful method of treatment, it did not appear to be strong enough in this particular case, which was of such long duration. The practitioner recalled a passage from chapter 73 of the *Miraculous Pivot*: "Moxibustion is proper for that which

needling cannot accomplish. Moxibustion warms and clears the 12 channels." Moxibustion was therefore combined with the acupuncture.

Because the eye is too tender an organ to be exposed directly to moxibustion, an indirect method was utilized whereby a layer of prepared walnut shell was interposed between the moxa cone and the eye. The walnut shell medium was used both to shield the eye from the excessive heat of moxibustion, and to promote the flow of Qi and invigorate the circulation of Blood locally.

The walnut shell medium was prepared as follows. A fresh walnut was cut in half, and the shell placed in a covered container together with 40g of Flos Chrysanthemi albi *(bai ju hua)* and 500ml of warm water. The solution was left to stand in a cool place for 24 hours. The effect of Flos Chrysanthemi albi *(bai ju hua)* was to penetrate the Liver channel, in order to clear the vision. The preparation strengthened the effect of moxibustion in warming the channels and vessels near the eye.

During treatment, the patient wore empty glasses frames to support the prepared walnut shell. The moxa cone was held by a piece of wire over the right eye. The heat was transmitted through the walnut shell. Treatment was administered once daily for 15-20 minutes. Acupuncture was also continued once daily, as described above.

RESULTS

After seven treatments, the patient felt relaxation in the right eye, with improvement in vision and diplopia. The right eyeball also began to abduct slightly. Vision was improved to 20/50. After ten treatments, the right eye returned to its normal central position, without retracting. After fifteen treatments, the right eye was completely normal, with vision of 20/16. The patient has been well ever since. □

Sudden Visual Failure

Bào Máng 暴盲

Zhang, male, 20 years old. The patient complained of constant headache, blurred vision and pain in the eyes. The symptoms began 20 days ago after drinking alcohol in a fit of anger. This was followed by a cold. He did not have a history of alcohol abuse or previous headache or eye problems. The headache and pain in the eyes were temporarily relieved by herbal medicine, but his vision remained seriously blurred. The patient was restless and irritable. His mouth was dry and bitter. Vitamin B complex and additional herbal medicines brought no relief. He therefore decided to try acupuncture.

Upon examination, the patient still had a slight headache, and his face was flushed. Urine was scanty and yellow. Stools were dry, and the patient was constipated. The tongue was red with a yellow coating. The pulse was wiry and rapid. Vision was 20/400 in the right eye, and finger-count was at 60cm in the left. Funduscopic examination revealed a hyperemic papilla with blurred margin and edema in the surrounding retina of the left eye.

SYNDROME DIFFERENTIATION

The Liver 'opens' externally through the eyes. The Gall Bladder channel originates at the outer canthus. The condition here arose after anger, which drives Qi upward, and alcohol, which is pungent and hot, produced Fire in the Liver and Gall Bladder that flared upward to the head and eyes. This was followed by an invasion of external Wind, which resulted in a struggle between Fire and Wind, thus further disturbing the eyes, and impairing the vision. The sudden onset of the condition indicated a pattern of excess. The upward-flaring of Liver Fire produced the flushed face, restlessness and irritability. Bile flowed upward with the Fire along the Gall Bladder channel, hence the bitter taste in the mouth. Fire destroys body Fluids, which accounts for the dry mouth, yellow urine, dry stools and constipation. The red tongue with yellow coating was a sign of Heat and excess. The rapid nature of the pulse likewise indicated a condition of Heat, and its wiry nature indicated a disorder of the Liver, and of Wind.

TREATMENT

Treatment was directed at clearing the Heat from the Liver and Gall Bladder, and clearing the vision by dispelling the Wind.

Points selected:

G-20 *(feng chi)*, Liv-2 *(xing jian)*, G-37 *(guang ming)*, LI-4 *(he gu)*, M-HN-9 *(tai yang)*, B-1 *(jing ming)*

Draining manipulation was applied at all points except M-HN-9 *(tai yang)* and B-1 *(jing ming)*. Treatment was administered once a day. The needles were retained for 30 minutes, and manipulated every 10 minutes.

Discussion of points:

G-20 *(feng chi)* is an important point for dispelling Wind and clearing the vision. Its effect is enhanced when combined with LI-4 *(he gu)*, which also dispels Wind. Liv-2 *(xing jian)* drains Liver Fire. G-37 *(guang ming)* is the connecting point of the Gall Bladder channel. Its name means 'brightness'. This point clears Fire from the Liver and Gall Bladder, and is an important point for treating eye diseases, and for clearing ('brightening') the vision. Pricking M-HN-9 *(tai yang)* with a pyramid needle to let 2-3 drops of blood acts to eliminate the pathogenic Heat, and to clear the vision. B-1 *(jing ming)* was selected as a local point in the vicinity of the eye. The combination of these points has the effect of driving the Fire downward, and of dispelling the Wind and clearing the vision.

M-HN-9 *(tai yang)* was bloodlet with a pyramid needle for three consecutive days, after which a filiform needle was substituted. Draining manipulation was then applied at this point. Bloodletting was discontinued because excessive use of this technique injures the Blood and Qi.

B-1 *(jing ming)* is located 0.1 unit medial to the inner canthus. It is usually needled to a depth of only 0.1-0.2 unit. However, deep insertion at this point has a very good therapeutic effect on diseases of the inner eye. In this case, the needle was therefore inserted to a depth of 1.0-1.2 units, and the needle sensation was transmitted to the back of the eye. Progression of the needle was slow along the medial margin of the orbit. When resistance was encountered, care was taken not to pierce the eyeball, but to continue directing the needle medially around the eyeball until the needle sensation was felt to have reached the back of the eye. Raise-thrust manipulation of the needle was avoided. The needle was withdrawn slowly, and a sterilized cotton ball was pressed over the needle opening for two minutes in order to prevent hemorrhaging.

RESULTS

The headache disappeared after one treatment, and a comfortably cooling sensation was felt in the eyes. Visual acuity began to improve after three treatments, together with amelioration of the other symptoms. After ten treatments with the same set of points, visual acuity had improved to 20/22 in the right eye, and 20/40 in the left. After twenty treatments, the patient felt that he had completely recovered. Vision was then 20/13 in the right eye, and 20/16 in the left. Retinoscopy found the papilla to be of normal color, and the surrounding retinal edema to have disappeared. The patient was still doing well on follow-up one-and-a-half years later. His vision was normal, as were the results of funduscopic examination. □

Tinnitus and Deafness
(Sudden Neural Deafness)

Ěr Míng, Ěr Lóng 耳鸣, 耳聋

Zhang, male, 24 years old. The patient complained of progressive tinnitus and hearing loss of about 5 months' duration. The symptoms first arose following a period of anxiety when the experienced occasional episodes of tinnitus, each lasting only a few minutes. About a month later, the tinnitus suddenly worsened, and became continuous; the sound was of a roaring nature. Loss of hearing was then experienced: total loss in the left ear, and from the right he could hear only when others shouted directly into the ear. Other symptoms included dizziness, headache, a dry and bitter taste in the mouth, irritability, restlessness, insomnia, scanty, yellow urine and dry stools. His condition was diagnosed by an otolaryngologist as sudden neural deafness. He took vitamins B$_{12}$ and E, but without effect. Hyperbaric therapy was also ineffective. He thereupon turned to acupuncture therapy.

Examination showed no inflammatory changes. There was also no tenderness over the mastoid process, and the eardrum was intact. The tongue was red with a thin, yellow coating, and the pulse was rapid and wiry.

SYNDROME DIFFERENTIATION

Acute onset of deafness in Chinese medicine is attributed to the obstruction of the ear by pathogenic influences. This patient's condition began with tinnitus, and progressed to deafness. Accurate differentiation is important if the condition is to be treated effectively. A discussion of the causes of tinnitus and deafness will therefore be useful. Deficient conditions include:

- Deficiency of the Spleen and Stomach, which causes insufficient Qi and Blood, and thus undernourishment of the ears. Other symptoms include a pasty complexion, lassitude, diminished appetite, watery stools, a thin and frail or big and weak pulse, and a tongue which is pale with a thin coating, and is tooth-marked.

- Deficiency of the Liver and Kidney, which causes insufficient Essence and Blood, and thus undernourishment of the sensory organs. Other symptoms include

225

dizziness, blurred vision, soreness of the lower back, spermatorrhea, a thin, frail pulse, and a red tongue. Alternatively, the symptoms may include weakness of the limbs, coldness in the lower back, impotence and premature ejaculation, a submerged, thin pulse, and a pale tongue with a thin coating.

- Fire of the Liver and Gall Bladder, which results when the emotions are so agitated that the Liver Qi loses its free-flowing nature and stagnates. Prolonged stagnation of Liver Qi transforms into Fire, which flares upward to engulf the ears. Symptoms include headache, flushed face, a bitter taste in the mouth, dry throat, restlessness, irritability, constipation, a wiry, rapid pulse, and a red tongue with a yellow coating.

- Stagnation of Phlegm and Fire in the ears, usually encountered only in obese persons. Symptoms include fullness in the chest, copious phlegm, a thin, greasy and yellow tongue coating, and a slippery, rapid pulse.

In the present case, the patient's symptoms clearly indicated that his condition was due to Fire of the Liver and Gall Bladder. The Liver, together with the Heart, regulates the emotions; emotional agitation, especially anger, causes stagnation of Liver Qi, which in turn gives rise to Liver Fire. The Gall Bladder and Liver are exterior-interiorly related, and an upward-flaring of Liver Fire may spread to the Gall Bladder. The Gall Bladder channel courses around the ear, and a branch enters the orifice. Upward-flaring of Fire from the Liver and Gall Bladder may thus involve the ear, leading to tinnitus, and when the ear is obstructed, to deafness.

This case was one of excess. The dizziness and headache arose as a result of Fire from the Liver and Gall Bladder flaring upward and attacking the head. Liver diseases are

characterized by irritability, which was also present in this case. Upward-flaring of Fire from the Liver affected the mind, giving rise to restlessness and insomnia. Fire often impairs the body Fluids, which here led to the dry mouth, scanty, yellow urine and dry stools. Upward-flaring of Fire from the Gall Bladder also caused the bitter taste in the mouth.

The red tongue with a yellow coating indicated an interior Heat syndrome. The wiry pulse pointed to Liver involvement, and the rapid pulse was a sign of Heat. In sum, this was a case of upward-flaring of Fire from both the Liver and Gall Bladder.

TREATMENT

Points on the Liver and Gall Bladder channels were selected, and local points were matched with remote ones. Draining manipulation was applied to clear the Heat and open the ear orifices.

Points selected:
G-2 *(ting hui)*, G-20 *(feng chi)*, G-34 *(yang ling quan)*, Liv-3 *(tai chong)*

All points were needled once daily with draining manipulation. The needles were raised-thrust and twirled with great amplitude, and then retained for 15 minutes during each session. The needles were withdrawn slowly, while being gently vibrated. After withdrawal of the needles, the needle holes were not pressed in order to allow the pathogenic influences to freely escape from the body.

Discussion of points:
G-2 *(ting hui)* and G-20 *(feng chi)* are points on the Gall Bladder channel. A branch of this channel enters the ear. G-2 *(ting hui)* and G-20 *(feng chi)* were selected as local points to remove the obstruction from the channels and ear orifices, as well as to relieve the dizziness and headache. TB-21 *(er men)* or SI-19

(ting gong) could have been substituted for G-2 *(ting hui)* with the same effect.

G-34 *(yang ling quan)* is the uniting point of the Gall Bladder channel. Uniting points are particularly useful in treating diseases of the Organs. This point was therefore selected to remove Fire from the Gall Bladder, and thus to dispel the bitter taste in the mouth. Liv-3 *(tai chong)* is the source point of the Liver channel. Source points are those at which the essential Qi of the Organs is stored. These points are used to treat disorders in their respective Organs. Since deficiency should be tonified and excess drained, Liv-3 *(tai chong)* in this case was drained to quell the Fire in the Liver. G-34 *(yang ling quan)* was combined with Liv-3 *(tai chong)* to enhance the effect of clearing the Heat from both the Liver and Gall Bladder. This was also an example of selecting points on the lower part of the body for disorders involving the upper part of the body. For disorders which are caused by the ascending of internally generated pathogenic influences (e.g., Liver Yang, Liver Fire, Heart Fire or Stomach Qi), it is a common practice to select points on the lower part of the body to guide the rebellious Qi downward. This is especially true for the upward-flaring of Fire and Heat. For this reason, local as well as remote points were selected to dispel the pathogenic influences both upward and downward.

RESULTS

The tinnitus was substantially reduced after ten treatments, but the patient's hearing remained poor. Loud noises could occasionally be heard near the left ear, but words could not be distinguished.

The tinnitus was completely alleviated after ten additional treatments with the same set of points. The ticking of a watch could then be discerned in the right ear, and loud speech could be heard in the left. The condition steadily improved. Hearing was finally restored to its original level after twenty-five treatments. The patient was followed up for one year, and there was no recurrence of tinnitus. □

Visual Disturbance
(Optic Neuritis)

Shì Lì Zhàng Ài 视力障碍

Ji, male, 10 years old. The patient was admitted for treatment of tubercular meningitis. After 3 months of treatment with both western and traditional Chinese medicine, there was significant improvement. However, within a period of 3 days, visual acuity suddenly deteriorated. This was accompanied by a dull frontal headache and tenderness of the eyeballs, as well as dizziness, blurred vision, tinnitus, redness of the lips and cheeks, dryness in the mouth with little desire to drink, disturbed sleep and excessive dreaming.

Ophthalmologic examination showed 20/200 eyesight in the left eye, and 20/100 in the right. Retinoscopy showed a hyperemic disc with blurred margin and some edema in the adjoining retina. The tongue was red, and the pulse was thin, wiry and rapid. The diagnosis was optic neuritis.

SYNDROME DIFFERENTIATION

The eyes are the 'opening' for the Liver. The functioning of the eyes is directly dependent on the supply of Blood to the Liver. When Blood supply is unsufficient, vision becomes blurred. Impaired vision may also occur when the Liver's spreading function is disturbed for prolonged periods of time, resulting in stagnant Qi, which transforms into Heat. Vision is also affected when the Kidney and Liver Yin are deficient.

In this case, the prolonged illness (tubercular meningitis) consumed Yin, and the remaining pathogenic factors attacked the Liver channel, causing the sudden blurring of vision. The other symptoms were also manifestations of Kidney and Liver Yin deficiency, and resulted from an upsurge of Fire from this deficiency.

TREATMENT

The principles of treatment were to nourish the Kidney and Liver Yin, and to clear the channels, thereby clearing the vision.

Points selected:

G-20 (feng chi), M-HN-8 (qiu hou), B-1 (jing ming), TB-23 (si zhu kong), B-23 (shen shu),

B-18 *(gan shu)*, K-7 *(fu liu)*, Sp-6 *(san yin jiao)*, Liv-8 *(qu quan)*

Treatment was administered once daily, with ten treatments comprising one course of therapy.

Discussion of points:

G-20 *(feng chi)* is a point on the Gall Bladder channel, which begins at the outer canthus of the eye. Because of the Yin/Yang relationship between the Liver and the Gall Bladder, this point was used to clear the head and vision. M-HN-8 *(qiu hou)*, B-1 *(jing ming)* and TB-23 *(si zhu kong)* are located in the vicinity of the eyeball, and were used as local points to clear the vision.

B-23 *(shen shu)* and B-18 *(gan shu)* are the associated points on the back for the Kidney and the Liver respectively. They were selected to nourish the Kidney and Liver Yin.

K-7 *(fu liu)* is the traversing point of the Kidney channel, and corresponds to metal. In this case, the mother-son tonifying principle was applied at this point, whereby K-7 *(fu liu)* (mother) was tonified in order to benefit the Kidney channel (son), which corresponds to water, since metal produces water according to the theory of the five phases. K-7 *(fu liu)* was thus used to nourish the Kidney Yin. Sp-6 *(san yin jiao)* is the point at which the three Yin channels of the leg intersect, and was selected to regulate the Liver and Kidney. Liv-8 *(qu quan)* was needled to quell the Fire and clear the Heat from the eyes.

G-20 (feng chi) was needled with the patient in a sitting position. The needle was inserted toward the tip of the nose to a depth of 1.0-1.5 units. The needle sensation was transmitted to the eyeball of the same side. The needle was retained for 15 minutes, and was then removed.

The other points were then needled with the patient lying down. When M-HN-8 *(qiu hou)* was needled, the eyeball was fixed in place with the thumb, while the needle was inserted slowly along the wall of the orbit to a depth of 1 unit. (If pain is encountered, the direction of the needle tip may be slightly altered.) There was a sensation of distention and soreness throughout the eye. Raise-thrust manipulation was not applied. B-1 *(jing ming)* was needled with the eye closed, and the eyeball gently pushed to the side; the needle was inserted slowly to a depth of 0.3 unit. Very slight twirling was applied. TB-23 *(si zhu kong)* was needled to a depth of 0.5 unit, directed posteriorly. These three points often bleed after needling, and it is therefore advisable to apply digital pressure for a few minutes after withdrawing the needles.

At K-7 *(fu liu)*, Sp-6 *(san yin jiao)*, Liv-8 *(qu quan)*, B-18 *(gan shu)* and B-23 *(shen shu)*, balanced tonifying-draining manipulation was used. The needles were retained for 30 minutes at all of the points except G-20 *(feng chi)*.

RESULTS

After one course of therapy, the patient's vision improved significantly. Ophthalmologic examination showed visual acuity of 20/100 and 20/50 in the left and right eyes respectively. Since the patient's general condition was improving satisfactorily, and because his eye condition was acute, treatment was increased to twice daily during the second course of therapy in order to accelerate recovery. By the end of this course, visual acuity was further improved to 20/30 in the left eye, and 20/20 in the right. After an intermission of five days, the frequency of needling was reduced to once daily to consolidate the effect. After fifteen more treatments with the same set of points, vision was 20/20 in both eyes. Treatment was then discontinued. The patient was followed up for one year, and his vision remained stable. □

CHAPTER FIVE
Disorders of the Skin

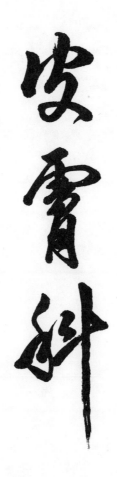

Damp Tinea-Like Rash
(Eczema)

Shī Xuǎn 湿癣

Zhao, female, 40 years old. The patient's chief complaint was itching of the skin, which began 20 days ago when she took a Chinese medication for chronic rhinitis called 'Special Pill for Tonifying the Brain' (bǔ nǎo dān). The following day she began to itch all over. At first she was able to cope with the itching, but later found it unbearable. Scattered, red eruptions appeared over her entire body. The patient discontinued use of the Chinese medication, and tried oral chlortrimeton and calcium gluconate injections, both of which were ineffective. A dermatologist prescribed oral dexamethasone and fluocinolone acetonide ointment; these two agents were also ineffective. The itching became so severe that the patient was unable to sleep at night. She then turned to acupuncture.

Upon examination, scattered small eruptions were still present, especially on the back and over the wrists and ankles. The eruptions had coalesced into red patches from which light yellow, clear fluid oozed upon scratching. The skin over the wrists and ankles was thickened from prolonged scratching and rubbing.

The patient was restless, and it was apparent that she had not slept well. She reported that her mouth was dry, but that she had no desire to drink. There was a bitter taste in her mouth. Her appetite was poor, and she complained of distention in the epigastrium. Her urine was yellow, and she was constipated. The tongue was red with a yellow, greasy coating. Her pulse was soggy and rapid.

SYNDROME DIFFERENTIATION

From the standpoint of western medicine, this patient had an allergic reaction to a medication. In Chinese medicine, the etiology of her condition can be deduced by understanding the causes of Damp tinea-like rash.

The condition was characterized by pruritus with small, red eruptions from which oozed a yellow, clear fluid upon scratching. Chinese medicine attributes Damp tinea-like rash to the confinement of pathogenic Wind, Dampness and Heat in the skin. Wind is characterized by its ambulatory nature, manifesting as wandering lesions or itching. Redness pertains to Heat; the red eruptions thus reflected the presence of Heat. The oozing of fluid upon scratching is a sign of Dampness. The accompanying symptoms of loss of appetite, gastric distention, constipation and yellow urine all indicated that Heat had accumulated in the Intestines. Heat impairs the body Fluids, hence the dryness in the mouth. However, the greasy tongue coating signifies Dampness, which reduced the patient's desire to drink. The condition was therefore one in which Damp-Heat in the Intestines became confined in the skin when dispersed outward, combined with the externally-contracted, pathogenic Wind, and resulted in stagnation of these pathogenic influences in the skin.

This patient took a Chinese medication which is sometimes prescribed for chronic nasal discharge. The traditional indications for this drug are deficiency of both Yin and Yang; its ingredients thus tonify Yang and nourish Kidney Yin. After taking the drug, the Damp tinea-like rash appeared. There are two explanations for this: either she took too much of the drug, leading to an accumulation of Damp-Heat; or she already had a condition of Damp-Heat, which was exacerbated by taking the drug. Because the patient exceeded the prescribed dosage, it can therefore be concluded that she had a preexisting condition of Damp-Heat. Indeed, one of the causes of chronic nasal discharge is Damp-Heat in the Spleen channel.

TREATMENT

Treatment was directed at clearing the Heat, resolving the Dampness, dispelling the Wind and arresting the itching.

Points selected:

LI-11 *(qu chi)*, TB-5 *(wai guan)*, Sp-10 *(xue hai)*, S-37 *(shang ju xu)*, Sp-9 *(yin ling quan)*

The points were needled once daily with draining manipulation, and the needles were retained for 15 minutes.

Discussion of points:

LI-11 *(qu chi)* is an important point for clearing Heat, and was thus chosen to clear the Heat from the Intestines. TB-5 *(wai guan)* functions to remove pathogenic influences (in this case Wind) from the exterior. Sp-10 *(xue hai)* is a point on the Spleen channel, and since the Spleen governs the circulation of Blood, this point acts to regulate and invigorate Blood circulation. Traditional Chinese medicine teaches that to control Wind, the Blood must first be regulated. Wind subsides by itself when normal Blood flow is restored, i.e., it is expelled naturally when it has nothing to cling to. Thus, although in this case there were no Blood symptoms per se, the strategy was to dispel the Wind indirectly by treating the Blood. The use of Sp-10 *(xue hai)* and TB-5 *(wai guan)* for invigorating the Blood and dispersing the Wind, combined with LI-11 *(qu chi)* for clearing the Heat, is an important combination of points for treating the itching due to stagnation of Wind and Heat in the skin.

Since this patient presented with Dampness in addition to Wind and Heat, the uniting point of the Spleen channel, Sp-9 *(yin ling quan)*, which also corresponds to water, was selected to resolve the Dampness. Furthermore, because the Damp-Heat arose from the Intestines before stagnating in the skin, the lower uniting point of the Large Intestine, S-37 *(shang ju xu)*, was needled to remove the Damp-Heat from that Organ.

Each of the Yang Organs which pertain to the arm channels (Large Intestine, Small Intestine and Triple Burner) has a uniting point on one of the leg Yang channels on the lower extremity: S-37 *(shang ju xu)* on the Stomach channel for the Large Intestine, S-39 *(xia ju xu)* on the Stomach channel for the Small Intestine, and B-39 *(wei yang)* on the Bladder channel for the Triple Burner. These are referred to as the lower uniting points. These points, as well as the uniting points of the Stomach, S-36 *(zu san li)*, the Gall Bladder, G-34 *(yang ling quan)*, and the Bladder, B-40 *(wei zhong)*, are located on the lower extremity, and are therefore referred to as the lower uniting points of the six Yang Organs. When these six points are used in treating diseases of the six Yang Organs, whether deficient or excessive in nature, satisfactory results are usually obtained. It was from such considerations that the lower uniting point of the Large Intestine, S-37 *(shang ju xu)*, was included in the prescription.

RESULTS

After the first treatment, the patient's sleep improved, the itching diminished, and there was normal bowel movement. After two treatments, the skin eruptions were greatly reduced, and the thickened skin over the wrists and ankles began to heal. Other symptoms, such as irritability, dryness of the mouth, distention in the stomach and poor appetite, were also much improved. After five treatments, the itching was completely arrested, the skin resumed its normal appearance, and the patient ceased to feel any discomfort. Three more treatments were administered to consolidate the therapeutic effect. The patient was advised to avoid taking similar herbal medication in the future. She was followed up for one year, and there was no recurrence of symptoms. □

Numbness of the Skin
(Lateral Femoral Cutaneous Neuritis)

Pí Fū Má Mù 皮肤麻木

Tang, female, 35 years old. Seven years ago, the patient was exposed to a draft in the hospital corridor following childbirth. At the time, she felt a transient, tingling pain on the lateral side of the left thigh. The pain later developed into local numbness, with an occasional sensation similar to that of ants running over the skin. Drugs and physical therapy were somewhat effective, but the patient did not continue therapy, and a complete cure was never realized. The condition was recently aggravated after a period of intensive work.

Examination revealed an area of numbness 12 x 8cm on the lateral side of the left thigh. The appearance of the skin was normal; there was no roughness or scaling. There was also no muscular atrophy. Limb motion and tendon reflexes were normal. The pulse was floating and weak, and the tongue was light red with a thin, white coating. The diagnosis was left lateral femoral cutaneous neuritis.

SYNDROME DIFFERENTIATION

In general, Qi and Blood are deficient in the post partum woman; normal nutrition and the natural resistance of the body are also disturbed. Pathogenic influences such as Wind, Cold and Dampness may take advantage of this condition to invade the body, thus causing dysfunction of the channels, and poor circulation of Qi and Blood. In chapter 43 of *Simple Questions*, it is observed that when obstruction of Qi and Blood occurs in the flesh, the result is numbness.

TREATMENT

The primary symptom in this case was local numbness of the skin. The disease was confined to the superficial tissues in that one area, and had not become a systemic condition. Therefore, only local points were selected to clear the channels and regulate the Qi and Blood. Radial needle manipulation was utilized.

A passage in chapter 7 of the *Miraculous Pivot* describes radial needling. It is performed by inserting one needle in the middle, and inserting four needles obliquely around the needle in the middle. This method is recommended for treating deep invasion of pathogenic influences over a wide area. Nowadays, it is used in the treatment of local numbness caused by obstruction in the flesh and skin.

Following these instructions, a needle was inserted to a depth of 2 units into the middle of the numb area, which in this case was located at G-31 *(feng shi)*. Four additional needles were then inserted in a radially symmetrical pattern, at a distance of 2-3 finger widths from the needle in the middle. Two of the four needles were inserted distal and proximal to the needle in the middle on the same channel. The other two needles were inserted on the remaining sides at an angle of 25⁰, directed toward the center of the affected area, to a depth of 2 units. Balanced tonifying-draining manipulation was utilized.

After the needle sensation was obtained, the needles were retained for 15 minutes.

Treatment was administered once daily, with seven sessions comprising one course of therapy. Between courses, there was an intermission of 2-3 days.

RESULTS

After one course of treatment, there was some sensory improvement. By the middle of the second course of treatment, definite improvement had occurred in the perception of pain and warmth. After the third course of treatment, tactile sensation returned, and after the fourth and last course, all sensations were restored. Follow-up for six months witnessed no recurrence of numbness. □

Purple Patches
(Thrombocytopenic Purpura)

Zǐ Bān 紫斑

Li, female, 40 years old. The patient had petechiae and ecchymosis (bleeding into the skin) on both legs for 2 years. Even though no apparent cause could be discerned, the patient thought mild trauma might have brought on the condition. The lesions appeared in patches and seemed to enlarge in size. During the past 6 months, there was also excessive uterine bleeding during menstruation, which lasted over 10 days. The blood was thin, light in color, and without clots. There was no dysmenorrhea. Associated symptoms included lack of appetite, general lassitude, dizziness, fitful sleep and excessive dreaming, a bland sensation in the mouth, and loose stools.

Physical examination found that the heart and lungs were normal, the abdomen was flat and without tenderness, and the liver and spleen were not palpable. Laboratory tests showed hemoglobin 10g/100ml, red blood cell count 3.50 million/cu mm, white blood cell count 6,000/cu mm, and blood platelets 42,000/cu mm. The western diagnosis was thrombocytopenic purpura. The tongue was pale, and the coating was thin. The pulse was thin and frail.

SYNDROME DIFFERENTIATION

Many names for this condition can be found in Chinese medical literature, including 'muscle bleeding', 'dark purple spots', 'purple marks', and the collective term, 'purple patches'. The criterion for this diagnosis is that the lesions are not raised above the surface of the skin, and therefore cannot be felt.

The lesions can be divided into two groups: Yang and Yin. The former pattern is one of Heat and excess. It is the Heat in the Blood that forces Blood to effuse into the skin. The onset is sudden, and the patient suffers from fever, thirst and restlessness. The tongue is red, and the pulse is rapid. On the other hand, the Yin pattern is usually caused by deficiency of Spleen Qi, which controls the flow of Blood. This pattern is characterized by a gradual onset and a prolonged course, and is accompanied by other symptoms of Spleen deficiency, such as listlessness and general debility.

In this case, the patient had repeated outbreaks of purple patches for two years (a comparatively protracted course), accompanied by lassitude, diminished appetite, loose stools, and a bland sensation in the mouth—all symptoms of Spleen deficiency. Further evidence was found in the lengthy menstrual period, and in the light colored flow. Because the Spleen is the primary source of Blood and Qi, its deficiency results in diminished supply of Blood and Qi to the Brain, hence the dizziness, fitful sleep and excessive dreaming. The pale tongue, and the thin, frail pulse confirmed the diagnosis.

TREATMENT

Points selected:

Sp-10 *(xue hai)*, Sp-6 *(san yin jiao)*, GV-14 *(da zhui)*

Treatment was administered once daily. After the arrival of Qi, the needles were retained for 20 minutes. Ten treatments comprised one course of therapy, and 2 days' rest was allowed between courses.

Discussion of points:

Sp-10 *(xue hai)* and Sp-6 *(san yin jiao)* were needled with tonifying manipulation. Warm needle moxibustion was applied at GV-14 *(da zhui)*. The point was first needled with tonifying manipulation. Then, while the needle was retained, a 2cm moxa stub was attached to the end of the handle of the needle. After the stub was burned, the needle was withdrawn.

Sp-10 *(xue hai)* is a point on the Spleen channel. Because the Spleen controls the flow of Blood, this point is frequently used in the treatment of various Blood diseases; hence its name, which means 'sea of Blood'. Sp-6 *(san yin jiao)* is the point of intersec-

tion of three channels: the Spleen, Kidney and Liver. The Liver stores Blood, and the Kidney stores Essence. Essence can be transformed into Blood. Therefore Sp-6 *(san yin jiao)* is used to strengthen Spleen Qi in order to invigorate the Kidney, and thereby enhance the production of Blood. GV-14 *(da zhui)* on the Governing vessel is the junction of all the Yang channels. Tonification of this point reinforces the Yang of the entire body, and when combined with Sp-6 *(san yin jiao)*, the Spleen is optimally tonified. Moxa is Yang-tonifying; its use in this case aided in the treatment of the deficiency syndrome.

RESULTS

After the third treatment of the first course of therapy, no new lesions appeared, and the old ones began to fade. Following the third treatment of the second course of therapy, menstruation began. Liv-1 *(da dun)* was then added to the prescription. Tonifying manipulation was used at this point, and the needle retained for 20 minutes. Daily treatment of Liv-1 *(da dun)* was continued until menstruation ended 5 days later. Liv-1 *(da dun)* is often used in the treatment of menstrual disorders because it regulates the menses and stops excessive bleeding. After the eighth treatment of the second course, every trace of hemorrhaging had disappeared. By the end of the second course, the patient was free of all symptoms. Laboratory tests then showed hemoglobin 10.5g/100ml, red blood cell count 4 million/cu mm, white blood cell count 6,000/cu mm, and blood platelets 86,000/cu mm. Follow-up after 3 months showed no relapse. □

Skin Rash

Pí Zhěn 皮疹

Han, female, 44 years old. The patient complained of rashes on her back. Red papules had first appeared about 2 years ago, and then affected her entire back. Itching was paroxysmal, especially at night. Yellow fluid oozed out upon scratching. She said that the itching always seemed to be present. Small, itching papules also appeared on the limbs for 7-10 days, before disappearing spontaneously. Other symptoms included insomnia and excessive dreaming during sleep, a sensation of heat in the chest, palms and soles, dryness in the mouth, and dry stools. Vitamin E, chlortrimeton and Chinese herbs, as well as local application of fluocinolone acetonide and hydrocortisone, proved to be ineffective, although these medications did not worsen the condition. She finally sought acupuncture treatment.

Examination revealed patches of dark red papules 8 x 10cm in size, which had merged into the surrounding skin. Elongated crusts along scratch lines were observed, but there was no exudation. The patient appeared listless, and had a pale complexion and undernourished nails. The tongue was pale and fissured, and the pulse was thin and wiry.

SYNDROME DIFFERENTIATION

In Chinese medicine, itching is related to Wind, which is characterized by mobility. Red papules are attributed to Heat confined in the skin. The itching rashes on this patient were therefore caused by Wind-Heat.

Further assessment was needed, however, to determine whether the condition was one of excess or deficiency, and of the exterior or the interior.

In general, conditions of excess and of the exterior are characterized by a rapid onset, a shorter course, and a sufficiency of normal Qi, while conditions of deficiency and of the interior are characterized by a slow onset, a longer course, and an insufficiency of normal Qi. The long course of this patient's condition (rashes on the back of two years' duration) indicated that it was of a deficient and interior nature. The other manifestations (insomnia, excessive dreaming, pale complexion, undernourished nails, listlessness, pale, fissured tongue, and wiry pulse) were all due to Blood deficiency.

Deficiency of Blood can give rise to internally generated Wind-Heat, which, when confined in the skin, manifests as itching rashes. The Heat generated by Blood deficiency also caused the hot sensation in the chest, palms and soles, as well as the dry mouth and dry stools. Deficiency of Blood also led to undernourishment of the skin; the rashes were thus dark red with scales. This case was therefore primarily caused by deficiency of Blood, resulting in the confinement of Wind-Heat in the skin.

TREATMENT

Treatment was directed at nourishing the Blood to relieve the internal Heat, and subduing the internally generated Wind to arrest the itching. Equal emphasis was placed on treating both the root cause as well as the manifestations of the condition by matching local points with remote ones, and by utilizing both tonifying and draining manipulation techniques.

Points selected:

B-13 *(fei shu)* and P-7 *(da ling)* were drained, B-17 *(ge shu)* was evenly tonified and drained, Sp-6 *(san yin jiao)* was tonified, and the plum-blossom needle was applied directly on the rashes.

Treatment was administered once daily, and the needles were retained for 30 minutes during each session.

Discussion of points:

Because the Lung is associated with the skin, B-13 *(fei shu)*, the associated point of the Lung on the back, was selected to remove the Wind-Heat that was confined in the skin. L-5 *(chi ze)* or L-10 *(yu ji)* could have been used to the same effect. The Pericardium is associated with Fire, and P-7 *(da ling)*, the 'son' point on the Pericardium channel, was chosen to relieve the internal

Heat in accordance with the mother-son, tonifying-draining method. The use of these two points served to relieve the Heat, subdue the Wind and arrest the itching; the manifestations of this condition were thus controlled.

B-17 *(ge shu)* is the meeting point of Blood. Balanced tonifying-draining manipulation at this point was intended to regulate the Blood system. Tonification of Sp-6 *(san yin jiao)*, the point of intersection of the Liver, Spleen and Kidney channels (all of which are associated with Blood), strengthened the effect of B-17 *(ge shu)* in regulating and nourishing the Blood. These points were used to correct the root cause of the patient's condition.

Plum-blossom needling was utilized to invigorate the local circulation of Qi and Blood, thus facilitating the elimination of the Wind-Heat. Each of the rashes was tapped with the needles, starting from the edges, and working along a spiral course toward the center. Each area was tapped 3-5 times before moving to the next one, about 1.0-1.5cm away. Percussion was light and regular, and the time of contact between the needle and skin was kept to a minimum.

RESULTS

The itching was somewhat relieved after ten treatments, and the patient was able to sleep at night. After fifteen treatments, the rashes were significantly reduced in size, with no more scaling. The patient experienced only slight itching during the night. After twenty treatments with the same points, the itching and all other symptoms were eliminated, with only scattered rashes remaining on the back. These disappeared completely after twenty-six treatments. The skin on the back resumed a normal appearance. Four more treatments were then administered to consolidate the effect. Follow-up one year later found no relapse. □

Snake-Creeping Red Papules
(Herpes Zoster)

Shé Dān 蛇丹

Zhou, male, 50 years old. Painful eruption of vesicles on the left side of the waist began 3 days prior to the patient's first visit to the clinic. He had a cold 10 days previously, and recovered after taking powdered form of Radix Isatidis seu Baphicacanthi (bǎn lán gēn). Three days ago, sudden pain was felt in the skin on the left side of the waist. At that time, the patient discovered a strip of vesicles at the site of the pain. The diagnosis was herpes zoster. Moroxydine and vitamins were prescribed, but without significant effect. The pain increased until even contact with the hands or clothing was intolerable, and his sleep was disturbed.

During the examination of the patient, a 3 x 9cm strip of vesicles was found to extend obliquely from just below the tip of the left 12th rib upward to the back. The demarcation with normal skin was clear. The vesicles ranged in size from that of peas to that of millet, and were clustered. At the upper end of the strip near the 12th thoracic vertebrae, small, scattered vesicles were found. Neither hemorrhage nor ulceration was evident.

The patient experienced intense pain, especially when the vesicles were touched. He seemed restless, and had a bitter taste in his mouth. His other symptoms included a flushed face, scanty and dark yellow urine, and dry stools. The sides and the tip of the tongue were red, and the tongue coating was dry and yellowish. The pulse was wiry and rapid.

SYNDROME DIFFERENTIATION

The phenomenon of herpes zoster is known in Chinese medicine as 'snake-creeping red papules' because of its shape and severe pain. Since quite a number of patients are affected in the waist region, it is also called 'fire papules around the waist' (chán yāo huǒ dān). The etiology of the disease is attributed to invasion of Wind-Heat into the body, and their subsequent entrapment in the skin.

This patient had just suffered from a cold, which provided the opportunity for the external pathogenic influences to invade the body. The painful eruptions were accompanied by restlessness, flushed face, and a bitter taste in the mouth, all of which are symptoms of vigorous internal Heat in the body, which had transformed into Fire poison. Fire-Heat is most apt to impair the body Fluids, as manifested by the scanty, dark yellow urine, and dry stools. The redness on the tip and sides of the tongue was caused by the spreading of the Heat. The yellow tongue coating and rapid pulse also pointed to Heat, while the wiry pulse indicated pain and Wind. The sudden onset of the disease was characteristic of Wind-borne disorders. All of the symptoms were those of excess.

TREATMENT

The principles of treatment were to dispel the Wind and Fire, arrest the pain and detoxify the body.

Points selected:

G-20 *(feng chi)*, B-40 *(wei zhong)*, P-7 *(da ling)*, LI-11 *(qu chi)*, and local needling at the affected site

Draining manipulation was applied using raise-thrust and twirling techniques, and the needles were retained for 15 minutes. Treatment was administered once daily.

Discussion of points:

G-20 *(feng chi)* is a point on the Gall Bladder channel. The Gall Bladder pertains to wood in the five phases. Wind is also associated with wood. Thus, G-20 *(feng chi)* is an important point for the treatment of Wind diseases. Needling G-20 *(feng chi)* disperses Wind.

LI-11 *(qu chi)* and B-40 *(wei zhong)* are important points for clearing Heat and detoxifying the body. P-7 *(da ling)* belongs to the Pericardium channel; the Pericardium pertains to fire. P-7 *(da ling)* is the earth or 'son' point on the Pericardium channel, and has a draining effect. When used in combination with LI-11 *(qu chi)* and B-40 *(wei zhong)*, the draining effect of P-7 *(da ling)* is strengthened for clearing Heat, quelling Fire, and detoxifying the body.

Local needling in the vicinity of the affected site invigorates the local Qi and Blood, relieves the inflammation and arrests the pain. The needling is performed as follows. The patient lies on the unaffected side. One needle is inserted at the 'head', and another at the 'tail' of the lesion. The needles are inserted obliquely, at an angle of 35-40⁰ to the skin surface, to a depth of 1.2 units. The tips of the needles are directed toward the body of the vesicles. More needles are then inserted 2cm apart along both sides of the lesion to a depth of 1.0-1.5 units, also obliquely toward the lesion. At the end of the session, the needles are removed slowly, and the needle openings are not pressed. The pathogenic Wind and Heat will follow the slow-moving needles out of the body. The reason for leaving the needle holes open is also to allow the pathogenic influences to exit freely.

RESULTS

After the first treatment, the patient reported that the local pain was markedly relieved, and that he could sleep much better; however, the vesicles showed no change. After three sessions, the pain disappeared completely, and the eruptions were also visibly reduced. The scattered vesicles disappeared, and the clustered ones became scattered. The skin was no longer painful to the touch, or upon contact with clothing. The symptoms of restlessness, flushed face, bitter taste in the mouth, and dry stools were all gradually resolved. After seven sessions, the patient had completely recovered.

Note: While herpes zoster itself is considered amenable to treatment, most acupuncturists in China believe that it is difficult to obtain more than temporary relief from postherpetic neuralgia. □

White Thorns
(Acne Vulgaris)

Fěn Cì 粉刺

Zhou, female, 28 years old. The patient complained of numerous brown papules on her cheeks. She first noticed them 3 years ago, following a period of emotional depression. The papules were about the size of grains of millet, and secondary infections were frequent, producing a white discharge upon squeezing. Slight edema surrounded the papules. The condition was diagnosed by a dermatologist as acne vulgaris. Treatment with oral tetracycline, muscular injection of vitamin B₆ and placental tissue fluid, and external application of sulfur solution were ineffective. She was then referred for acupuncture therapy.

On examination, the patient was found to have a flushed face and dry mouth. Her tongue was red, and her pulse was rapid.

SYNDROME DIFFERENTIATION

Acne are red follicular papules, with a predilection for the face, chest and upper back. According to Chinese medicine, acne usually results from Heat in the Lung, Stomach or Blood. Acne due to Heat in the Lung appears when the Heat is blocked by external Wind from releasing, and thus remains confined in the skin. Dryness of the mouth and nose, a thin tongue coating and a floating pulse are symptoms commonly associated with this pattern. Acne due to Heat in the Stomach results when overeating of rich food impairs the functioning of the Yang Brightness (Stomach) channel, such that Heat from the Stomach and Spleen is confined in the skin. Overeating, foul breath, constipation, aversion to heat, thirst and a preference for cold beverages are indicative of this pattern. Acne due to Heat in the Blood is found when emotional trauma harms the Qi and causes it to stagnate. The resulting Heat is confined in the nutritive and blood levels. Symptoms include a flushed face marked with scattered, red papules.

In this case, there were no signs of Wind-Heat involvement, nor were there any indications of Heat in the Spleen and Stomach. However, the patient did have a history of emotional disturbance, and the resulting obstruction to the flow of Qi gave rise to Heat stagnation, which was manifested on the face in the form of flushed cheeks and red papules. Other signs of Heat included the red tongue and rapid pulse.

TREATMENT

Treatment was directed at dispelling the Heat from the Blood.

Points selected:

Sp-10 *(xue hai)*, LI-11 *(qu chi)*, B-17 *(ge shu)*, Sp-6 *(san yin jiao)*, LI-4 *(he gu)*, GV-14 *(da zhui)*

Treatment was administered once daily, and the needles were retained for 20 minutes during each session.

Discussion of points:

Sp-10 *(xue hai)* is indicated for diseases involving the Blood system. Among the eight meeting points, B-17 *(ge shu)* is the one associated with Blood, hence its use in all Blood-related diseases. LI-11 *(qu chi)*, LI-4 *(he gu)* and GV-14 *(da zhui)* are among the points commonly used to dispel Heat. Sp-6 *(san yin jiao)* is the point of intersection of the three Yin channels of the leg, and was selected here for regulating the Qi and Blood.

All of the points except GV-14 *(da zhui)* were drained by using raise-thrust and twirling manipulation. When needling GV-14 *(da zhui)*, the patient sat in a chair with her head bowed slightly forward. The needle was inserted to a depth of 1 unit, and then twirled; raise-thrusting of the needle was avoided. The needle was withdrawn immediately after the patient reported that the feeling of Qi had arrived.

RESULTS

After 20 treatments, the facial flush was slightly reduced, but no change in the papules was observed. Reevaluation of the symptoms suggested involvement of the Lung, since the Lung controls the superficial layers of the body, and is associated with most skin diseases. Therefore, B-13 *(feishu)*, B-15 *(xin shu)* and B-17 *(ge shu)* were pricked with a pyramid needle to eliminate the Heat from the Blood.

To perform this technique, the patient sat on a chair with her back exposed. After disinfection with iodine and alcohol, the skin surrounding each of the points was held between the fingers and the point was pricked open with a pyramid needle, making an incision approximately 1-2cm across. The skin was spread apart to expose a few white fibers. These fibers were picked up and severed, one by one. The wound was then swabbed with iodine, and covered with sterile gauze. Pricking was administered only once at each of the points: B-13 *(fei shu)* the first week, B-15 *(xin shu)* the second, and B-17 *(ge shu)* the third week. The papules began to subside after the second pricking, and only a few remained after the third. Treatment with the pyramid needle was then terminated.

In the meantime, treatment of the points in the original prescription was continued every other day, except that GV-14 *(da zhui)* and LI-11 *(qu chi)* were discontinued because of the reduction in facial papules. The papules disappeared entirely, and the patient's face recovered its normal appearance one month after the last treatment. □

CHAPTER SIX
Women's Disorders

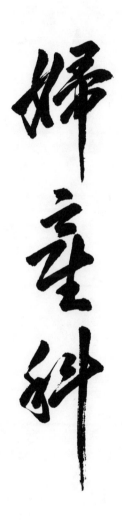

Abdominal Mass
(Inflammation of the Adnexa Uteri)

Zhēng Jiǎ 癥瘕

Lin, female, 35 years old. The patient had a miscarriage 2 years ago. Since that time, she suffered from intermittent, dull pain on both sides of the lower abdomen. At the same time, there was an increase in vaginal discharge, which was yellow in color and sticky in consistency. Her menstrual cycle was regular, but the flow had increased and was often mixed with clots. During menstruation, there was also an increase in pain, associated with a down-bearing feeling in the lower abdomen. Other symptoms included soreness in the lower back, lack of strength and spirit, and drowsiness. The tongue was red with reddish purple spots along the edges. The pulse was wiry and rapid.

Pelvic examination found a multiparous introitus, a normal vaginal canal, smooth cervix, and an anteflexed uterus, which was normal in size. A tender mass about the size of a walnut was found on the left adnexa. The right adnexa was moderately thickened and tender. The diagnosis was chronic inflammation of the adnexa. Treatment included antibiotics and physical therapy, but was without effect. The patient was therefore referred for acupuncture therapy.

SYNDROME DIFFERENTIATION

Masses in the abdomen have been recognized since ancient times, despite the fact that intraabdominal surgery was not performed then. In the classical literature, masses are discussed under the general categories of immobile abdominal masses (zhēng), and mobile abdominal masses (jiǎ). An immobile abdominal mass is fixed in one location, as is its associated pain. It is palpable and solid. A mobile abdominal mass does not have a fixed location, nor is its pain fixed. Upon palpation, the mass seems to 'roam'. When it occurs in women, the cause of an abdominal mass in usually related to the four physiological processes peculiar to the female: menstruation, pregnancy, labor and leukorrhea.

In this case, the patient first experienced lower abdominal pain about one month after a miscarriage. It can be surmised that there was a cause-and-effect relationship between the pain and the miscarriage. According to

Chinese medicine, if the normal Qi is not impaired, external pathogenic influences cannot prevail. The miscarriage, which resulted from the general weakness of normal Qi, must have precipitated the invasion of pathogenic influences, which injured the Penetrating channel and Conception vessel and caused the stagnation of Qi and Blood. The stagnation interfered with the flow of Qi and Blood in the channels, and thus gave rise to pain. Because the Penetrating channel and Conception vessel were damaged, Damp-Heat poured downward and caused an increase in vaginal discharge that became yellow and sticky. The blood clots and reddish purple spots on the tongue were signs of Blood stasis. The pulse was wiry because of the pain, and rapid because of the Heat. In short, the syndrome was one of stagnant Qi and Blood, with Damp-Heat pouring downward.

TREATMENT

The principles of treatment were to regulate the Qi and invigorate the Blood, and to clear the Dampness and cool the Heat. Points on the Conception, Spleen and Stomach channels were selected.

Because the Penetrating channel is the 'sea of Blood' and regulates the Qi and Blood of the twelve primary channels, it is indicated for menstrual disorders, leukorrhea and lower abdominal pain. The Conception vessel governs the Womb and is indicated for menstrual disorders, leukorrhea and lower abdominal masses. Because the Stomach and Spleen channels interconnect with the Penetrating channel and Conception vessel, points on the Stomach and Spleen channels of the lower abdomen are effective in treating abdominal pain and masses. Stimulation of these points also invigorates digestion, promotes the regeneration of Qi and Blood, and clears stagnation from the channels.

Points selected:

CV-4 *(guan yuan)*, CV-3 *(zhong ji)*, S-28 *(shui dao)*, S-29 *(gui lai)*, Sp-8 *(di ji)*, Sp-13 *(fu she)*, Sp-6 *(san yin jiao)*, S-36 *(zu san li)*

All points were needled bilaterally. Treatment was administered once daily, with 20 treatments comprising a single course of therapy.

Discussion of points:

CV-4 *(guan yuan)* and CV-3 *(zhong ji)* are points on the Conception vessel. When these two points are drained, the Damp-Heat is cleared. The needles were inserted to a depth of 1 unit. When the needle sensation was obtained, the needles were raised to just beneath the skin, and then redirected downward at an oblique angle to a depth of 1 unit. Draining manipulation through twirling was applied until the needle sensation was transmitted down to the perineum.

S-28 *(shui dao)* and S-29 *(gui lai)* are located just above S-30 *(qi chong)*, which intersects the Penetrating channel. Because S-30 *(qi chong)* is an inconvenient location for needling, S-28 *(shui dao)* and S-29 *(gui lai)* were chosen instead to produce the same therapeutic effects: cooling the Damp-Heat, regulating the Qi, and invigorating the Blood. These two points were needled perpendicularly to a depth of 1 unit, and were drained with raise-thrust and twirling manipulation. The needle sensation was felt in the adnexal area. Sp-8 *(di ji)* was also drained to cool the Damp-Heat, invigorate the Blood, and resolve the stagnation. This point is effective in treating abdominal masses, leukorrhea and dysmenorrhea. Sp-13 *(fu she)* is another point which is traditionally indicated for the treatment of lower abdominal masses.

S-36 *(zu san li)* and Sp-6 *(san yin jiao)* are frequently used in the treatment of women's diseases. As supplementary points, their use enhances the actions of the other points. They were needled with balanced tonifying-draining manipulation.

With the exception of CV-4 *(guan yuan)* and CV-3 *(zhong ji)*, after obtaining the needle sensation, warm needle moxibustion was applied at the points to break up the Blood stasis and mass. (Note that moxibustion can be used in some Heat conditions, as in this case.) The needles were then retained for 20 minutes.

RESULTS

After ten treatments, the pain was somewhat alleviated. By the completion of the first course of therapy, the pain had disappeared, vaginal discharge had decreased, and the patient's spirit and strength had begun to improve. Three days into the intermission between the first and second courses of therapy, menstruation started. The period lasted five days, and only mild pain was experienced.

When the period ended, two more courses of therapy were administered. Treatment was discontinued during the next menstrual period because the needle sensation at CV-4 *(guan yuan)*, CV-3 *(zhong ji)*, S-28 *(shui dao)* and S-29 *(gui lai)* was rather strong, and needling these points might have caused an increase in the flow. The patient reported that no pain was experienced during this time, and with the exception of a few small clots, the flow was normal.

After completing three courses of therapy, the patient underwent another pelvic examination. The mass in the lower abdomen had resolved. Needling was therefore discontinued. A follow-up after one year showed no relapse. The results of another pelvic examination at that time were normal. □

Abnormal Menstruation

Yuè Jīng Shī Tiáo 月经失调

Xu, female, 32 years old. Over 2 years ago, the patient's first child had been delivered by forceps because of failure to progress with labor. The patient became worried about the mental development of the child, and had been anxious and depressed ever since. Six months after childbirth, menstruation resumed. The flow was heavy and lasted 14 days. After that, every period was about 10 days early, with profuse flow of dark purple blood with clots. Pain in the lower abdomen was also present. Diethylstilbestrol, progestogen and testosterone propionate were prescribed, but to no avail. Curettage and Chinese herbal decoctions were then tried, but still without effect. The patient became emaciated, weak, spiritless and dizzy, slept poorly yet dreamed excessively, and lost her appetite. In spite of various hemostatics and hormones, menorrhagia persisted, with each period lasting about 12 days.

Examination found the patient to be pale, depressed, restless and irritable. She also suffered from pain and fullness in the hypochondria, and experienced dryness and a bitter taste in the mouth. Her tongue was pale, with a thin, yellow coating. The pulse was thin and wiry. Laboratory tests showed blood platelet count 110,000/cu mm, hemoglobin 9.5g, red blood cell count 3 million/cu mm, and white blood cell count 6,000/cu mm.

SYNDROME DIFFERENTIATION

This case was characterized by excessive duration of menstruation, and a shortening of the interval between cycles. Menstruation is a physiological function governed by the Conception vessel and the Penetrating channel. Both are influenced by the Liver because the Penetrating channel is the 'sea of Blood' which the Liver stores, and the Liver channel communicates with the Conception vessel in the lower abdomen. Thus, stagnation of Liver Qi, which in this case was caused by emotional upset, disturbed the functions of the Conception vessel and Penetrating channel, and resulted in an abnormal menstrual cycle.

Qi is the driving force behind the flow of Blood. Since the Qi had become stagnant, Blood stasis occurred. This resulted in the dark purple menstrual blood containing clots, and lower abdominal pain. Blood is the 'mother of Qi'. Because of the great loss of blood, Qi also became deficient. Deficiency of both Qi and Blood was manifested in the systemic symptoms of emaciation, general weakness, lack of spirit, pallor, dizziness and dream-disturbed sleep. Other symptoms, such as the fullness and pain in the hypochondria, reflected stagnant Liver Qi. The irritability, restlessness and yellow tongue coating likewise resulted from the transformation into Heat of constrained Qi. The pale tongue was a sign of deficiency of Qi and Blood, and the thin, wiry pulse signified deficiency and disease of the Liver.

These symptoms presented a pattern of a mixed nature, because both excess and deficiency were simultaneously present in the form of stagnant Qi and Blood stasis in the Liver, and deficiency of Qi and Blood.

TREATMENT

To regulate the Qi in the Conception vessel and the Penetrating channel, the stagnant Qi was dispersed, and the flow of Blood invigorated, by balanced tonifying-draining manipulation through raise-thrust and twirling techniques. To strengthen the Qi and Blood, tonifying manipulation alone was applied through raise-thrust and twirling techniques.

Points selected:

CV-17 *(tan zhong)*, P-6 *(nei guan)*, G-34 *(yang ling quan)*, Liv-3 *(tai chong)*, Sp-6 *(san yin jiao)*. These points were evenly tonified and drained. CV-4 *(guan yuan)* and S-36 *(zu san li)* were only tonified.

All of the above points were needled once daily. The needles were retained for 20 minutes during each session.

Discussion of points:

CV-17 *(tan zhong)* is the meeting point of

Qi. It functions to expand the chest and regulate Qi. P-6 *(nei guan)* also expands the chest and relieves fullness. G-34 *(yang ling quan)* is the lower uniting point of the Gall Bladder channel. Because the Gall Bladder and Liver are exterior-interiorly related, combining G-34 *(yang ling quan)* with Liv-3 *(tai chong)*, the source point of the Liver channel, soothes the Liver and resolves stagnation. Because Sp-6 *(san yin jiao)* is the point of intersection of the three Yin channels of the leg (Kidney, Liver and Spleen), and the Conception vessel is the 'sea of the Yin channels', needling Sp-6 *(san yin jiao)* regulates Qi in the Conception vessel. Sp-6 *(san yin jiao)* also supplements Liv-3 *(tai chong)* in spreading Liver Qi. Although it is true that L-7 *(lie que)* is the meeting point of the Conception vessel, Sp-6 *(san yin jiao)* was chosen instead because it regulates the Liver, Spleen and Kidney channels. Most gynecological problems involve these three Organs, and in this case, it was the Liver that was the root of the problem. All of the aforementioned points were involved in treating the menstrual disorder.

CV-4 *(guan yuan)* is an important point for invigoration. It nourishes the Kidney and restores Yang, and promotes the digestive function of the Stomach and Spleen. S-36 *(zu san li)* is the lower uniting point of the Stomach channel. It regulates the Spleen and Stomach, and when combined with CV-4 *(guan yuan)*, replenishes Qi and Blood.

RESULTS

After ten treatments, menstruation began on the twenty-sixth day from the beginning of the previous period, but the flow was still excessive. This was a sign that Heat was still present in the Blood. Sp-10 *(xue hai)* and Liv-1 *(da dun)* were therefore added. The former cools Heat, while the latter is the well point of the Liver channel. This point regulates the menses, and stops abnormal bleeding. On the fourth day of menstruation, the bleeding began to diminish. On the seventh day, the period ended. The patient reported that the flow was only about one-third of the amount before acupuncture treatment began. Needling of Sp-10 *(xue hai)* and Liv-1 *(da dun)* was then stopped, but treatment of the original points continued on a daily basis in order to resolve the root problem.

The patient's next menstrual period occurred 28 days after the previous one. Because the bleeding was still somewhat excessive, needling of Sp-10 *(xue hai)* and Liv-1 *(da dun)* was resumed. This period lasted 6 days, and the total loss of blood was markedly reduced. All of the other signs and symptoms also showed significant ameliora-

tion. Her appetite improved, and color began to appear in her cheeks; she gained 2.5kg. Laboratory tests indicated hemoglobin 11.5g, and red blood cell count 4 million/cu mm. Treatment continued with the original points as before.

The third menstrual period occurred 28 days after the previous one, and the flow was moderate. Treatment was then suspended for observation. For 7 months, menstrual records showed menstruation lasting 5-7 days, and a cycle of 28-30 days, with moderate bleeding and no clots. The other symptoms also disappeared, except for a slight feeling of heaviness in the lower abdomen during menstruation. □

Breast Abscess
(Acute Mastitis)

Rǔ Yōng 乳痈

Zhao, female, 26 years old. Seven days post partum, the patient suddenly developed pain in her left breast, with elevation of temperature to 37.5°C. She was nursing at the time, and measures were taken to suppress lactation. There was no history of breast problems. Conservative treatment consisting of parenteral penicillin, oral sulfonamides and fomentation was administered for 3 days, but was ineffective. The breast became red and swollen, and the patient suffered from nausea, fever and chills. On the 4th day, she was referred for acupuncture therapy.

Examination showed a temperature of 38.2⁰C. The left breast was inflamed. Under the nipple, a mass of about 5 x 5cm was palpated. The mass was tender, but was not fluctuant. The tongue was red with a yellow, slightly sticky coating. The pulse was wiry and rapid. Inquiry also revealed constipation and thirst, with a desire to drink. Laboratory tests showed a white blood cell count of 14,600/cu mm.

SYNDROME DIFFERENTIATION

Traditionally, the Chinese have advocated rich foods and medicinal tonics for the post partum woman, which was the case with this patient. When taken in excess, however, stagnation results, and Heat arises in the Stomach. The toxic Heat obstructs the flow of Blood and Qi in the Stomach channel, and since the breast lies in the path of this channel, the obstructed Blood and Qi causes retention of milk. The retained milk and toxic Heat in turn collect in the breast and cause redness, swelling and pain of the gland. Heat in the Stomach also causes fever, thirst with desire to drink, and constipation. Nausea is a sign of rebellious Stomach Qi, i.e., the Qi flows in the wrong direction. A red tongue with a yellow coating is an indication of Heat. A rapid pulse is also an indication of Heat, while a wiry pulse denotes pain.

TREATMENT

The objective was to clear the Heat and thereby disperse its accumulation in the Stomach channel.

Points selected:

G-21 *(jian jing)*, S-36 *(zu san li)*, P-6 *(nei guan)*, GV-14 *(da zhui)*, and bloodletting on the back

The first three points were needled bilaterally, and draining manipulation was used at all of the points. In needling G-21 *(jian jing)*, only twirling technique was applied; raise-thrust was avoided in order to prevent pneumothorax resulting from puncturing the lung apices. Twirling technique alone was also applied at GV-14 *(da zhui)* because of its location between two spinal processes. P-6 *(nei guan)* and S-36 *(zu san li)* were needled with both twirling and raise-thrust manipulation. The needles were retained for one hour, and manipulated for one minute once every five minutes.

Bloodletting on the back is traditionally used in the treatment of breast abscesses. This is done by first locating spots, pinpoint in size, which are bright red in color, and do not fade upon pressure. They are not elevated above the surface of the skin. These spots are found on the back, usually in the area between the 7th cervical and 12th thoracic vertebrae. In this case, three such spots were found at the level of the 5th and 6th thoracic vertebrae — two spots 2-3 units left of the spine, and one spot 2.5 units to the right. After pricking the points, a few drops of blood were squeezed from each. Because these spots do not reappear after bloodletting, they were pricked only once, during the first visit. All of the other points were needled on a daily basis.

Discussion of points:

G-21 *(jian jing)* is often used in treating breast abscesses. It is also a point of intersection of the Gall Bladder, Stomach, Triple Burner and Yang Linking channels, all of which course through the chest and/or breast. Needling this point regulates the flow of Qi in these channels, clears the Heat, and disperses accumulations so that the swelling is reduced, and the pain is relieved. GV-14 *(da zhui)* was chosen in this case for its Heat-reducing function. S-36 *(zu san li)* was drained in order to clear the Heat which had accumulated in the Stomach channel, which courses through the breasts. S-36 *(zu san li)* is also a point for general invigoration, and was chosen to increase the body's detoxifying ability. P-6 *(nei guan)* was selected to pacify the Stomach and suppress the rebellious Qi.

Bloodletting through pricking drains the toxic Heat when the disease has reached its climax.

RESULTS

After the first treatment, the pain, swelling and redness diminished, and the patient's temperature was reduced to 37.5°C. After three treatments, the pain, swelling and redness disappeared; only negligible tenderness remained below the left nipple. Other symptoms also showed marked improvement. When the temperature returned to normal (36.5°C) on the fourth day, the use of GV-14 *(da zhui)* was discontinued, and the retention of needles was reduced to thirty minutes for the next three treatments. After a total of six treatments, the symptoms were completely resolved, the white blood cell count was down to 6,500/cu mm, and the patient was discharged. She was followed-up for one month, and the mastitis did not recur. She did not resume nursing because lactation had been suppressed.

Note: Acute mastitis should be treated as soon as pain and disturbance of milk flow are observed. Early treatment may prevent the formation of abscesses. □

Breast Masses
(Fibrocystic Breast Disease)

Rǔ Pǐ 乳癖

Wang, female, 45 years old. Masses were present in both breasts for 2 years. There was painful distention that radiated to the axillae and back, and which intensified during menstruation, or upon emotional upset. Examination revealed a mass of 1 x 2cm in the upper lateral part of the right breast, and a mass of 2 x 3cm in the same location of the left breast. The masses were of moderate consistency, with distinct and smooth margins. There was tenderness but no adhesion to the skin, which appeared normal in color. The condition was diagnosed by a surgeon as fibrocystic breast disease. The patient thereupon sought acupuncture therapy.

The four examinations of traditional Chinese medicine revealed that both breasts felt distended and painful. The patient complained of distention and constriction in the chest, which she tried to relieve by heaving deep sighs. She reported that she had a short temper, and complained of forgetfulness and excessive dreaming during sleep. She had a bitter taste in her mouth, and her throat felt dry, but she had no desire to drink. Urine was scanty. Menstruation was excessive, and deep red in color. The tongue was red and dry, with a thin, yellow coating. The pulse was wiry, thin and rapid.

SYNDROME DIFFERENTIATION

In Chinese medicine, breast masses are attributed primarily to emotional disturbance, which leads to stagnation of Liver Qi. Stagnation of Qi and stasis of Blood then develop into masses. Breast masses may also be caused by deficiency of Qi and Blood, the retarded circulation of which causes them to aggregate and form masses.

Clinically, the symptoms may be those of either excess or deficiency. There are two patterns of excess: Liver Fire and stagnant Liver Qi. There are likewise two patterns of deficiency: deficiency of Liver and Kidney Yin, and deficiency of Qi and Blood.

In addition to painful distention of the breasts, symptoms of Liver Fire include local tenderness and a sensation of heat, a bitter taste in the mouth, dry throat, congested and aching eyes, restlessness and irritability, yellow urine, and a red tongue with a yellow coating. The pulse is wiry and rapid.

Symptoms of stagnant Liver Qi include painful distention of the breasts (exacerbated during menstruation), and emotional disturbance. Menstrual irregularities are not uncommon. In the control cycle of the five phases, metal (Lung) controls wood (Liver). When Liver Qi is stagnant, this relationship can reverse. This can lead to a sense of constriction in the chest, relieved by deep sighing. The pulse is wiry.

Symptoms of deficiency of Liver and Kidney Yin include dizziness, dryness of the eyes, soreness in the lower back and weakness in the knees, and a sensation of heat in the chest, palms and soles. The tongue is red with little coating, and the pulse is wiry, thin and rapid. Deficiency of Qi and Blood is manifested as facial pallor, poor appetite and persistent fatigue. The tongue is pale with a thin, white coating, and the pulse is frail.

In this case, the symptoms of oppression in the chest and deep sighing, short temper, and painful distention of the breasts all indicated stagnant Liver Qi. On the other hand, the bitter taste in the mouth, dry throat, red, dry tongue with a thin, yellow coating, and the wiry, thin and rapid pulse were all manifestations of Heat from deficiency, caused by depletion of Liver Yin after a long bout of Fire which had arisen from stagnant Liver Qi.

TREATMENT

The principles of treatment were to eliminate the stagnant Liver Qi and restore normal function to the Liver, replenish the Liver Yin and suppress the Liver Fire, and clear the channels that traverse the breasts.

Points selected:

CV-17 *(tan zhong)*, SI-1 *(shao ze)*, G-21 *(jian jing)*, LI-4 *(he gu)*, Liv-3 *(tai chong)*, Liv-8 *(qu quan)*, S-36 *(zu san li)*

Treatment was administered once daily, and was continued through menstruation because of the menstrual irregularity.

Discussion of points:

CV-17 *(tan zhong)* regulates the movement of Qi. Its stimulation invigorates the flow of Qi, and eliminates stagnation. Liv-3 *(tai chong)* is the source point of the Liver channel. It is used to eliminate stagnation of Liver Qi, and to restore normal function to the Liver. Liv-8 *(qu quan)* is the uniting point of the Liver channel; its nature pertains to water. In the generation cycle of the five phases, water generates wood, with which the Liver is associated. Needling this point thus has the effect of nourishing Liver Yin. SI-1 *(shao ze)* and G-21 *(jian jing)* relieve stasis, which clears the channels and resolves breast masses; they are often used in the treatment of masses. S-36 *(zu san li)* is a point on the Yang Brightness channel of the leg, which courses through the breasts. This point regulates the Qi and Blood, and is often used for stagnant Liver Qi. LI-4 *(he gu)* is a point on the Yang Brightness channel of the arm. Because S-36 *(zu san li)* and LI-4 *(he gu)* both belong to Yang Brightness channels, needling them regulates the Qi of these channels so that the stagnation is reduced, and the masses are resolved.

Stagnant Liver Qi is a condition of excess. Deficient Liver Yin is a condition of deficiency. In accordance with the principle of draining excess and tonifying deficiency, this condition was therefore treated with both draining and tonifying manipulation. Tonifying manipulation was used at Liv-8 *(qu quan)* to replenish the deficient Yin Fluids. Balanced tonifying-draining manipulation was used at S-36 *(zu san li)* and LI-4 *(he gu)*. Draining manipulation was used at the remaining points, except at SI-1 *(shao ze)*, which was quickly pricked.

CV-17 *(tan zhong)* was needled by downward, transverse insertion to a depth of 1.5 units, which produced a local sensation of soreness and distention. G-21 *(jian jing)* was needled with a perpendicular insertion to a depth of 1.0 unit, which produced soreness and distention that radiated to the back of the shoulder. LI-4 *(he gu)* and Liv-3 *(tai chong)* were needled obliquely, in a proximal direction, to a depth of 0.6-0.8 unit. The needle sensation was transmitted to the elbow and knee respectively. Liv-8 *(qu quan)* and S-36 *(zu san li)* were needled perpendicularly to a depth of 1.0 unit, eliciting a strong sensation of soreness and distention. Except at SI-1 *(shao ze)*, all needles were retained for 30 minutes.

RESULTS

After 15 treatments, the painful distention of the breasts was markedly reduced, but the masses remained. Moxibustion at S-18 *(ru gen)* was therefore added to the prescription. S-18 *(ru gen)* is located on the mamillary line in the 5th intercostal space. Its stimulation has the effect of clearing the channel locally. A moxa stick was held above, and moved constantly around the point, heating the area for 20 minutes during each treatment. The skin was flushed, but care was taken not to blister the skin.

Ten days later, the masses had diminished in size to 0.5 x 0.7cm in the right breast, and 1.0 x 0.8cm in the left. Daily treatment was continued for one more month, by which time the masses had completely disappeared. Another week's treatment was administered to consolidate the effect. On follow-up two years later, there was no evidence of masses. □

Eye Pain During Menstruation
(Periodic Keratitis)

Xíng Jīng Mù Tòng 行经目痛

Wang, female, 29 years old. Over the past 6 months, the patient suffered from eye pain, sensitivity to light, tearing and blurred vision during every menstrual period. The symptoms appeared with the onset of menstrual flow, and ended when the flow stopped. Her periods were late by several days, and the flow was scanty, diluted and bright red. They usually lasted 4 days. At other times, she also experienced dizziness, palpitations and a flushed face, and was irritable. Steroids and antibiotics were tried, but without effect. She finally came to the acupuncture clinic during a flare-up of the eye symptoms upon onset of menstruation.

When the patient's eyes were examined, her vision was found to be 20/66. There were areas of mixed injection in the conjunctiva, and densely concentrated, pinpoint epithelial exfoliations in both corneas. The fundus was normal. The condition was diagnosed as periodic keratitis.

SYNDROME DIFFERENTIATION

According to traditional Chinese medicine, it is the Essence of the Yin and Yang Organs that nourishes the eyes. Of all the Organs, the Liver is particularly important because it 'opens' through the eyes. When the Liver functions smoothly, the eyes can see and distinguish colors, i.e., the normal functioning of the eyes depends on nourishment from the Liver. A dysfunction of the Liver thus impairs the normal functioning of the eyes.

The eye symptoms occurred during the patient's menstrual period, which indicated a relationship with the dysfunctioning of the Liver. Because of insufficient Blood in the Liver, menstruation was delayed, and was scanty.

Because the Liver and the Kidney have the same source, a deficiency of Liver Yin is sometimes accompanied by a deficiency of Kidney Yin. Deficiency of Yin leads to Fire. The patient was therefore irritable, and experienced palpitations and a flushed face, as well as a lean stature, a red tongue, and a thin, rapid pulse. All of these symptoms pertained to deficiency of Liver and Kidney Yin, which resulted in a flare-up of Fire from deficiency.

TREATMENT

The principles of treatment were to replenish the Liver and tonify the Kidney so as to nourish the Yin and reduce the Fire.

Points selected:

B-18 *(gan shu)*, B-23 *(shen shu)*, Liv-8 *(qu quan)*, Sp-6 *(san yin jiao)*, K-2 *(ran gu)* and Liv-2 *(xing jian)*. Local points in the vicinity of the eye included B-1 *(jing ming)*, B-2 *(zan zhu)* and M-HN-9 *(tai yang)*.

Treatment was administered once daily, with six treatments comprising one course of therapy.

Discussion of points:

B-18 *(gan shu)* and B-23 *(shen shu)* are the associated points on the back for the Liver and Kidney respectively. These two points function to nourish the Liver and the Kidney. Liv-8 *(qu quan)* is the uniting point of the Liver channel. This point pertains to water, which generates wood in the generation cycle of the five phases. Wood pertains to the Liver; hence tonifying Liv-8 *(qu quan)* strengthens the Liver. Sp-6 *(san yin jiao)* is the point at which the three Yin channels of the leg intersect; this point regulates the Liver and Kidney. K-2 *(ran gu)* is the gushing point of the Kidney channel, and Liv-2 *(xing jian)* is the gushing point of the Liver channel. Stimulation of the gushing points regulates body temperature, and can reduce Fire in the body. The local points in the vicinity of the eyes, B-1 *(jing ming)*, B-2 *(zan zhu)* and M-HN-9 *(tai yang)*, were used to regulate the local flow of Qi and Blood.

Following the principle of tonifying deficiency and draining excess, B-18 *(gan shu)*, B-23 *(shen shu)*, Liv-8 *(qu quan)* and Sp-6 *(san yin jiao)* were needled with tonifying manipulation, using raise-thrust and twirling techniques. Liv-2 *(xing jian)* and K-2 *(ran gu)* were drained. B-1 *(jing ming)*, B-2 *(zan zhu)* and M-HN-9 *(tai yang)* were needled with balanced tonifying-draining manipulation.

Filiform needles 1-unit in length were used for the points in the vicinity of the eyes. At B-1 *(jing ming)* the needle was inserted perpendicularly, and very slowly, 0.1 unit medial to the inner canthus, to a depth of 0.5-0.8 unit. Needle twirling was minimal, and raise-thrust techique was not utilized. At B-2 *(zan zhu)* the needle was directed toward B-1 *(jing ming)* to a depth of 0.3 unit. M-HN-9 *(tai yang)* was needled perpendicularly to a depth of 0.5 unit.

RESULTS

The eye symptoms improved significantly after one week of therapy. Treatment was then suspended for observation of the patient. However, eye pain and sensitivity to light recurred on the first day of her next menstrual period. The symptoms were relieved after another course of needling. In order to prevent another relapse, prophylactic needling was begun about one week before the anticipated date of her next period, and treatment was continued on a daily basis until the period ended. The eye symptoms of pain, tearing and sensitivity to light recurred, but only very slightly. After another two months of similar prophylactic treatment, the eye symptoms did not recur during a follow-up of one-and-a-half years. During this time, her menstrual cycle also remained normal. □

Infertility
(Tubal Occlusion)

Bú Yùn Zhèng 不孕症

Li, female, 30 years old. The patient came for acupuncture treatment when she had failed to conceive for 6 years, despite a normal sexual life, and the apparent good health of both herself and her spouse. She was a sentimental person, and was easily depressed. She began menstruating at age 16, with each period being about 8-15 days late. Fullness of the breasts and lower abdominal pain usually began 3-5 days before each period. The cramps were so intense that ibuprofen was required. The scanty flow was light in color, and contained a small number of clots. Each period lasted 3-5 days. Following an X-ray examination 3 years after her marriage, she was diagnosed as having bilateral tubal occlusion by insufflation. Three years of treatment with Chinese herbs was ineffective. She suffered from fatigue, dizziness, insomnia, poor appetite, abdominal distention and leukorrhea.

The four examinations of Chinese medicine found the patient to have a pale complexion, a pale tongue with a thin, white coating and purple spots, and a thin and wiry pulse. Gynecological examination revealed a slightly eroded cervix, a normal uterus slightly displaced anteriorly, but with good mobility, and adnexa of normal size. Another X-ray again revealed bilateral occlusion of the tubes.

SYNDROME DIFFERENTIATION

In Chinese medicine, infertility is closely related to menstruation. This patient had a menstrual disorder; treatment therefore began by regulating her menstruation. Infertility of six years' duration, late menstruation, dysmenorrhea, and the accompanying symptoms suggested the following analysis.

Mental depression led to stagnation of Liver Qi and the malfunctioning of the Liver in storing Blood, thus resulting in late periods. Since the Liver channel courses through the breasts and lower abdomen, stagnation in this channel caused the pain in those areas. Poor circulation of Blood due to stagnation of Liver Qi gave rise to such symptoms as dysmenorrhea, clots in the menstrual flow, and purple spots on the tongue. When the Liver malfunctions, its spreading function is disturbed. The Spleen's transporting function is in turn affected, and Dampness accumulates, which in this case was manifested by leukorrhea. The Spleen and Stomach are the source of nutrients for growth and development. Disruption of the Spleen's function resulted in such local symptoms as the scanty and light-colored menstrual flow, as well as general manifestations, which included the pale complexion, lassitude, dizziness, insomnia, pale tongue and thin pulse. The other pulse characteristic — wiry — is often associated with pain, and also indicates a Liver problem.

In summary, this was a case of stagnation of Liver Qi leading to stasis and deficiency of both Qi and Blood, with resulting malnourishment of the Penetrating channel and Conception vessel. In Chinese medicine, the Penetrating channel and Conception vessel pertain to menstruation and fertility. As the 'reservoir of Blood', the Penetrating channel is closely related to the Liver, which stores Blood. Thus, dysfunction of the Liver may affect the Penetrating channel. The Conception vessel governs conception, and the infertility in this case occurred as a result of malnourishment of the Conception vessel due to the deficiency of Qi and Blood.

TREATMENT

The principles of treatment were to soothe the Liver, strengthen the Spleen, replenish the Qi, and regulate the Penetrating channel and Conception vessel. Points on the Liver, Spleen, Stomach and Conception channels were selected. Regulation of these channels was the goal of treatment. Since this case involved excess and deficiency, balanced tonifying-draining manipulation was applied.

Points selected:
CV-4 *(guan yuan)*, S-28 *(shui dao)*, S-29 *(gui lai)*, S-36 *(zu san li)*, Sp-6 *(san yin jiao)*, Liv-3 *(tai chong)*

Treatment was administered once daily, and the needles were retained for 20 minutes during each session.

Discussion of points:
CV-4 *(guan yuan)* is the point of intersection of the three Yin channels of the leg on the Conception vessel. Because both the Conception vessel and Penetrating channel originate in the Womb, this point was used to facilitate the flow in the Liver, Spleen, Kidney, Conception and Penetrating channels, as well as to replenish the Qi. S-28 *(shui dao)* and S-29 *(gui lai)*, which are located on the lower abdomen, served to regulate menstruation. S-36 *(zu san li)* and Sp-6 *(san yin jiao)* were selected to invigorate the Spleen and to replenish the Qi, in order to correct the deficiency of Qi and Blood. Liv-3 *(tai chong)*, the source point of the Liver channel, was chosen to soothe and regulate the Liver.

RESULTS

Menstruation began after the ninth treatment, and Sp-10 *(xue hai)*, a point on the Spleen channel, was added to nourish the Blood, and to invigorate its circulation. The addition of Sp-10 *(xue hai)* during menstruation was indicated because the Blood needs nourishment to replace the Blood that is lost in menstruation, and the circulation needs to be invigorated so that the flow is smooth. If this point had not been added, menstruation may not have been smooth and regular; and if this point had been used when there was no flow, its best effect may have been lost (although there would not have been any adverse effects).

Menstruation stopped five days later, and the patient reported reduced pain in her breasts and lower abdomen during her period. Treatment was continued with the original point prescription, and Sp-10 *(xue hai)* was dropped. After twenty-five more treatments, the patient's spirit and appetite improved, and her complexion turned ruddy. The abdominal distention disappeared, and the leukorrhea was reduced.

The next period began 28 days after the previous one. The flow was red and without clots, and was increased in volume. The patient experienced no discomfort. Treatment, including the use of Sp-10 *(xue hai)*, was continued through this period, and was then stopped.

When the patient returned to the clinic about seven weeks later, she complained that she had not menstruated for fifty days. She was tired, had a poor appetite, and suffered from occasional nausea. Examination showed a red tongue with a thin, white coating, and a wiry and slightly slippery pulse. Pregnancy was suspected, and confirmed by a pregnancy test. The patient gave birth about nine months later. □

Itching of the Vulva
(Senile Vaginitis)

Yīn Yǎng 阴痒

Wang, female, 56 years old. The patient complained of intense itching over the vulva, associated with burning and dryness in the vaginal canal, of 8 years' duration. The condition was worse before going to bed, and also disturbed her sleep. During the day, the patient was irritable and restless. Onset of menses was at the age of 15, and her cycle had been regular. She had twice been pregnant. Menopause occurred at about the age of 45.

Gynecologic examination showed withering of the mucous membrane over the vulva, and thickening of the skin, with scaling and scratch marks. The vaginal mucosa was atrophied, red and congested, with the folds flattened. Leukoplakia of the vulva was not present. Exfoliative cytology of the vaginal secretion led to a diagnosis of senile vaginitis. The patient's tongue was dark red, and her pulse was rapid.

SYNDROME DIFFERENTIATION

Three syndromes can be distinguished for this condition: Damp-Heat, Yin deficiency, and Heat in the Blood. In addition to the itching over the vulva, the Damp-Heat type is characterized by profuse vaginal discharge that is yellow, foamy and sticky. Associated symptoms are a bitter taste in the mouth, restlessness, thirst, a dry tongue, and dark yellow urine; frequency and urgency of urination with a burning sensation in the urethra is sometimes also present. Other symptoms include a yellow, greasy tongue coating and a rapid, wiry pulse.

The symptoms of Yin deficiency type are dryness, itching and wrinkles around the vulva, dizziness, vertigo, soreness and weakness of the lower back and knees, hot palms and soles, red cheeks and afternoon fever. The tongue is red, and the pulse is rapid and thin.

The Heat in the Blood type is characterized by itching and other symptoms of dryness, since Heat in the Blood leads to internal Dryness. Thus, such symptoms as thirst, irritability, a scarlet tongue and a rapid pulse may also be present.

In this case, the symptoms included a burning sensation in the vagina, itching, and thickened, coarse skin with excoriation.

These were clearly signs of an insufficiency of Fluids due to the patient's advanced age, since Fluids (Yin) are essential for lubricating and nourishing the skin and orifices. (The introitus and vulva are regarded as an orifice.) The color of the tongue, as well as the nature of the pulse, also pointed to Heat in the Blood. In summary, this case was one of Heat in the Blood, resulting in manifestations of internal Dryness.

TREATMENT

The principles of treatment were to cool the Blood and clear the Heat in order to lubricate the skin and other areas affected by dryness, and to alleviate the itching.

Points selected:

Liv-11 *(yin lian)*, Liv-8 *(qu quan)*, CV-1 *(hui yin)*, Sp-10 *(xue hai)*

All points were needled once daily with draining manipulation, utilizing raise-thrust and twirling techniques. Ten treatments comprised one course of therapy, with three days' rest between courses.

Discussion of points:

The Conception vessel is the 'sea' of the Yin channels. CV-1 *(hui yin),* a point on the Conception vessel, is effective in treating leu-

korrhea and genital itching. Liv-11 *(yin lian)* regulates the Blood, nourishes the Womb and lubricates the sinews, and is also used for leukorrhea and itching of the vulva. Liv-8 *(qu quan)* clears and cools Damp-Heat along the path of the Liver channel, and in this case was chosen to treat the vaginitis, leukorrhea and itching. It should be noted that because the Liver channel winds around the external genitalia, these Liver points are effective in treating itching of the vulva due to either Heat in the Blood, or Damp-Heat. Sp-10 *(xue hai)* cools Heat in the Blood, and arrests itching. It can therefore be used for any type of itching due to Heat in the Blood.

RESULTS

After five treatments, the itching diminished, and the intravaginal burning sensation disappeared. By the conclusion of the first course of therapy, the itching had stopped altogether. Nevertheless, a second course of therapy with the same set of points was administered to consolidate the therapeutic effect. A follow-up three months after cessation of treatment showed no relapse. Examination found that the vaginal congestion and excoriation of the skin of the vulva had disappeared. □

Menopausal Syndrome

Gēng Nián Qī Zōng Hé Zhèng 更年期綜合症

Lin, female, 48 years old. The patient had suffered from menstrual irregularities for 2 years, with menstruation occurring from twice a month, to once every 3 months. The flow also varied, and was sometimes heavy. For the past 2 months, she had low-grade fevers in the afternoons. The patient reported frequent hot flushes, restlessness and irritability, emotional tension, dizziness, blurred vision, tinnitus, palpitations, insomnia, forgetfulness, and hot palms and soles. The lower back and knees were sore and weak. She experienced itching all over her body, even though there was no sign of rash or desquamation.

The patient's tongue was red and without coating. Her pulse was wiry, thin and rapid. Blood pressure was 180/110mm Hg. The diagnosis was menopausal syndrome.

SYNDROME DIFFERENTIATION

All the symptoms reflected menstrual disturbances after middle age. According to Chinese medicine, menstruation is related to the functions of the Penetrating channel and Conception vessel. The Penetrating channel is the reservoir of Blood, and the Conception vessel controls the Womb and fetus. These channels regulate the amount of flow and timing of menstruation, gestation and lactation. The Conception vessel joins the Kidney channel in the abdomen. The Penetrating channel starts in the interior of the lower abdomen and descends to the perineum, then travels forward and to the surface of the body at S-30 *(qi chong)*, and ascends through the abdomen with the Kidney channel. The Penetrating channel and Conception vessel communicate with the Kidney; thus, menstruation is related not only to the Penetrating channel and the Conception vessel, but also to the abundance of Kidney Qi.

In *Simple Questions* (chapter 1), it is noted: "When a girl is 7 years of age, her Kidney begins to flourish; at 14 years, the Conception vessel opens up and the Penetrating channel flourishes, resulting in regular menstruation and the ability to conceive. . . . At 49 years, the Conception vessel becomes depleted and deficient, the Blood in the Penetrating channel is exhausted, and menstruation ceases."

This patient was approaching 49 years of age, the stage of menopause. By this time, the Kidney Qi is deficient, as are the Penetrating channel and Conception vessel, resulting in irregular menstruation. Kidney Qi includes both Kidney Yang and Kidney Yin. Generally speaking, deficiency of Kidney Yin leads to manifestations of Heat from deficiency, and deficient Kidney Yang leads to manifestations of Cold from deficiency. This patient had afternoon fevers, hot flashes, hot palms and soles, a red tongue without coating, and a rapid pulse. These were all symptoms of Heat from deficiency, and the diagnosis was accordingly deficiency of Kidney Yin. The Kidney resides in the lumbar region and 'opens' to the outside through the ears; thus, the patient experienced soreness in the lower back and weakness in the knees, as well as tinnitus.

The Kidney also controls the Yin Fluids of the five Yin Organs. Deficiency of Kidney Yin leads to deficiency of Heart Yin, and the generation of Heart Fire; hence the palpitations, insomnia and forgetfulness. Deficiency of Kidney Yin also leads to deficiency of Liver Yin, and the generation of Liver Fire; hence the irritability, restlessness, emotional tension, dizziness and blurred vision. A wiry pulse is a sign of blazing Liver Fire, and a thin pulse is a sign of Heart Yin deficiency. Deficiency of Yin Fluids in the Organs leads to malnourishment of the skin, and causes itching.

In sum, this case was one of Kidney Yin deficiency, deficiency of the Penetrating channel and the Conception vessel, and blazing Fire of the Heart and Liver.

TREATMENT

The principles of treatment were to tonify the Kidney and nourish the Yin, and to regulate the Penetrating channel and Conception vessel, in order to quell the Fire in the Heart and Liver.

Points selected:

Group 1: K-6 *(zhao hai)*, K-3 *(tai xi)*, Sp-4 *(gong sun)*, Sp-10 *(xue hai)*, P-6 *(nei guan)*

Group 2: K-7 *(fu liu)*, Sp-6 *(san yin jiao)*, CV-4 *(guan yuan)*, P-7 *(da ling)*, Liv-3 *(tai chong)*

The two groups of points were used in rotation. Treatment was administered once daily, with eight treatments comprising one course of therapy. Three days' rest was allowed between courses.

Discussion of points:

K-6 *(zhao hai)*, K-7 *(fu liu)* and K-3 *(tai xi)* belong to the Kidney channel, and their primary function is to tonify the Kidney and nourish the Yin. Sp-6 *(san yin jiao)* is the point of intersection of the Kidney, Spleen and Liver channels. This point is accordingly used in the treatment of diseases of the three Yin channels of the leg, and is effective in treating irregular menstruation. CV-4 *(guan yuan)* is a point on the Conception vessel, and Sp-4 *(gong sun)* is one of the confluent points of the eight miscellaneous channels, joining the Penetrating and Spleen channels. These two points regulate the Conception vessel and the Penetrating channel. All of the above points were needled with tonifying manipulation to resolve the deficiency of Kidney Yin, and the deficiency of the Conception vessel and Penetrating channel.

P-6 *(nei guan)* and P-7 *(da ling)* belong to the Pericardium channel. These two points act to eliminate Heart Fire. Liv-3 *(tai chong)* is a Liver channel point, and was used to quell the Liver Fire. Sp-10 *(xue hai)* is indicated for irregular menstruation and itching of the skin. With the exception of Sp-10 *(xue hai)*, which was needled with balanced tonifying-draining manipulation, the other three points were drained in order to quell the Fire in the Heart and Liver.

It is important that the two point groups be used in rotation. In general, treatment should not involve too many points at one time. The points selected for this patient were all compatible points on related channels. Tonification was supplemented with draining manipulation in order to replenish the deficiency, and to simultaneously reduce the excess. In so doing, the efficacy of the treatment was raised, and the patient was better able to tolerate the therapy.

RESULTS

After four sessions, the afternoon fevers subsided, and the dizziness, blurred vision and palpitations were also ameliorated. After eight sessions, the patient felt improvement in all respects. She was then allowed to rest for three days before the second course of therapy was begun.

By the end of the second course, all of the symptoms had basically disappeared, and treatment was therefore discontinued. On follow-up three months later, the patient reported that two weeks after cessation of acupuncture therapy, menstruation resumed with normal flow for three days. After that, normal menstruation occurred during the ensuing two months. There was no recurrence of symptoms. □

Painful Menstruation

Tòng Jīng 痛经

Zhang, female, 22 years old. This woman complained of painful menstruation of about 1 year's duration. The patient was generally in low spirits. She had started menstruating at age 13. Her cycle was 28-30 days, and the flow lasted 4-5 days. Cramps began 1 week before menstruation, and radiated to the lower back, and occasionally to the hypochondria. Clots were found in the flow, which was moderate in volume, and dark purple in color. The pain subsided upon onset of menstruation, and everything returned to normal when her period ended.

No obvious abnormality was revealed through physical examination, which included a pelvic exam. However, the tongue was dark with a thin, white coating and purple spots, and the pulse was wiry.

SYNDROME DIFFERENTIATION

Painful menstruation is a common complaint in women. Chinese medicine distinguishes two types, excess and deficiency. Symptoms of excess are usually caused by stagnation of Liver Qi, or an attack by external Cold on the Womb. Symptoms of deficiency usually result from deficiency of the Liver and Kidney, or of Essence and Blood. They may also result from a weak constitution, or from too many childbirths, which harms the Liver, Kidney, Essence and Blood.

It is important to distinguish between these two types. The duration and nature of the pain provide important clues. In cases of excess, the pain begins several days before onset of the period, and ceases upon the end of menstruation. In cases of deficiency, the pain does not appear until after the menstrual period has begun. The pain from excess is more intense and fitful, and is aggravated by pressure, whereas the pain from deficiency is more continuous, and may be relieved by pressure. In this patient, the pain started a week before the onset of menstruation, and was fitful in nature; there were no symptoms of deficiency, and it was therefore diagnosed as a case of excess.

Further analysis was then necessary to distinguish whether the condition was related to the Liver, or was caused by an attack of external Cold on the Womb. In the absence of Cold symptoms (e.g., an aversion to cold and preference for warmth, relief of pain by warmth, and aggravation of pain by cold), it was concluded that the condition was related to the Liver.

The Liver soothes and regulates the flow of Qi and Blood. It also regulates emotions. Mental stress, and anger which results from it, may interfere with the function of the Liver. The low spirits of this patient were associated with stagnant Liver Qi, which resulted in dysfunction of the Liver. Menstruation is regulated by the Penetrating channel and the Conception vessel. The Penetrating channel is the reservoir of Blood, and since one of the functions of the Liver is to store Blood, there is an intimate relationship between the Penetrating channel and the Liver. With dysfunction of the Liver, the flow of Blood in the Penetrating channel is impaired, and the stagnation of Liver Qi leads to stasis of Blood in the Womb, causing pain.

The symptoms in this case, including low spirits and pain in the hypochondria, were consistent with this diagnosis. Because the circulation of Blood depends on the motivating force of Qi (the 'commander' of Blood), the stagnation of Qi also caused stasis of Blood in the Womb, hence the dark menstrual flow with clots. This conclusion was supported by the relief of pain upon discharge of the blood clots. The dark tongue with purple spots was evidence of Blood stasis, and the wiry pulse indicated Liver involvement. In summary, this was a case of stagnant Liver Qi with stasis of Blood.

TREATMENT

The principles of treatment were to soothe the Liver, regulate the Qi and invigorate the Blood to relieve the pain.

Points selected:

Liv-14 *(qi men)*, Liv-3 *(tai chong)*, CV-6 *(qi hai)*, Sp-6 *(san yin jiao)*

Daily treatment commenced one week before onset of the menstrual period, and the needles were retained for 20 minutes during each session. All points were drained.

Discussion of points:

Liv-14 *(qi men)* is the alarm point of the Liver. Liv-3 *(tai chong)* is the source point of the Liver channel. The combined use of these two points serves to soothe the Liver and regulate the flow of Qi. In needling Liv-14 *(qi men)*, caution must be exercised. The needle should be inserted obliquely toward the posterior axillary line, until the patient reports the arrival of the needle sensation. Twirling manipulation alone should be used; raise-thrust technique should not be used in order to avoid penetrating the thoracic wall.

CV-6 *(qi hai)*, a point on the Conception vessel, leads to the Womb. Draining this point promotes the flow of Qi, invigorates the Blood and regulates the Conception vessel and Penetrating channel. Sp-6 *(san yin jiao)* is the point of intersection of the three Yin channels of the leg. In this case, Sp-6 *(san yin jiao)* was combined with CV-6 *(qi hai)* to regulate the flow of Qi and Blood in the lower Burner, which includes the Womb.

RESULTS

After three treatments, the pain began to diminish, and was much less severe at the onset of menstruation than it had been during the previous period. All of the other symptoms also showed improvement. Treatment was stopped when the period ended, thus completing the first course. One week before the next period, treatment was resumed using the same points. This time no pain was reported, except for slight discomfort over the lower abdomen, and the flow was normal in color. Follow-up for six months showed no relapse. □

Vaginal Bleeding

Bēng Lòu 崩漏

Feng, female, 32 years old. The patient had a weak constitution. Four months prior to her first visit, she experienced intermittent vaginal bleeding on a daily basis, presumably induced by overworking. The bleeding occurred 2-6 times each day, and her daily blood loss was estimated to be 20-100ml. Other symptoms included dizziness, blurred vision, excessive dreaming, lassitude, restlessness, loss of appetite and dull pain in the lower abdomen. She began menstruating at age 15, and her cycle was 25-29 days, with each period lasting 3-6 days. However, ever since the vaginal bleeding began, her menstrual periods had stopped.

Gynecological examination found the uterus to be in a normal position. It was moderately soft, mobile, and without mass or tenderness. The adnexa on the right was thickened. The diagnosis was functional uterine bleeding.

Prior treatment included vitamin K, Adrenosin, Agrimonium (prepared Chinese herb), progesterone, testosterone propionate and Chinese herbal decoctions. All were ineffective. Blood transfusion and curettage were then tried, but were also ineffective. She was finally referred to the acupuncture clinic.

The four examinations of Chinese medicine showed pallor, a thin and poorly nourished body, a low voice, and vaginal blood that was pale and mixed with clots. The tongue was pale and had tiny, purple eruptions along the edges. The coating was thin and white. The pulse was thin on the left side, and submerged and frail at the middle position on the right.

SYNDROME DIFFERENTIATION

According to traditional Chinese medicine, strain injures Qi. In this case, vaginal bleeding occurred upon overworking in a woman with a weak constitution. This was accompanied by a lack of spirit, strength and appetite, all of which were signs of deficient Qi. The overworking injured the Spleen Qi, which then lost control of the flow of Blood. The prolonged bleeding naturally led to deficiency of Blood. With deficiency of both Qi and Blood, the entire body was deprived of nutrition; hence the pallor, low voice, dizziness and blurred vision. The Heart houses the Spirit. Since the Heart was undernourished, her sleep was disturbed, and she dreamed excessively. Deficiency of Blood caused malnourishment of the Womb, and gave rise to lower abdominal pain. Because deficiency of Qi slowed the flow of Blood, Blood stasis resulted, which caused clots to form in the expelled blood, and purple eruptions to appear along the edges of the tongue. The pale tongue, and the thin pulse on the left side, were consistent with deficiency of both Qi and Blood. The submerged and frail pulse at the middle position on the right especially reflected deficiency of Spleen Qi.

TREATMENT

The principal points were those on the Spleen and Stomach channels. These points were tonified to invigorate the Qi and control the Blood.

Points selected:

GV-20 *(bai hui)*, CV-4 *(guan yuan)*, Sp-10 *(xue hai)*, S-36 *(zu san li)*, Sp-6 *(san yin jiao)*

Treatment was administered once daily, and the needles were retained for 30 minutes during each session.

Discussion of points:

GV-20 *(bai hui)* is the point of intersection of the Governing vessel with the Bladder channel, and is the point at which all the Yang channels intercommunicate. It has the function of strengthening and elevating Qi. In this case, it was selected in accordance with the principle of treating diseases of the lower part of the body with points on the upper part. CV-4 *(guan yuan)* intercommunicates with all three Yin channels of the leg, and is one of the important points for strengthening source Qi, which supplies the energy for all activities of the body. To en-

hance the therapeutic effect, warm needle moxibustion was applied. Sp-10 *(xue hai)* tonifies and invigorates the Blood, and is therefore useful in treating deficiency of Blood, complicated by stasis.

S-36 *(zu san li)* is an important point for tonifying deficiency conditions. Warm needle moxibustion was also applied at this point. Needling Sp-6 *(san yin jiao)*, the point of intersection of the three Yin channels of the leg, not only strengthens the Spleen, but also tonifies the Kidney, thus further buttressing the underlying support of the Spleen.

This combination of points was therefore chosen to tonify the Qi and stop the bleeding, and at the same time to regenerate Qi and Blood.

RESULTS

After four treatments, the frequency of bleeding was reduced to 2-4 times daily. After six treatments, the bleeding stopped, and the other symptoms began to subside. The dizziness, blurred vision and disturbed sleep all disappeared. Her appetite improved, and her spirit was restored. The pulse also became moderately strong, indicating the restoration of Stomach Qi. After twenty treatments, regular menstruation resumed. Treatment continued during menstruation in order to resolve the clots. Following her period, CV-4 *(guan yuan)* and GV-20 *(bai hui)* were dropped from the prescription, as the deficiency of Qi was resolved. Ten more treatments with the remaining points were then administered to consolidate the therapeutic effect.

Follow-up for three months showed no recurrence of abnormal bleeding. Her menstrual cycle was 28-30 days. Each period lasted 5-7 days. The flow was moderate, normal in color, and without clots. □

Vaginal Discharge

Bái Dài 白带

Chen, female, 32 years old. The patient had suffered from profuse vaginal discharge for more than a year. The discharge was white, watery and odorless, and trickled incessantly. The patient became spiritless and weak, and developed a poor appetite. She had begun menstruating at age 14, with a cycle of 28-30 days. There was no correlation between her period and the discharge. She was examined 10 days after the onset of her most recent period.

The four examinations of Chinese medicine showed a lackluster face, and a pale tongue with a thick, greasy coating. The pulse was moderate, soggy and floating. Gynecological examination showed mild cervical erosion, but no other positive findings. Papanicolaou test was also negative.

SYNDROME DIFFERENTIATION

In Chinese medicine, vaginal discharge is usually ascribed to an impairment of the Conception vessel. Syndrome type is differentiated by the color and quality of the discharge. If the discharge is white, thin and odorless, and trickles incessantly, it is attributed to deficient Spleen Qi. In this syndrome, the Spleen is unable to properly transform and transport water and Dampness, which then descend and injure the Conception vessel. If the discharge is yellow, thick and foul, then the syndrome is one of Damp-Heat pouring downward and injuring the Conception vessel.

In this case, the white, watery and odorless discharge, which trickled incessantly, was characteristic of deficient Spleen Qi. Other symptoms, such as the lack of spirit, loss of appetite and lassitude, were all evidence of Spleen dysfunction due to Dampness. The paleness of the tongue was a sign of deficient Spleen Qi, and the greasy coating was an indication of Dampness. The soggy, floating pulse was also consistent with the presence of Dampness distressing the Spleen.

TREATMENT

The principles of treatment were to tonify the Spleen Qi and resolve the Dampness.

Points selected:

CV-4 *(guan yuan)*, Sp-9 *(yin ling quan)*, Sp-6 *(san yin jiao)*, B-31 *(shang liao)*, G-26 *(dai mai)*

All points were tonified using raise-thrust and twirling manipulation. Treatment was administered once daily. Seven treatments comprised one course of therapy, with three days' rest between courses.

Discussion of points:

All three Yin channels of the leg intersect at CV-4 *(guan yuan)*, which is an important point for general strengthening of deficient Qi. The use of this point therefore tonifies the Spleen and resolves Dampness. Needling Sp-9 *(yin ling quan)* likewise tonifies the Spleen and resolves Dampness. The Spleen, Kidney and Liver channels also intersect at Sp-6 *(san yin jiao)*, which is an important point for treating many gynecological disorders. B-31 *(shang liao)* regulates the lower Burner. G-26 *(dai mai)* regulates the Girdle channel, which intersects the Gall Bladder channel at this point. It has traditionally been used for vaginal discharge. Li Shizhen of the Ming dynasty wrote in his *Studies of the Eight Miscellaneous Channels:* "When Dampness moves into the lower Burner and disrupts the Girdle channel, vaginal discharge will be profuse."

RESULTS

After three treatments, the discharge began to abate, and by the end of the first course of therapy, it was substantially reduced. Needling was continued until the discharge totally ceased at the end of three courses. The patient's appetite and spirit also showed much improvement. Follow-up six months later found no relapse. □

Vomiting During Pregnancy

Rèn Shēn Ǒu Tù 妊娠呕吐

Jian, female, 26 years old. The patient began suffering from nausea and vomiting about 50 days after her last menstrual period. There were no fever or chills, nor other symptoms of systemic infection. She had no desire to eat, and any food ingested would be immediately thrown up. The vomitus consisted of only what had been eaten. Sometimes vomiting occurred even when nothing had been eaten, and then only mucus and sour fluid would be brought up. The patient quickly became spiritless, weak, dizzy and drowsy.

Gynecological examination revealed enlargement of the uterus commensurate with a pregnancy of two months. Aschheim-Zondek test for pregnancy was positive. Since the patient could not tolerate oral antiemetics, intravenous fluids and tranquilizers were administered. Even this was ineffective, however, and the patient was referred for acupuncture therapy.

The four examinations of Chinese medicine revealed a yellow, lackluster complexion. The abdomen was bloated. Her tongue was pale with a thin, white coating. The pulse was moderate in rate yet slippery, and collapsed when pressed with force.

SYNDROME DIFFERENTIATION

According to Chinese medicine, the Stomach is a receptacle for food, and is responsible for advancing the preliminarily digested food. The direction of the movement of Stomach Qi should therefore always be downward. Vomiting results whenever Stomach Qi rebels in the opposite direction. This can be attributed to several causes, among which are stagnation of Liver Qi, and stagnation of Phlegm-Dampness.

When the vomiting occurs during the early stages of pregnancy, however, another cause is indicated. During pregnancy, menstruation ceases and the Blood that would ordinarily be drained from the body is retained in the Womb, which is controlled by the Penetrating channel. When the Blood flows normally, the Qi flows smoothly. Yet in this case when the Blood was retained, an over-abundance of Qi in the Penetrating channel resulted. Because the Penetrating channel is controlled by the Yang Brightness

(Stomach) channel, an over-abundance of Qi in the Penetrating channel harms the Stomach, and causes its Qi to rebel in the opposite direction. That is what occurred here.

Vomiting during pregnancy can be either mild or severe. The mild form may subside spontaneously in a few weeks. The severe form, however, may be harmful to both the mother and fetus. This was clearly a severe case of vomiting that was caused by both a deficiency of Stomach Qi prior to pregnancy, and an over-abundance of Qi in the Penetrating channel after pregnancy began. The pale face, dizziness, lack of strength, bloated abdomen, loss of appetite, pale tongue, and pulse which collapsed when pressed were all signs of deficiency of Stomach Qi.

TREATMENT

Since the condition involved the rebellion of Stomach Qi, as well as an over-abundance of Qi in the Penetrating channel, treatment was aimed at calming the Stomach and pacifying the Penetrating channel in order to correct the direction in the flow of Qi, and thereby stop the vomiting.

Points selected:

S-36 *(zu san li)*, P-6 *(nei guan)*, Sp-4 *(gong sun)*

All points were needled once daily. The needles were retained for 20 minutes, during which time they were manipulated once.

Discussion of points:

S-36 *(zu san li)* is the lower uniting point of the Stomach. When needled with tonifying manipulation, the Stomach Qi is strengthened. P-6 *(nei guan)* is the connecting point of the Pericardium channel. It is also one of the confluent points of the eight miscellaneous channels, communicating with the Yin Linking channel, which courses through the abdomen. Needling this point pacifies the Stomach, expands the chest and

regulates Qi, hence its importance in the treatment of vomiting. Sp-4 *(gong sun)* is the connecting point of the Spleen channel, and is useful in the treatment of disorders of the Spleen and Stomach. This point is also one of the confluent points of the eight miscellaneous channels, communicating with the Penetrating channel. Needling Sp-4 *(gong sun)* regulates the Qi of the Penetrating channel. Since morning sickness can be a normal incident of the physiologic process of pregnancy, an over-abundance of Qi in the Penetrating channel does not require the use of draining manipulation. Instead, balanced tonifying-draining manipulation should be used at P-6 *(nei guan)* and Sp-4 *(gong sun)*.

Acupuncture during pregnancy should be administered with caution. For women with a history of miscarriage, avoid needling if possible. In all cases, points that usually elicit a strong response, such as LI-4 *(he gu)* and Sp-6 *(san yin jiao)*, should be avoided. For pregnancies of less than three months, points on the lower abdomen and sacral region must not be used. After three months, neither points on the abdomen nor those on the lower back should be used.

RESULTS

After one treatment, the patient had fewer episodes of vomiting, and was able to hold down a small amount of food. After two treatments, the vomiting ceased, her appetite increased, and the bloating was markedly improved. After four treatments, the patient's appetite had returned to normal, and the dizziness and bloating had disappeared. Although there was still some mild nausea, treatment was discontinued because the patient was satisfied with the results. Followup revealed that the nausea had completely resolved about one week after the last treatment, and that there were no further episodes of nausea or vomiting. □

CHAPTER SEVEN
Children's Disorders

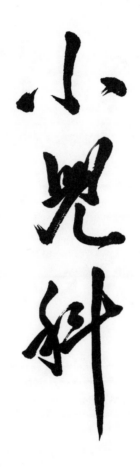

Childhood Hyperactivity

Xiǎo Ér Duō Dòng Zhèng 小儿多动症

Luo, male, 8 years old. This child was mentally well-developed. Signs of hyperactivity became evident at the age of 4, and the condition worsened after he started school. He was unable to concentrate, and was always looking about and fidgeting, such as playing with his pencil box, or cutting the desk with his pen knife. During recess, he would run and jump on the playground, and was the most active of all the children. At home, he was more concerned with what was occurring outside his window than he was with his studies. He went to sleep late, and dreamed excessively. Consequently, his record at school was poor, and he failed many examinations. The advice and admonitions of his teacher and parents did not help. Sedatives prescribed by a doctor were also ineffective.

Examination found the boy to be of small and weak stature. His mouth was dry, and his tongue was pale with red edges and tip. The tongue coating was yellow and dry.

SYNDROME DIFFERENTIATION

Childhood hyperactivity is characterized by overactivity that leaves the child unable to concentrate and remain still for the period of time expected of children of that age. According to Chinese medicine, hyperactivity is due to a disturbance in the functions of the Heart and Liver. The Heart controls the Spirit and emotions. When the Heart loses its ability to control the Spirit, restlessness sets in. When the Heart Yin is deficient, Fire from deficiency flares upward, causing redness of the tongue, excessive dreaming, and dryness in the mouth.

The Liver has the function of smoothing and regulating the flow of Qi and Blood. The nature of the Liver pertains to wood. Wind is the primary characteristic of the spring season, which also pertains to wood. The Liver is thus associated with wind. The nature of wind is one of motion. In this case, the yellow and dry tongue coating indicated deficiency of Liver Yin, causing Liver Yang to transform into internal Wind, which in turn induced the hyperactivity. The child was therefore diagnosed as suffering from internal disturbance of Liver Wind, and deficient Heart Yin.

TREATMENT

Treatment was directed at calming the Heart, subduing the ascendant Liver Yang, and tonifying the Yin.

Points selected:

GV-20 *(bai hui)*, M-HN-1 *(si shen cong)*, P-6 *(nei guan)*, H-7 *(shen men)*, Liv-8 *(qu quan)*, Liv-3 *(tai chong)*, Sp-6 *(san yin jiao)*

Treatment was administered once daily for 20 minutes. Ten sessions comprised one course of therapy, and 2-3 days' rest was allowed between courses.

Discussion of points:

GV-20 *(bai hui)* belongs to the Governing vessel, and is located on the head at the vertex. Its stimulation has the effect of subduing Wind, and calming the Spirit. M-HN-1 *(si shen cong)* is a group of four points located 1 unit anteriorly, posteriorly, and bilaterally to GV-20 *(bai hui)*. These points are also used for calming the Spirit.

P-6 *(nei guan)* is the point of confluence of the Pericardium and Yin Linking channels, and is used to treat diseases of the Heart, chest and Stomach. H-7 *(shen men)* is the source point of the Heart channel. Source points are especially useful in the treatment of diseases of the Organs. In this case, H-7·*(shen men)* was used to nourish the Heart Yin, soothe the Heart, and calm the Spirit.

Liv-8 *(qu quan)* is the uniting point of the Liver channel. Its nature pertains to water, and it acts to nourish the Liver Yin. Liv-3 *(tai chong)* is the source point of the Liver channel. It is used for regulating the Liver and restraining ascendant Liver Yang. Sp-6 *(san yin jiao)* is the point of intersection of the three Yin channels of the leg. It was selected in this case for nourishing the Liver and Kidney to control the disturbance caused by ascendant Liver Yang.

Since this case was a combination of Liver Yin deficiency and Liver Wind (excess), both tonifying and draining techniques were utilized. Draining manipulation was used at Liv-3 *(tai chong)* in order to extinguish the Wind. The other points were tonified, as the root of the problem was Yin deficiency.

At GV-20 *(bai hui)* and M-HN-1 *(si shen cong)* the needles were inserted obliquely to a depth of 0.6 unit. At P-6 *(nei guan)*, H-7 *(shen men)* and Liv-3 *(tai chong)* the needles were inserted perpendicularly to a depth of 0.8 unit, and at Liv-8 *(qu quan)* and Sp-6 *(san yin jiao)*, to a depth of 1 unit.

RESULTS

After four courses of therapy, the child was less hyperactive, and could sleep better, with less dreaming. H-7 *(shen men)* was therefore dropped from the prescription, and B-18 *(gan shu)*, B-15 *(xin shu)* and GV-14 *(da zhui)* were added. B-18 *(gan shu)* and B-15 *(xin shu)* are the associated points on the back for the Liver and Heart respectively. They serve to regulate the functions of these Organs. GV-14 *(da zhui)* on the Governing vessel controls the Yang of the entire body. Needling GV-14 *(da zhui)* regulates the equilibrium of the body's Yin and Yang, especially in cases of hyperactive Yang.

Treatment with this modified prescription was continued for four more courses, by which time the symptoms of hyperactivity had substantially improved. The frequency of treatment was then reduced to two sessions per week for another month. Observation of the child at that time found that his hyperactivity was under control, and treatment was therefore discontinued. During a follow-up for one year, the child's concentration, school work and physical development all improved.

Note: The use of acupuncture in the treatment of mental disorders is a new area of exploration. Chinese doctors believe that acupuncture can be effective to a certain extent. But because there are as yet no published reports, it is difficult to assess its true value, or to generalize about what kinds of disorders will respond well to treatment. It is, however, agreed that acupuncture should be used in conjunction with other therapies, such as counseling and special education. □

Enuresis

Yí Niào 遗尿

Dai, female, 8 years old. The patient complained of bed-wetting for 5 years. At the age of 3, she began wetting the bed about twice a week. Other symptoms that appeared at about the same time included lassitude, a tendency to be silent, poor appetite, loss of weight, sweating upon slight exertion, and a propensity for catching colds. Treatment with traditional and modern medicines was ineffective.

Examination revealed a pale complexion, a pale tongue with a white coating, and a thin, weak pulse. No organic cause for the condition could be found.

SYNDROME DIFFERENTIATION

Descriptions of enuresis are found in the ancient literature (e.g., chapter 23 of *Simple Questions*). Bed-wetting results primarily from a deficiency of Yang, which leads to a loss of control of body Fluids (here urine) by the Bladder. There are two clinical types, one due to deficiency of Kidney Yang, and the other to deficiency of Qi in the Lung and Spleen. The former, found mainly in children with a weak natural constitution, occurs when the body Fluids cannot be driven upward by the fire of the 'gate of vitality' because of deficiency of Kidney Yang. Impair-ment of the Triple Burner leads to a loss of control of body Fluids by the Bladder. Deficiency of Kidney Yang is always associated with a Cold pattern, with such symptoms as a cold sensation in the limbs, intolerance of cold, a slow and weak pulse, and aggravation of symptoms by cold. On the other hand, Qi deficiency of the Lung and Spleen is due to a general decline in health, or to impairment of ancestral Qi after a serious illness; in both of these conditions, the weakened Qi is unable to drive the body Fluids upward. As a result of the loss of control over water, enuresis appears, together with other symptoms of Qi deficiency of the Lung and Spleen.

This patient had a poor appetite and was emaciated. Both symptoms were manifestations of deficiency of Spleen Qi in metabolizing nutrients and water. Moreover, her tendency to be silent, and her propensity for catching colds, indicated a deficiency of

Lung Qi. The thin, weak pulse, together with the pale tongue and white coating, were also signs of deficiency. In sum, this was a case of Qi deficiency of the Lung and Spleen leading to a loss of control over water.

TREATMENT

The principles of treatment were to strengthen the Lung by invigorating the Spleen, and to stabilize the Bladder.

Points selected:
GV-20 *(bai hui)*, B-13 *(fei shu)*, B-20 *(pi shu)*, S-36 *(zu san li)*, Sp-6 *(san yin jiao)*, CV-6 *(qi hai)*, CV-4 *(guan yuan)*. Moxibustion was also administered at the latter two points.

Discussion of points:
GV-20 *(bai hui)*, a point on the Governing vessel, was chosen to tonify Yang, and to stabilize the Bladder. The Qi of the Lung and the Spleen flow to B-13 *(fei shu)* and B-20 *(pi shu)* respectively. These two points were needled to regulate the Lung and Spleen.

CV-4 *(guan yuan)* is the point at which source Qi is stored, and CV-6 *(qi hai)* is the 'sea of Qi'. Both points were chosen to replenish Qi and to warm the Kidney in order to invigorate Yang. While either of these two points may be used for conditions of deficient Qi, in this case both points were used to enhance the therapeutic effect. The use of these points also helped treat the deficiency of Qi of the Lung and Spleen. According to Chinese medicine, the Kidney is the origin of source Qi. In order for the Organs to function properly, they must be warmed and stimulated by source Qi. Needling and applying moxibustion at CV-4 *(guan yuan)* and CV-6 *(qi hai)* replenishes the source Qi, thus strengthening the Spleen and Lung.

S-36 *(zu san li)* is an important point for replenishing Spleen Qi. Sp-6 *(san yin jiao)* is traditionally used for treating enuresis.

All of the points were tonified since this was a deficiency syndrome. Warming cylinder moxibustion was applied at CV-6 *(qi hai)* and CV-4 *(guan yuan)* after the needles were inserted. At GV-20 *(bai hui)* the needle was inserted obliquely forward until the needle sensation was obtained. At B-13 *(fei shu)* and B-20 *(pi shu)*, needling was performed with the patient in a sitting position; needle insertion was oblique to a depth of 0.5 unit, at which point an intense needle sensation was experienced. The scraping method was used at these two points to help conduct and spread the Qi in the channels. This technique was accomplished by scraping the handle of the needle several times with the nail of the index finger, from the lower end of the handle upward. The needles were withdrawn five minutes after scraping. S-36 *(zu san li)* and Sp-6 *(san yin jiao)* were tonified through raise-thrust manipulation.

Scraping was applied at B-13 *(fei shu)* and B-20 *(pi shu)*, but not at the other points, because the needle sensation is conducted more readily at the other points through raise-thrust manipulation (except at GV-20 *[bai hui]*, where the sensation is best conducted through twirling manipulation). At B-13 *(fei shu)* and B-20 *(pi shu)*, only twirling manipulation can be used, and the needle sensation is not propagated so readily; scraping thus enhances the sensation.

RESULTS

During the first ten days of daily treatment, bed-wetting occurred only once. The child's spirits also improved. Treatment was continued for fifteen sessions, during which no further bed-wetting episodes occurred. The patient's complexion turned ruddy, and her appetite improved. Examination then revealed a pale tongue and a thin pulse. Treatment was discontinued for five days. One evening, however, she drank too much, and wet the bed that night. The effect was still considered to be unstable, and treatment was therefore resumed twice a week. After one more month of treatment with the same set of points, the condition was completely resolved. Examination showed the tongue to be slightly redder than before, and that the pulse was still thin. The patient's parents were advised to give her a more nutritious diet in order to strengthen her constitution. On follow-up one year later, the child was found to be healthy, and had not experienced any more episodes of bed-wetting. □

Excessive Childhood Salivation

Xiǎo Ér Liú Xián   小儿流涎

Wang, male, 3 years old. The patient had experienced excessive salivation since early infancy. The flow was so voluminous that his mother had to put a padded napkin under his chin to catch the overflow. The child had a dull, sallow complexion, and his hair was lusterless. He was inactive, and his appetite was poor. His stools were not well-formed, and his urine was often milky. Because of the continuous wetting by saliva, white erosion of the skin was found at the angle of the mouth, over and under the chin, and on the front of the neck. His tongue was pale with a thin coating, and his pulse was thin and weak.

SYNDROME DIFFERENTIATION

Salivation is controlled by the Spleen. The mouth is the 'opening' for the Spleen. Excessive salivation and failure of the mouth to close properly can be attributed to insufficiency of Spleen Yang.

Because of congenital weakness and postnatal malnutrition, the patient in this case had a sallow complexion and lusterless hair, and was inactive. Because of the insufficiency of Spleen Yang, the Fluids were not properly transported. Instead, they accumulated and traveled upward, causing excessive salivation. The soft or semi-fluid stools, as well as the milky urine, pale tongue and weak pulse, were all signs of insufficient Spleen Yang.

TREATMENT

The principle of treatment was to invigorate the Spleen and Stomach, and thereby restrain the excessive salivation.

Points selected:
S-36 *(zu san li)*, CV-12 *(zhong wan)*, CV-6 *(qi hai)*, S-4 *(di cang)*, CV-24 *(cheng jiang)*, CV-23 *(lian quan)*

Treatment was administered once daily. Because the Blood of young children is limited, and the Qi is weak, the needles were inserted quickly, and superficially. Only a few raise-thrust and twirling manipulations of the needles were required. The needles were then quickly withdrawn, and the openings were immediately pressed with a finger to prevent the loss of Qi.

Discussion of points:

S-36 *(zu san li)* is an important point for general strengthening of various weak and deficient conditions. CV-12 *(zhong wan)*, the alarm point of the Stomach, regulates the Qi of the Spleen and Stomach. CV-6 *(qi hai)* is another important point for strengthening, as it raises the Yang and tonifies the Qi. These three points were, in this case, chosen as remote points (from the mouth) for the overall supplementation of Spleen and Stomach Qi.

The other three points in the prescription were selected as local points. They are all traditionally used for excessive salivation. In fact, their Chinese names intimate their functions. S-4 *(di cang)* means 'earth granary'. This point is helpful in treating excessive salivation, as earth controls water in the control cycle of the five phases. CV-24 *(cheng jiang)* means 'container of saliva'. Needling this point therefore helps to control salivation. CV-23 *(lian quan)* means 'ridge spring'. It is at this point that the ancients believed that the Fluids (here saliva) sprang forth. Needling this point controls the 'spring'.

RESULTS

After 15 daily treatments (excluding Sundays), significant improvement was obtained. There was a marked decrease in salivation and an increase in appetite. To see if the therapy had been effective, and to facilitate the healing of the skin lesions, treatment was suspended for 1 week, and the cotton-padded napkin removed. Upon resumption of treatment, the skin lesions were found to have healed, but some overflow of saliva at the corner of the mouth was still evident. Treatment was therefore continued for 20 days, after which the excessive salivation stopped. The child's complexion had also improved, and he had gained some weight. He was followed up at his day-care center for 6 months. There was no relapse, and he was found to be more alert and responsive. □

INDICES

Point Index

BLADDER CHANNEL

CONCEPTION VESSEL

Index